Exploring Electronic Health Records

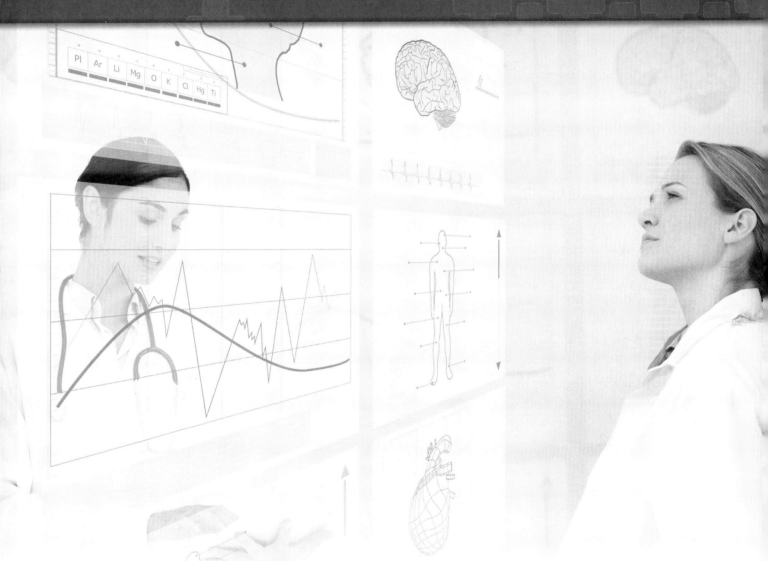

Darline Foltz, RHIA • Karen Lankisch, PhD, RHIA

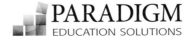

PARADIGM
EDUCATION SOLUTIONS

St. Paul

Director of Editorial: Christine Hurney
Managing Editor: Brenda M. Palo
Developmental Editor: Stephanie Schempp
Director of Production: Timothy W. Larson
Senior Production Editor: Lori Michelle Ryan
Cover and Text Designer: Jaana Bykonich
Production Specialists: Jaana Bykonich and Tammy Norstrem
Copy Editors: Kristin Melendez and Sherri Damlo of Damlo Edits
Proofreader: Laura Nelson
Indexer: Terry Casey
Senior Product Manager: Lara Weber McLellan
Health Careers Product Manager: Selena Hicks

ISBN 978-0-76385-724-0 (text)
ISBN 978-0-76385-729-5 (text and Course Navigator)
ISBN 978-0-76386-003-5 (eBook and Course Navigator via mail)
ISBN 978-0-76386-004-2 (eBook and Course Navigator via email)

© 2015 by Paradigm Publishing, Inc.
875 Montreal Way
St. Paul, MN 55102
Email: educate@emcp.com
Website: www.ParadigmCollege.com

Brief Table of Contents

Table of Contents

Chapter 11: The Personal Health Record and the Patient Portal   256

Chapter 12: Implementation and Evaluation of an EHR System   294

Exploring Electronic Health Records is an up-to-date, accurate, and approachable text that introduces students to the concepts and features of electronic health record systems. This textbook was designed to help students learn about the functionality of the electronic health record (EHR) as it applies to the many careers within the fields of health information management, health information technology, and allied health. Students gain an awareness of how the electronic health record supports efficiencies and accuracy within both inpatient and outpatient facilities, and how EHRs contribute to the goals of increased patient safety and security.

This book also integrates activities from Paradigm's EHR Navigator, a live, web-based application. Paradigm designed and developed this system based on the best features of many industry EHR systems. The EHR Navigator first provides students with plentiful practice through interactive tutorials that teach the principals of EHR software. These tutorials supply a depth of activity practice to ensure that students build skills that are transferable to the variety of EHR systems they will encounter in their careers. Students are then assessed on these important EHR activities within the EHR Navigator.

The EHR Navigator interactive tutorials and assessments can be found on Paradigm's Course Navigator. The Course Navigator is a learning management system that contains many interactive learning tools, such as quizzes, assessments, and flashcards.

Chapter Features: A Visual Walk-Through

Each chapter contains features that aid student learning. These features, as outlined below, teach students the fundamentals of EHRs, challenge them to think critically, and give them additional online learning opportunities. The features of each chapter are designed to address different learning styles and stress the importance of professionalism and soft skills.

Engaging **two-page openers** provide students with learning opportunities that supplement each chapter's core content. This feature includes fun facts about EHRs, historical background, quotations from government officials, notes from workers in the field, and professionalism tips to prepare students for careers in health information technology or management, and allied health.

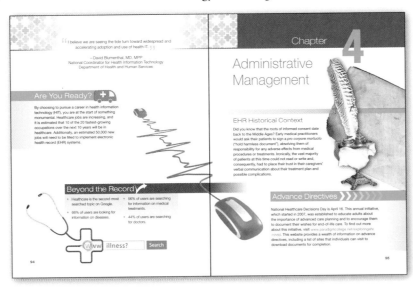

1 Learning Objectives establish a clear set of goals for each chapter.

2 Key terms are set in bold.

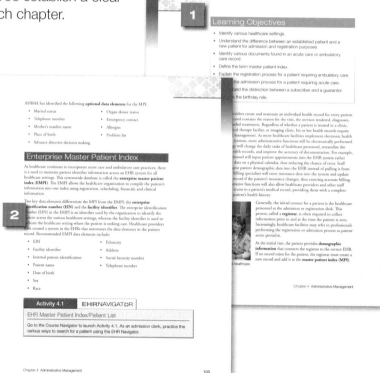

3 Expand Your Learning margin feature speaks to digitally savvy students and integrates Internet resources and online learning opportunities.

4 Consider This provides real-life scenarios and challenges students to think critically.

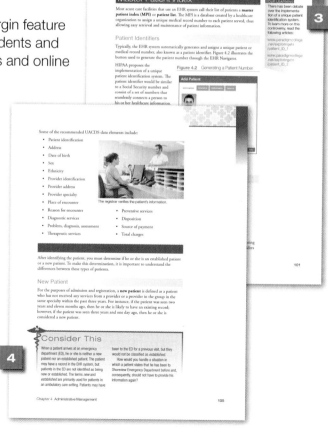

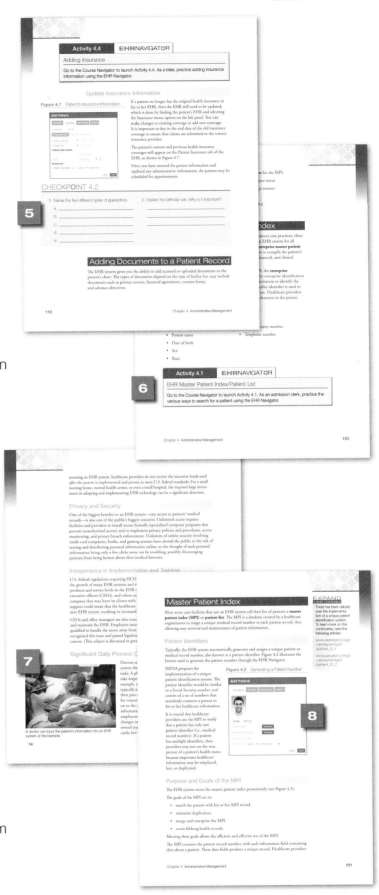

5 Checkpoint gives students periodic stopping points to test their learning within each chapter. The answers to the chapter Checkpoints are located in Appendix A.

6 Activities from the EHR Navigator point students to the Course Navigator learning management system to launch interactive tutorials. These activities give students hands-on practice in an EHR system.

7 Photographs reinforce the text and help students to visualize EHR concepts and real-world patient interactions.

8 Screenshots from the EHR Navigator illustrate key components of an EHR system as they relate to chapter content.

9 Figures in the form of flow charts help students understand crucial work flow concepts.

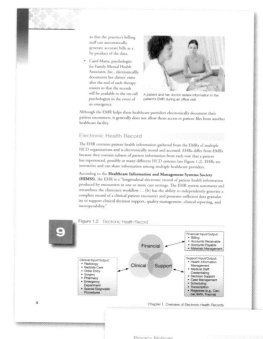

10 Figures in the form of healthcare documents and forms provide additional detail and visual reinforcement of chapter topics.

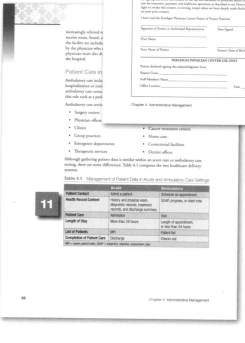

11 Tables encapsulate pertinent information related to the chapter and serve as a study aid for students.

12 Chapter Summary offers an overview of the key points of the chapter.

13 EHR Review provides multiple-choice and true/false questions and a list of acronyms from the chapter, and directs students to flash cards available on the Course Navigator.

14 EHR Application supplies short answer and critical-thinking questions.

15 EHR Evaluation provides an opportunity for students to create a presentation, perform online activities, and take the EHR Navigator assessments that are located on the Course Navigator.

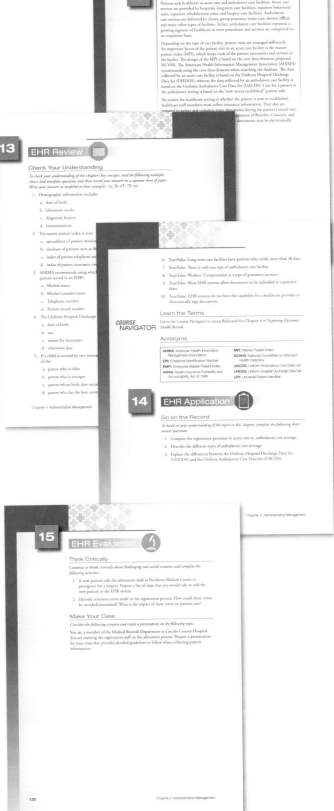

Components

To support their study of the textbook, students have access to additional print and electronic resources. These resources enhance students' skills and develop their ability to apply these skills within a range of healthcare roles. Paradigm provides all students, regardless of their preferred learning styles, a variety of exercise types.

Appendices

Appendix A contains the answers to chapter Checkpoints.

Appendix B contains a handwritten medical record that illustrates the components of a typical paper record and is referenced as a learning tool in end-of-chapter and online activities.

COURSE NAVIGATOR

Course Navigator

The Course Navigator is a learning management system that contains the EHR Navigator activities and assessments, as well as flash cards, quizzes, and other interactive learning materials from the text. Through the Course Navigator site at www.paradigmcollege.net/coursenav, instructors can set up an *Exploring Electronic Health Records* course. The Course Navigator site requires students to log in with an enrollment key, which students will receive from instructors, and a passcode, which can be purchased with the textbook.

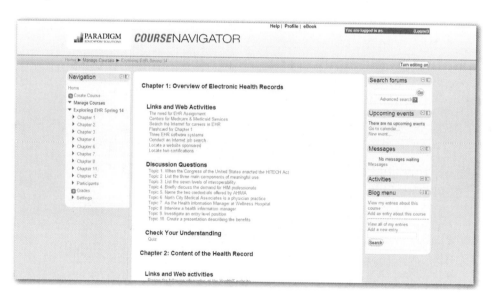

EHR Navigator

Access to the EHR Navigator is included with this textbook. It is a live program that replicates professional practice and prepares students for today's workplace.

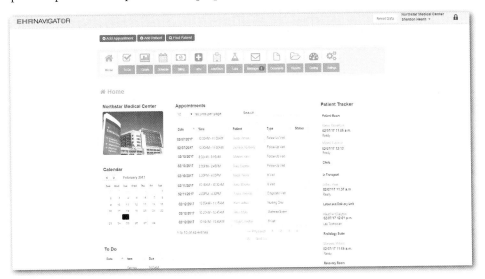

The EHR Navigator provides experience in all areas of EHRs, including adding and scheduling patient appointments, adding clinical data to patient charts, coding, and e-prescribing. The EHR Navigator gives students practice in both inpatient and outpatient settings.

The EHR Navigator's interactive tutorials offer students practice in a format that is easy to navigate, colorful, and user friendly. Each chapter contains interactive tutorials based on the core content and EHR system principals. The tutorials train students by stepping them through a variety of inpatient, outpatient, and personal health records activities.

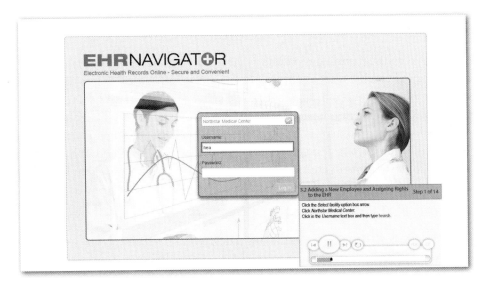

The EHR Navigator also includes assessments that are graded and reported to the instructor.

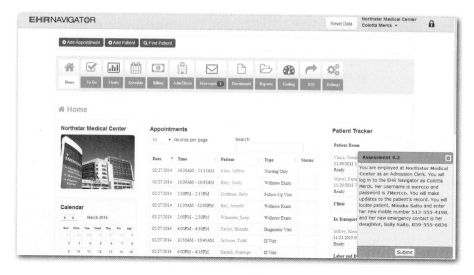

eBook

For students who prefer to study with an eBook, this text is available in an electronic form. The Web-based, password-protected eBook works on all devices and features dynamic navigation tools, including bookmarking, a linked table of contents, and the ability to jump to a specific page. The eBook format also supports helpful study tools, such as highlighting and note taking.

Additional Resources for the Instructor

Exploring Electronic Health Records provides instructors with helpful tools for planning and delivering their courses and assessing student learning.

Instructor's Guide with Instructor Resources CD

In addition to course planning tools and syllabus models, the *Instructor's Guide* provides chapter-specific teaching hints and answers for all end-of-chapter exercises. The *Instructor's Guide* also offers ready-to-use chapter tests and midterm and final examinations. Included in the package is the Instructor Resources CD, which offers PowerPoint® presentations as well as the ExamView® Assessment Suite. ExamView® is a full-featured, computerized test generator that provides both print and online tests and the option for instructors to create customized tests using the chapter item banks.

Instructor Internet Resource Center

Many of the features that appear in the printed *Instructor's Guide* also are available on the password-protected instructor section of the Internet Resource Center for this title at www.paradigmcollege.net/exploringehr.

Distance Learning Cartridges

Distance learning cartridges are available for this program. They provide Web-based teaching and learning tools, including course delivery, assessment, and content management.

About the Authors

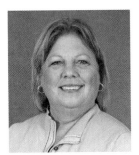 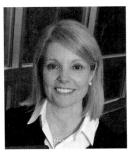

Darline Foltz, RHIA   Karen Lankisch, PhD, RHIA

Darline Foltz is an assistant professor at the University of Cincinnati–Clermont College. She holds bachelor's degrees in both Health Information Management and Information Processing Systems, and is currently working to achieve her master's degree in Educational Studies. Foltz has more than 30 years of experience in the health information field and has held multiple hospital management positions. As owner and president of Foltz & Associates, Healthcare Consulting Firm, Foltz has provided health information management and information systems consulting services to many clients, including hospitals, long-term care facilities, dialysis clinics, and mental health agencies. Active in professional and community service, she is a past-president of the Ohio Health Information Management Association and former chairperson of the long-term care section of the American Health Information Management Association (AHIMA). She is an approved AHIMA ICD-10 Trainer.

Dr. Karen Lankisch is a professor and program director of Health Information Systems Technology at the University of Cincinnati–Clermont College. She is certified through the American Health Information Management Association (AHIMA) as a Registered Health Information Administrator and has more than 10 years of experience in the field of health information. In addition, she serves as a support faculty member for the Instructional Design Technology Graduate Program, as well as an external mentor in the University of Cincinnati's New Faculty Institute Initiative. Dr. Lankisch is a Quality Matters Master Peer Reviewer and has completed reviews both nationally and internationally. In addition to being an author, she has served as a national consultant for Paradigm Education Solutions, giving workshops and presentations to instructors on Paradigm's technology learning solutions. In 2013, she received the University of Cincinnati Faculty Award for Innovative Use of Technology in the Classroom.

Authors' Acknowledgments

Co-authoring *Exploring Electronic Health Records* with Dr. Karen Lankisch has been a unique and rewarding experience. Without Karen's help and support, this endeavor would not have been possible and I am truly indebted to her for her confidence and mentoring. Together we brainstormed, created, wrote, rewrote, stressed, and laughed. Special thanks to our editor, Stephanie Schempp, whose patience and expertise are unmatched. Our programmer for the EHR Navigator, Jessica Lindfors, saved us at a time when I thought this project would not come to fruition. As a bonus, I even learned a little Swedish along the way! Thanks again, Stephanie and Jessica, for guiding me through this project. Thanks to my children, Jeff, Matt, and Jen, for listening to my authoring stories with love and support and to Carrie, my daughter-in-law and enthusiastic cheerleader. I have a feeling they are happy that this project is finished. Special thanks to my 3-year-old granddaughter, Emma, who provided laughter and play when it was most needed! To my parents, Dan and Ann, the most wonderful parents, I owe everything. Their lifelong love, support, and work ethic has instilled in me the belief that a life lived with love, faith, and hard work will result in special things. How right they are!

Darline Foltz

To complete a project of this scope requires a network of support. I am indebted to many people. I am especially grateful to my husband, Paul, my children, Michelle and son-in-law William, Brian, Becca, and Molly, and my mother, Irene, to whom I owe everything. Even more important, I would not have completed this project without all of their continued support, love, and encouragement. To my co-author, Darline, thanks for sharing your expertise, insight, and talents on this book. We persevered through tears and laughter to accomplish this project. Stephanie, Brenda, Jessica, and Chuck–thank you for never giving up and for believing in this project. Special thanks to all of the wonderful people at Paradigm Education Solutions who have enriched my life: John, Todd, Kevin, Jeff, April, Lara, and Laurie. Thank you to production, editorial, and the reviewers for your work and feedback on this project. Finally, to my University of Cincinnati–Clermont colleagues, Ron, Jeff, Tracey, and Sue, and the rest of my department, thank you for your encouragement along the way.

Karen Lankisch

Acknowledgments

The quality of this body of work is a testament to the feedback we have received from the many contributors and reviewers who participated in the development of *Exploring Electronic Health Records*.

We would like to thank the following reviewers who have offered valuable comments and suggestions on the content of this textbook.

Rosann M. O'Dell, D.H.Sc., MS, RHIA, CDIP
Johnson County Community College
Overland Park, KS

Desantila Sherifi, MBA, RHIA
Devry University
Ambler, PA

Corinne Smith, MBA, RHIA, CCS, CDIP
Montgomery College
Annapolis, MD

Special thanks also go to William Hervey, JD, LL.M., from Middle Georgia State College in Macon, GA, for his review of Chapter 6, and to the members of Paradigm's Health Information Technology Advisory Board for providing valuable and thoughtful advice throughout the development of this text.

Additional thanks go to the ExamView and PowerPoint writers and testers, as well as to the programmers, writers, and testers of the EHR Navigator software. In particular, we thank Jessica Lindfors, Jeri Kedrowski, Chuck Bratton, and Christine Hurney.

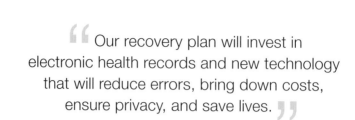

" Our recovery plan will invest in electronic health records and new technology that will reduce errors, bring down costs, ensure privacy, and save lives. "

—President Barack Obama during his address to the Joint Session of Congress, February 24, 2009

Are You Ready?

The demand for health information management (HIM) professionals is predicted to increase 20% by 2018. A myriad of careers is available for those individuals with an HIM background, including hospital chief executive officers, coders, system analysts, and electronic health record project managers.

What aspect of the field most interests you?

Beyond the Record

- Outpatient facilities that adopt and use electronic health records (EHRs) for 15 years could save as much as $42 billion each year.

- Inpatient facilities that adopt and use EHRs for 15 years could experience a net savings of $371 billion.
- In 2012, nearly 40% of U.S. primary care physicians and 35% of hospitals used EHRs. Still, these statistics are much lower than figures reported from other countries. For example, in the Netherlands, 98% of health records are stored electronically.

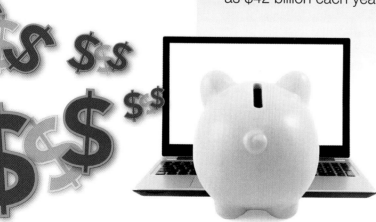

1

Overview of Electronic Health Records

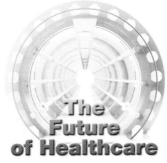

The Future of Healthcare

How will implementing electronic health records (EHRs) change the healthcare field? Patient safety is likely to improve because EHRs eliminate one of the most common causes of medical errors: illegible handwriting. EHRs will also improve communication between patients and the healthcare team once healthcare providers are able to more easily access their patients' complete medical histories.

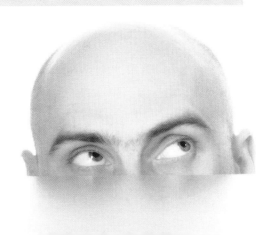

Learning Objectives

- Define the terms *electronic medical record (EMR)* and *electronic health record (EHR)* and understand their distinctions.

- Explain the concept of interoperability and its importance in the EHR environment.

- Define the terms *syntactic interoperability level* and *semantic interoperability level*.

- Define computer protocol and discuss the most common communication protocol, HL7.

- Describe the Health Information Technology for Economic and Clinical Health Act and the federal incentive program for implementing EHRs.

- Understand the concept of meaningful use and identify its three main components.

- List and discuss the benefits and barriers to implementing EHRs.

- List and discuss the evolving roles of the health information manager in the EHR environment.

EXPAND YOUR LEARNING

U.S. President Barack Obama highlighted the need for electronic health records. To hear what he had to say, visit

www.paradigmcollege.net/exploringehr/obama_video

The United States is entering a new era of healthcare, requiring providers to use **electronic health records (EHRs)** to improve healthcare delivery. EHRs replace traditional paper medical records that have been used for centuries, making health information accessible to healthcare providers across the world with only a few keystrokes. This nearly instantaneous access to health information is expected to significantly increase facility efficiency, improve patient outcomes, and result in a healthier population.

Never before have healthcare delivery and technology met at such a pivotal point. U.S. federal regulations and incentives are motivating many hospitals, physicians, dentists, nursing homes, outpatient clinics, and other providers to begin implementing EHRs. Starting January 1, 2015, the U.S. government will begin reducing Medicare payments to healthcare providers without an EHR system that complies with federal standards. (The specifics of these regulations and the healthcare providers affected will be discussed later in this chapter.) These dramatic changes, and the consequences of falling behind, may leave some healthcare facilities scrambling to fulfill federal requirements. However, more proactive providers are well along in the process of implementing EHRs and are training current staff members and pushing schools to educate future employees so that they are capable and ready to meet such transitional challenges.

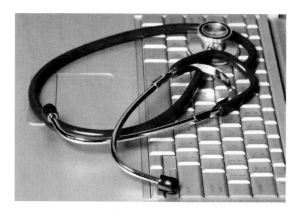

EMR vs. EHR

The terms *electronic medical record (EMR)* and *electronic health record (EHR)* are often confused with one another. EMRs and EHRs are similar concepts but different in both scope and relationship. The EMR belongs to a single healthcare provider or organization, whereas the EHR integrates EMRs from multiple providers. In other words, EMRs are individual data sources that inform and populate collected patient information from the global EHR system.

Electronic Medical Record

An **electronic medical record (EMR)** is an electronic version of patient files within a single organization, and it allows healthcare providers to place orders, document results, and store patient information for one facility, commonly called the **healthcare delivery (HCD) system**. For example, Hope Hospital in Cincinnati, Ohio, might implement an EMR to replace its separate order entry, results reporting, and documentation computer systems. Implementing a complete EMR will replace the paper medical record and can be used by physicians, nurses, other clinicians, and clerical staff. The EMR becomes the facility's legal record of the treatment course provided to the patient while he or she is in the care of the facility. The EMR is owned by the HCD system, a concept that is discussed further in Chapter 2. Figure 1.1 represents an EMR, and illustrates how each facilities' EHR is a separate, stand-alone record.

Figure 1.1   Electronic Medical Records from Different Healthcare Facilities

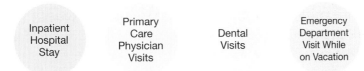

The scenarios below indicate possible EMR usage:

- Dr. Schwartz enters an order at the bedside terminal of patient Ellie Smith for a complete blood count laboratory test to rule out anemia.

- Nurse Holloway scans the bar code on patient Susan Miller's identification band followed by the bar code on the medication prior to administering the drug. This procedure helps to guarantee the accuracy of the medication's type, dose, and route of administration and helps verify that the patient is not allergic to this medication.

- Admission Clerk Shika Nadal registers a patient for admission, creating a new account number that links to the patient's EMR.

- Dental Hygienist Sarah Alvaro obtains dental X-rays of patient Lashonda Johnson with a camera that interfaces with the dental office's EMR.

- Dr. Blatt enters his hospital patient visits into his mobile device as he performs patient rounds and then syncs the device with his practice's EMR.

- Linda Agee, practice manager for Cardiology Associates, ensures that all physicians and staff members document services provided and co-pays collected so that the practice's billing staff can automatically generate accurate bills as a by-product of the data.

- Carol Matta, psychologist for Family Mental Health Associates, Inc., electronicallly documents her clients' visits after the end of each therapy session so that the records will be available to the on-call psychologists in the event of an emergency.

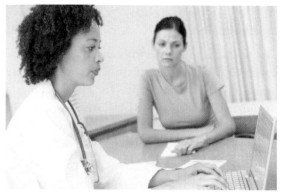

A patient and her doctor review information in the patient's EMR during an office visit.

Although the EMR helps these healthcare providers electronically document their patient encounters, it generally does not allow them access to patient files from another healthcare facility.

Electronic Health Record

The EHR contains patient health information gathered from the EMRs of multiple HCD organizations and is electronically stored and accessed. EHRs differ from EMRs because they contain subsets of patient information from each visit that a patient has experienced, possibly at many different HCD systems (see Figure 1.2). EHRs are interactive and can share information among multiple healthcare providers.

According to the **Healthcare Information and Management Systems Society (HIMSS)**, the EHR is a "longitudinal electronic record of patient health information produced by encounters in one or more care settings. The EHR system automates and streamlines the clinician's workflow.... [It] has the ability to independently generate a complete record of a clinical patient encounter and possesses sufficient data granularity to support clinical decision support, quality management, clinical reporting, and interoperability."

Figure 1.2 Electronic Health Record

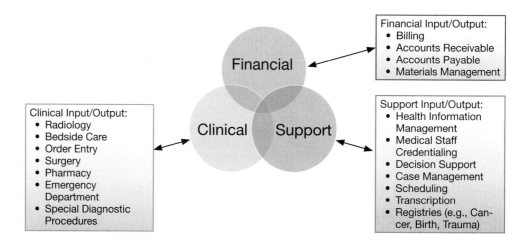

Financial Input/Output:
- Billing
- Accounts Receivable
- Accounts Payable
- Materials Management

Clinical Input/Output:
- Radiology
- Bedside Care
- Order Entry
- Surgery
- Pharmacy
- Emergency Department
- Special Diagnostic Procedures

Support Input/Output:
- Health Information Management
- Medical Staff Credentialing
- Decision Support
- Case Management
- Scheduling
- Transcription
- Registries (e.g., Cancer, Birth, Trauma)

Financial

Clinical   Support

CHECKPOINT 1.1

1. What is the definition of an electronic medical record (EMR)? _____

   _____

   _____

2. What is the definition of an electronic health record (EHR)? _____

   _____

   _____

   _____

3. List three major differences between EMR and EHR.

   a. _____

   b. _____

   c. _____

The term **longitudinal** indicates that a patient's EHR will continue to develop over the course of care. Every medical event and document can be accessed within the EHR, regardless of facility, country, or time period.

Consider This

Kim Singh visits the emergency department of Hope Hospital complaining of chest pain. Kim mentions that she had echocardiography and an electrocardiogram (ECG) performed at the office of cardiologist Dr. Carruthers approximately one month ago. The emergency department physician is able to immediately view Kim's echocardiographic and ECG results.

Kim's health record is located in a central repository of health information in which Hope Hospital, Cincinnati Dental Care, Dr. Carruthers' office, and Happy Knoll Nursing Home all participate. How might Kim's care have differed if the emergency department and the cardiologist did not have electronic health records that communicate with one another? How might her care have differed in a paper health record environment?

Kim Singh's longitudinal EHR is represented in Figure 1.3 and now contains both her visit to Dr. Carruthers' office and her emergency department visit to Hope Hospital. Notice that patient information can be freely shared among different HCD settings. This patient's longitudinal EHR will continue to grow as she has additional encounters with providers such as an optometrist, surgeon, outpatient surgery center, nursing home, dentist office, or mental health professional.

In the preceding example, the EHR Central Data Repository stores all patient data for the participating healthcare facilities on a privately owned server, which is one method of storing EHRs.

Figure 1.3 Longitudinal Electronic Health Record

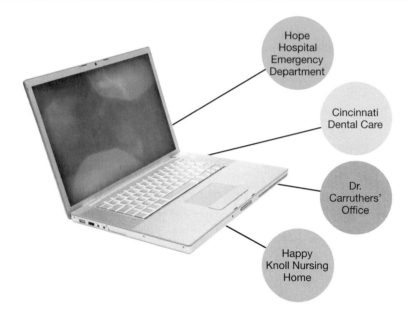

Interoperability

The success of the EHR primarily rests on **interoperability**, which is the ability of one computer system to communicate with another computer system. There are six different levels of interoperability, demonstrating a range of communication ability. Computer systems unable to exchange information are considered Level 0, whereas computer systems with Level 6 interoperability can share and manipulate data to the highest degree possible. Each level is defined as follows:

- **Level 0:** Stand-alone systems have **no interoperability**.

- **Level 1:** A communication infrastructure is established that allows systems to exchange bits and bytes of data.

- **Level 2:** The **syntactic interoperability level** introduces a common data format for information exchange, but the meaning of the data cannot be interpreted.

- **Level 3:** At the **semantic interoperability level**, the meaning of the data is shared and the information is interpreted.

- **Levels 4–6:** The higher the level, the greater the amount of data manipulation and conceptualization achieved.

Research at the Virginia Modeling, Analysis and Simulation Center (VMASC) defined the hierarchy of interoperability with its **levels of conceptual interoperability model (LCIM)**, which was developed in 2003. Since then, this model has undergone some changes, but the basic concept remains the same. Figure 1.4 illustrates the LCIM model.

Most of the focus when referring to interoperability in relation to the EHR is on syntactic and semantic interoperability (Levels 2 and 3). A minimally successful EHR system must at least use a common data format that can exchange information, and that format must meet the definition of syntactic interoperability (Level 2). However, ideally

Figure 1.4 Levels of Conceptual Interoperability Model

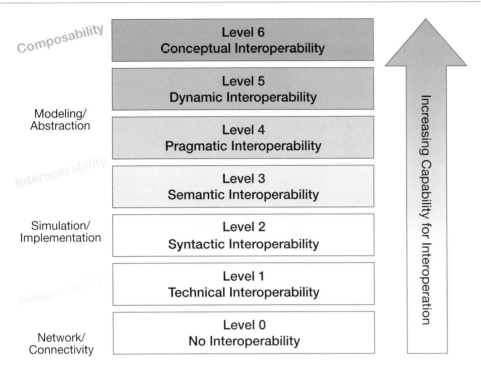

an EHR system will meet the definition of semantic interoperability (Level 3), so that health information can be understood and interpreted, not merely shared.

For example, if the EMR of Children's Hospital wants to share data with the EMR of Dr. Allen, a primary care physician, then both EMR systems must have a common technical foundation and, at the very least, syntactic interoperability. Syntactic interoperability facilitates the basic communication and exchange of information between EMRs, enabling the EMR system at Children's Hospital to send the laboratory reports of a patient to Dr. Allen's EMR system. The semantic interoperability of both EMRs allows Dr. Allen to understand the meaning of the laboratory results.

The concept of interoperability is not unique to EHRs. For example, fire and police communication systems must have interoperability to effectively communicate with each other and to respond to emergencies in a fast, organized fashion.

Computer Protocols

For EHRs to be useful and beneficial, *all* participating EMRs need one standard set of interoperability computer protocols. A **computer protocol** is a standardized method of communicating or transmitting data between two computer systems. For example, if three people who speak different languages want to effectively communicate, they will need to use one common language to speak to one another. It does not matter which language they choose; they just have to agree on one.

This is the challenge facing the health information technology (HIT) profession today—choosing one language or set of protocols that all EMRs will use, thereby making all EMRs interoperable and, thus, creating one standard EHR system. Many groups and organizations are working on different protocols, hoping to establish a universal set of standards. The most common communication protocol in use today is called **Health Level Seven International (HL7)**, which focuses on the exchange of clinical and administrative data. HL7 is also the name of an international group of collaborating healthcare subject-matter experts and information scientists. Figure 1.5 provides an example of an immunization record written using HL7 protocol.

The **U.S. Department of Health & Human Services (HHS)** has also undertaken efforts to create and adopt health informatics standards through the **Consolidated Health Informatics (CHI)** standards, which, although not required by law, have been voluntarily adopted by federal agencies and healthcare vendors doing business with the U.S. federal government to ensure efficient communication among agencies and EHR systems. CHI standards are also pursued by private medical facilities to improve communication and ensure interoperability during Medicare and Medicaid transactions.

Some of the adopted CHI standards include HL7, the **Institute of Electrical and Electronics Engineers 1073** (IEEE 1073; addresses the interoperability of medical devices), **Logical Observation Identifiers Names and Codes** (LOINC; sets standards for the electronic transfer of clinical laboratory results), and **Digital Imaging and Communications in Medicine** (DICOM; allows images and associated information to be accessed and transferred from manufacturers' devices and medical staff workstations). Ultimately, the decision to adopt a universal set of interoperability communication protocols rests with the U.S. federal government and any future mandates it proposes.

The **Office of the National Coordinator for Health Information Technology (ONC)** is the U.S. federal body that recommends policies, procedures, protocols, and standards for interoperability. The ONC is part of the HHS and was created by the **American Recovery and Reinvestment Act of 2009 (ARRA)**. The mission of the ONC is "to improve health and healthcare for all Americans through use of information and technology." The EHR system is at the center of plans for accomplishing this mission. Implementation plans span many years and will require billions of dollars. To put that estimate into perspective, the budget of the ONC for 2012 was $78.4 million.

The ONC has funded a number of health IT programs, including the development of the **Nationwide Health Information Network (NwHIN)**. The NwHIN is a set of standards, services, and policies that enables health information to be securely exchanged over the Internet and that will help create an environment where healthcare

Figure 1.5 Health Level Seven International Protocol

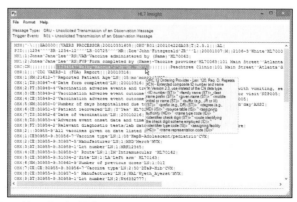

Courtesy of Steve Hart, Senior IT Consultant, HL7 2.X Certified, http://www.hartsteve.com

Chapter 1 Overview of Electronic Health Records

information is stored and shared securely and electronically. To help facilitate the move from paper medical records to an EHR, the ONC created a forum, the S&I Framework (Standards and Interoperability Framework), in which healthcare providers and stakeholders can focus on solving real-world interoperability challenges.

CHECKP◉INT 1.2

1. What is the definition of interoperability?

   _____

   _____

2. What level of interoperability is needed for electronic health records to interpret data?

   _____

   _____

3. What is the most common type of communication protocol in use today?

   _____

Federal Regulations

Members of the U.S. Congress demonstrated their commitment to a nationwide implementation of EHR technology by enacting the **Health Information Technology for Economic and Clinical Health (HITECH) Act** in February 2009, which was part of the ARRA. This legislation set aside $19.2 billion to achieve the following goals:

- To encourage physicians, hospitals, and other providers to implement the EHR by offering financial incentives. The HITECH Act defines different stages of EHR implementation and funding to healthcare providers. For example, physicians can receive up to $44,000 in incentive payments under Medicare and even more if they treat Medicaid patients. A hospital can receive up to $2 million as a base payment.

- To create the Health Information Technology Extension Program, which is designed to help small- and medium-sized physician practices implement an EHR system

- To establish a national Health Information Technology Research Center (HITRC) and Regional Extension Centers (RECs) to work with each other to share best practices for implementing EHRs and act as resources for physicians and other healthcare providers

After a provider implements an EHR system that meets the established government requirements, that provider must submit applications to receive incentive funds under the Medicare and/or Medicaid programs. Eligible healthcare providers implementing "meaningful use" of a certified EHR can receive up to $44,000 over five years under the Medicare EHR Incentive Program and up to $63,750 over six years under the Medicaid EHR Incentive Program. Figure 1.6 illustrates the the professionals eligible for the Medicare EHR Incentive Program and the Medicaid EHR Incentive Program.

Those providers who do not implement an EHR system by January 1, 2015, will receive reduced reimbursement from Medicare. For example, physicians who have not adopted certified EMR/EHR systems or cannot demonstrate "meaningful use" by the beginning of 2015 will see Medicare reimbursements reduced by 1%, a rate that will increase by 2% in 2016, 3% in 2017, 4% in 2018, and up to 5%, depending on future adjustments. Obviously, most healthcare facilities desire full reimbursement and cannot afford to delay their implementation of EMR/EHR systems.

EXPAND YOUR LEARNING

You can find more information regarding meaningful use and incentive programs on the Centers for Medicare & Medicaid Services website at

www.paradigmcollege.net/exploringehr/EHR_Incentive_Programs.

Figure 1.6 Eligible Professionals Under Medicare and Medicaid EHR Incentive Programs

Eligible professionals under the Medicare EHR Incentive Program include:

- Doctors of medicine or osteopathy
- Doctors of dental surgery or dental medicine
- Doctors of podiatry
- Doctors of optometry
- Chiropractors

Eligible professionals under the Medicaid EHR Incentive Program include:

- Physicians (primarily doctors of medicine and doctors of osteopathy)
- Nurse practitioners
- Certified nurse-midwives
- Dentists
- Physician assistants who furnish services in a federally qualified health center or rural health clinic led by a physician assistant

Meaningful Use

Meaningful use is the set of standards defined by the **Centers for Medicare & Medicaid Services (CMS)** Incentive Programs that governs the use of EHRs and allows eligible providers and hospitals to earn incentive payments by meeting specific criteria. Healthcare providers must prove that they have implemented EHR technology and are thus eligible for incentive funds by meeting the requirements of meaningful use. Meaningful use is included in the HITECH Act and defines the accepted levels of EHR implementation and qualifications to receive federal incentives. These definitions can be measured in quality and quantity.

Meaningful use requirements evolve in three stages. Stage 1 requirements focus on data capture and sharing and were implemented during 2011–2012. Stage 2 requirements focus on advancing clinical processes and are being implemented in 2014. Looking toward the future, Stage 3 requirements will focus on improved outcomes and are planned for implementation in 2016.

There are three main components of Stage 1 meaningful use:

- Use of certified EHR technology in a meaningful manner, such as e-prescribing

- Use of certified EHR technology for the electronic exchange of health information to improve the quality of healthcare

- Use of certified EHR technology to submit clinical quality measures (CQM) and other measures

Benefits of EHRs

The transition to EHRs will require monumental effort on the part of doctors, healthcare staff, regulators, government officials, and everyone working in the healthcare industry. The final goals of the transition are higher quality healthcare services, more effective and efficient communication, and healthier patients. Advocates of the transition cite many potential and already realized benefits as reasons to approach this future work with excitement and a sense of opportunity. The most obvious benefits (all leading to improved patient care and safety) include:

- Improved documentation

- Streamlined and rapid communication

- Immediate and improved access to patient information

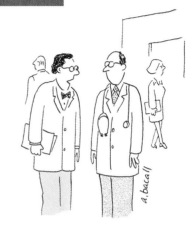

"Another advantage of switching to electronic health records is that it will make your indecipherable handwriting obsolete."

Improved Documentation

A classic complaint about doctors is their terrible handwriting. Many medication errors are the result of illegible and misinterpreted physician notes. Staff members waste time and become frustrated trying to read and interpret clinician notes, and the clinician often needs to be contacted to clarify meaning. Figures 1.7 and 1.8 illustrate the difference between handwritten and electronic progress notes, respectively.

EHRs use standardized templates that capture data by typing, scanning, and utilizing drop-down menus, among other features. Physicians can enter complex prescriptions,

Figure 1.7 Handwritten Progress Note

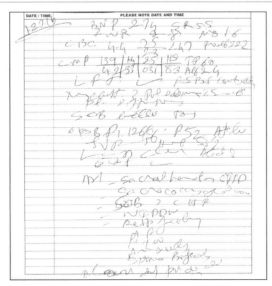

Figure 1.8 Electronic Progress Notes

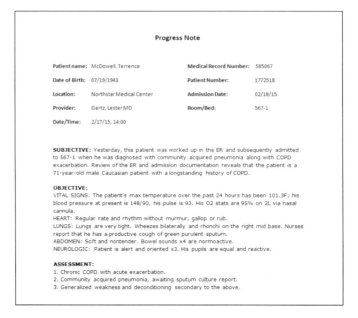

and, typically, patients can electronically fill out forms and questionnaires without incident. A doctor can record patient visit notes directly into the EHR without transcribing tape-recorded or handwritten notes. Not only will daily documentation be more accurate, but medical studies may also be more effectively conducted. For example, a new drug can be closely monitored, and a hospital's effort to track patterns like smoking cessation or overall diet improvement may be much easier. Data can be collected, identified, and sorted within a single database, leading to more accurate and innovative research.

Streamlined and Rapid Communication

The implementation of an EHR system streamlines the patient documentation process. The provision of patient care in any HCD system is complex due to the coordination of staff members and workflow processes in such areas as medications, procedures, testing, decision making, and communication. When documenting patient care using a paper record, healthcare personnel must enter patient information multiple times on multiple forms. However, when documenting patient information electronically, personnel enter the information once, whiich saves time, allows an easy database search, and helps maintain the consistency and integrity of the patient record.

EHR technology also allows for streamlined and rapid communication of information. For example, instead of waiting for a patient's test results to pass among several staff members, healthcare providers using an EHR system can be automatically alerted when the laboratory technicians file the reports.

EHR technology also streamlines the medication dispensing process and improves medication safety. For example, a patient's paper prescription typically travels from the doctor to the nurse, from the nurse to the clerk, and then from the clerk to the pharmacist. An EHR system allows a physician to use e-prescribing, a process that transmits the prescription directly to the pharmacist. This transmittal process eliminates the need for a nurse or other staff member to enter the medication order into the computer, a clerical step that impedes patient care. E-prescribing also allows direct communication between the pharmacist and the prescriber to resolve any prescription errors. An EHR system also has an automatic feature that alerts prescribers to drug incompatibilities, a step that may take several hours to determine in the paper prescription-filling process.

Immediate and Improved Access to Patient Information

With a robust, interoperable EHR system, healthcare organizations can nearly instantaneously access a patient's entire health history by viewing a patient's dental records, home healthcare visits, psychiatry records, and any other necessary history. The significance of this ability cannot be overstated. Healthcare staff can spot medical errors and inconsistencies more quickly and can instantly view the results of medical procedures performed across the globe. They can easily track and measure years of patient outcomes without having to search for misplaced records.

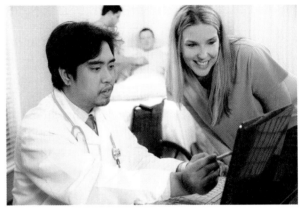

Staff members access a patient's information quickly and efficiently when using an EHR system.

Healthcare facilities are not the only ones benefitting from this access. Patients who cannot remember past procedures, diagnoses, or even allergies can be protected from hasty and underinformed medical decisions. Patients can monitor personal health goals and even report glucose readings or progress during their exercise routines from home, and patients with an allergic reaction or injury presenting to a different hospital while on vacation will not have to worry. All of their health records will be accessible, thus allowing any healthcare provider the ability to make informed and safe choices.

Barriers to EHR Implementation

To best assist with the transition to EHRs and to ensure an efficient, successful program, it is important to understand the reservations held by some patients, physicians, staff, and agencies. Many of these barriers are valid concerns in the emerging EHR field, and overcoming such barriers will be critical to developing effective policies, technologies, and education for everyone within the healthcare industry. Some common criticisms of the EHR system include:

- High cost
- Privacy and security
- Inexperience in implementation and training
- Significant daily process changes

High Cost

High cost is the most common barrier described by healthcare leadership. Whether the cost is $50,000 to implement an EHR system for a small physician or dental practice, or several million dollars for a large hospital, the costs can be a relative burden for most healthcare providers. Although federal financial incentives help offset the costs of implementing an EHR system, healthcare providers do not receive the incentive funds until *after* the system is implemented and proven to meet U.S. federal standards. For a small nursing home, mental health center, or even a small hospital, the required large investment in adopting and implementing EHR technology can be a significant deterrent.

Privacy and Security

One of the biggest benefits to an EHR system—easy access to patients' medical records—is also one of the public's biggest concerns. Unlimited access requires facilities and providers to install secure firewalls (specialized computer programs that prevent unauthorized access) and to implement privacy policies and procedures, access monitoring, and privacy breach enforcement. Violations of online security involving credit card companies, banks, and gaming systems have alerted the public to the risk of storing and distributing personal information online, so the thought of such personal information being only a few clicks away can be troubling, possibly discouraging patients from being honest about their medical histories.

Inexperience in Implementation and Training

U.S. federal regulations requiring HCD systems to implement EHRs have spawned the growth of many EHR systems and vendors. Faced with a great variability of the products and service levels in the EHR market, physicians, dentists, hospital chief executive officers (CEOs), and others are justifiably reluctant to select an EHR company that may leave its clients with little to no support. Such lack of software support could mean that the healthcare provider would have to implement an entirely new EHR system, resulting in increased costs and disruption of services.

CEOs and office managers are also concerned about hiring the right staff to implement and maintain the EHR. Employers must ensure that new staff members will be qualified to handle the move away from paper records. The U.S. federal government recognized this issue and passed legislation to create certification programs for HIT careers. (This subject is discussed in greater detail later in this chapter.)

Significant Daily Process Changes

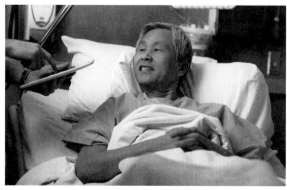
A doctor can input the patient's information into an EHR system at the bedside.

Doctors and staff may also be reluctant to embrace a system that requires an overhaul of their daily duties and tasks. A physician might argue that using EHRs will take *longer* to process patients and their information. For example, after a patient checkup, the physician might typically jot down notes or dictate into a tape recorder, then pass that information along to a staff member for transcription. With the EHR, the doctor must log on to the system, locate the patient's chart, enter the information, and then save it to the patient's files. All employees of a healthcare facility will experience similar changes to a system they might have been using for several years or decades. This change in

Chapter 1 Overview of Electronic Health Records

routine could easily feel frustrating and unnecessary, thus creating barriers to change and difficulties in the successful implementation of an EHR system. It may take years for staff members to buy in to the new technology. Offices might also see staff turnover as a result of duty and task changes.

CHECKP◆INT 1.3

1. List three benefits of implementing an electronic health record (EHR) system.

   a. _____

   b. _____

   c. _____

2. List four barriers to successfully implementing an EHR system.

   a. _____

   b. _____

   c. _____

   d. _____

Moving Forward

In the same way that building a new subway system or highway is expensive to implement and may cause traffic delays while being built, investment in the EHR is a temporary burden. The savings from replacing inefficient paper medical records will inevitably pay off the initial investment, as well as free healthcare providers from the inefficiencies of paper systems.

Privacy and security problems are not specific to EHRs; rather, these problems are similar with any company or industry that maintains an online presence. Although efforts must—and will—be made to protect personal health records, the world is just beginning to understand the true risks of managing personal information online. Due to more awareness of identity theft, many people have learned not to post the names and birth dates of their children on personal websites, and others have learned not to email credit card and Social Security numbers based on unsolicited requests. In the same way, industries are using significant resources to create security programs and procedures to address past breaches and anticipate future issues. Chapter 6 will discuss privacy and security issues in greater detail.

Having adequate support for the EHR system, both from the EHR vendor and from qualified staff, will be an important piece of the puzzle for healthcare facilities. Given time, quality EHR vendors are likely to rise to the top, giving healthcare providers confidence in their chosen EHR companies. As the field of HIT grows, more and more students will graduate with the appropriate knowledge and experience to implement, use, and maintain an EHR system. The inconveniences experienced by doctors and other clinical staff early on in the process are essential steps toward the dramatic improvement in benefits to the U.S. healthcare system.

Evolving Roles in the EHR Environment

Managing the transition from paper to electronic records requires individuals with special skills and education. The U.S. Department of Labor, Bureau of Labor Statistics, reports that the demand for **health information management (HIM)** professionals will increase 20% by 2018, and it acknowledges that the "increasing use of electronic health records will continue to broaden and alter the job responsibilities of health information technicians. For example, with the use of EHRs, technicians must be familiar with EHR computer software, maintaining EHR security, and analyzing electronic data to improve healthcare information."

The **American Health Information Management Association (AHIMA)** provides many opportunities for credentialing health information professionals interested in implementing and managing EHRs, such as:

> **RHIT: Registered Health Information Technician (Associate's Degree)**
>
> **RHIA: Registered Health Information Administrator (Bachelor's Degree)**
>
> **CHTS: Certified Healthcare Technology Specialist** (intended for professionals with various educational backgrounds, interested in working with EHRs)

Certified Professional in Healthcare Information & Management Systems (CPHIMS) is a certification offered by HIMSS. Eligibility for the CPHIMS examination requires a bachelor's degree, along with five years of associated information and management systems' experience, three years of which must be in healthcare. There are approximately 1,500–2,000 individuals credentialed as CPHIMSs and, of these professionals, 37% work as a chief information officer (CIO) or vice president of an information technology or information security department.

In addition to well-established certification programs, the U.S. federal government set aside $32 million in grants through the HITECH Act for universities to train individuals in an abbreviated health information management course. Individuals who trained under these programs sponsored by the federal government were eligible to take the HIT Pro competency examination in one of the following specialties:

- Practice Workflow & Information Management Redesign Specialist
- Clinician/Practitioner Consultant
- Implementation Manager
- Implementation Support Specialist
- Technical/Software Support Staff
- Trainer

As of July 29, 2013, these HIT Pro certifications converted to a CHTS.

Employee positions at an HCD provider include CIO, systems analyst, systems administrator, database administrator/specialist, EHR project manager, and EHR trainer. These positions are explained in more detail on the Internet Resource Center at www.paradigmcollege.net/ehr and are primarily available at either a healthcare provider or an EHR software vendor. Other health-related entities such as insurance companies, durable medical equipment companies, medical billing companies, and so forth, continue to create positions to work with EHRs for healthcare facility customers. For example, an insurance company adopts policies and procedures for accessing clients' EHRs, so it will need staff to develop and implement these standards.

EXPAND YOUR LEARNING

Search the Internet for EHR careers and prepare a presentation on different career opportunities.

Chapter Summary

Creating a national (and international) record-keeping system will not be simple, but this task is a testament to the scope and vision of electronic health record (EHR) implementation. Although the current generation may experience struggles as the EHR is implemented, the resulting nationwide EHR system will provide future healthcare providers with a more reliable, efficient, and cost-effective healthcare system. As healthcare and technology evolve together, new jobs and career opportunities will be created; patient outcomes will improve; and healthcare delivery will see gains in efficiency, communication, and overall quality.

EHR Review

Check Your Understanding

To check your understanding of this chapter's key concepts, read the following multiple-choice and true/false questions and then record your answers on a separate sheet of paper. Write your answers as modeled in these examples: 1a; 2b; 6T; 7F; *etc.*

1. What is the most common communication protocol?

   a. Syntactic

   b. Semantic

   c. Health Level Seven International

   d. NwHIN

2. What is the U.S. federal body that recommends policies, procedures, protocols, and standards for interoperability?

   a. Office of the National Coordinator for Health Information Technology

   b. Centers for Medicare & Medicaid Services

   c. Health Information Technology for Economic and Clinical Health

   d. U.S. Department of Health and Human Services

3. What is an EHR that continues to develop over the lifelong course of care?

   a. Vertical EMR

   b. Longitudinal EHR

   c. Personal health record

   d. Interoperable health record

4. Interoperability is

   a. a communication protocol.

   b. the ability of one computer system to communicate with another system.

   c. a longitudinal protocol.

   d. another name for an EMR.

5. The individual data sources that inform and populate the collected patient information of the global EHR are

   a. personal health records.

   b. physician office billing records.

   c. hospital records.

   d. EMRs.

6. True/False: The abbreviations EHR and EMR can be interchangeably used because they represent the same type of electronic record.

7. True/False: Electronic health records (EHRs) are interactive and can share information among multiple healthcare providers.

8. True/False: The ONC has funded the Nationwide Health Information Network (NwHIN) for the secure exchange of health information over the Internet.

9. True/False: The S&I Framework is a forum of healthcare providers and stakeholders.

10. True/False: Healthcare providers that do not implement an EHR system by 2014 will be assessed fines by the U.S. federal government.

Learn the Terms

Go to www.paradigmcollege.net/exploringehr/Chapter1_Flash_Cards to access flash-cards for Chapter 1 of *Exploring Electronic Health Records*.

COURSE
NAVIGATOR

Acronyms

AHIMA: American Health Information Management Association

ARRA: American Recovery and Reinvestment Act of 2009

CHI: Consolidated Health Informatics

CMS: Centers for Medicare & Medicaid Services

CPHIMS: Certified Professional in Healthcare Information & Management Systems

DICOM: Digital Imaging and Communications in Medicine

EHR: Electronic Health Record

EMR: Electronic Medical Record

HCD: Healthcare Delivery System

HHS: U.S. Department of Health & Human Services

HIM: Health Information Management

HIMSS: Healthcare Information and Management Systems Society

HIT: Health Information Technology

HITECH: Health Information Technology for Economic and Clinical Health

HITRC: Health Information Technology Research Center

HL7: Health Level Seven International

IEEE 1073: Institute of Electrical and Electronics Engineers 1073

LCIM: Levels of Conceptual Interoperability Model

LOINC: Logical Observation Identifiers Names and Codes

NwHIN: Nationwide Health Information Network

ONC: Office of the National Coordinator for Health Information Technology

REC: Regional Extension Center

RHIA: Registered Health Information Administrator

RHIT: Registered Health Information Technician

VMASC: Virginia Modeling, Analysis and Simulation Center

EHR Application

Go on the Record

To build on your understanding of the topics in this chapter, complete the following short answer questions.

1. When members of the U.S. Congress enacted the HITECH Act, they set specific goals the act would accomplish. List and briefly explain these goals.

2. List the three main components of Stage 1 meaningful use.

3. List the six levels of interoperability.

4. Briefly discuss the demand for health information management professionals that will be created by the increased use of EHRs.

5. Name two credentials offered by AHIMA for health information professionals.

Navigate the Field

To gain practice in handling challenging situations in the workplace, consider the following real-world scenarios and then use the guiding questions to help you formulate your responses.

1. North City Medical Associates is a physician practice that has struggled over the past 10 years with a tremendous growth in new patients and a lack of technology to keep up with the additional record keeping, billing, and scheduling. Jackie Lee, office manager at North City Medical Associates, decided to take advantage of incentive funds offered by the U.S. federal government and implemented an EHR system 18 months ago. Jackie now reports that the EHR system has paid for itself several times over through practice efficiency and cost savings. Describe some specific ways in which you believe North City Medical Associates made its practice more efficient and may have experienced cost savings following its implementation of the EHR system.

2. As the health information manager at Wellness Hospital, you have been asked to research what the hospital must prove to meet meaningful use guidelines. Describe what the hospital can do to meet these guidelines.

EHR Evaluation

Think Critically

Continue to think critically about challenging real-world scenarios and complete the following activities.

1. Interview a health information manager at a hospital regarding the challenges of managing a health information department in a hospital that uses an EHR system.

2. Investigate an entry-level position on www.paradigmcollege.net/ehr/HICareers.

   a. Select an entry-level position that you might be interested in pursuing.

   b. Describe the position along with the promotional and transitional career pathways.

Make Your Case

Consider the following scenario and create a presentation on the following topic.

Create a presentation describing the benefits of and barriers to EHR implementation.

Explore the Technology

To expand your mastery of EHRs, explore the following online activities.

1. Perform an Internet search and name three EHR software systems commonly used by physician offices.

2. Conduct an Internet job search to identify five different types of EHR positions located in your area.

3. Locate a website sponsored by the U.S. federal government that provides information and resources regarding EHRs.

4. Locate two certifications other than RHIT and RHIA that can be awarded to individuals in the EHR field.

Are You Ready?

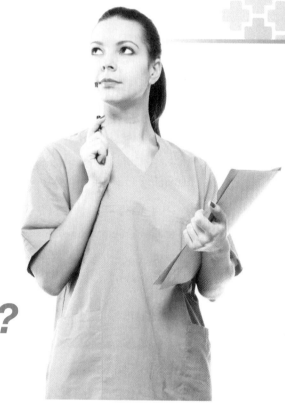

The workflow of a paper-based medical office is more employee-intensive than an office that uses an electronic health record (EHR) system.

How do EHRs change the day-to-day responsibilities if you are part of the health administrative staff?

How might your role evolve as more of your duties are electronically performed?

Beyond the Record

- Each patient visit requires approximately 10–13 pieces of paper.

- The healthcare industry uses thousands of tons of paper every year.

- A physician accumulates approximately 975 new pages of paperwork each week and spends about eight hours per week processing it.

EHR Time Line

- **Between 206 BCE and 8 ADE**—Chunyu Yi keeps the first known medical record.

- **Between 1790 and 1821**—some of America's earliest hospitals began keeping patient records, including the New York Hospital, Pennsylvania Hospital, and Massachusetts General Hospital.

- **1860s**—Physicians treating Civil War soldiers keep standardized records.

- **1917**—The American College of Surgeons (ACS) develops a hospital standardization program.

Chapter 2

Content of the Health Record

Maintaining a Legal Health Record

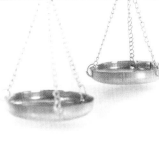

The health record, whether paper or electronic, is the legal record for a healthcare organization. Thus, there are many standards a health record should follow to protect the healthcare organization.

For a health record to be used as evidence in a court case, it needs to follow four basic principles. The record must:

- be documented following normal routines.
- be kept in the regular course of healthcare business.
- be recorded during or close to the time the event happened.
- be recorded by a person with knowledge of the events.

Healthcare facilities must routinely assess policies and procedures regarding record keeping to ensure their records are legally sound.

- **1970s**–Dr. Lawrence L. Weed and Jan Schultz develop a medical record software program called PROMIS (Problem-Oriented Medical Information System).

- **1990s**–The U.S. Veterans Health Administration's Computerized Patient Record System (CPRS) is the first large-scale deployment of an electronic health record (EHR).

- **2009**–The American Recovery and Reinvestment Act of 2009 (ARRA) outlines federal incentives for adopting EHRs.

Learning Objectives

- Define the term *health record* and examine its multiple purposes.
- Explain ownership of the health record.
- Describe the requirements and standards for the health record.
- Describe the paper health record's purpose, format, and features.
- Differentiate the types of data in the health record.
- Explain the importance of proper documentation in the health record.
- Describe the purpose, format, and features of the electronic health record (EHR).
- Compare and contrast the workflow of the paper health record versus the EHR.

The concept of electronic health records (EHRs) has emerged from the growing partnership between healthcare and technology. The integration of EHRs in the healthcare practice is built on the foundation of health record content. Health records contain essential elements of clinical, administrative, financial, and legal information that play key roles in a patient's current and future healthcare. The healthcare field uses health records to manage and research improvements and innovations. Healthcare settings are required to maintain health records for every patient, and they must all follow the licensing, accrediting, and other regulatory body requirements.

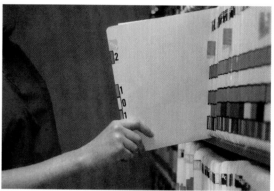

Whether on paper or in an electronic system, health records play key roles in a patient's current and future healthcare.

History of the Health Record

According to the U.S. National Library of Medicine, a **healthcare facility** "includes hospitals, clinics, dental offices, outpatient surgery centers, birthing centers, and nursing homes." Each facility creates individual health records for its patients. These records reflect all episodes of care that patients receive.

Hippocrates, considered one of the most important figures in medical history, and his followers were among the first to describe and document many diseases and medical conditions. However, Chunyu Yi, a famous Chinese physician of the Han dynasty who died around 8 ADE, kept the first known health record. He tracked his patients' residences, their names, occupations, disease information, diagnoses, and prognoses. This record provides valuable historic data.

Between 1790 and 1821, some of America's earliest hospitals began keeping patient records, including the New York Hospital, Pennsylvania Hospital, and Massachusetts General Hospital. Health records, historically restricted by the documentation habits of each individual healthcare provider, began to evolve in the United States during the Civil War. During this time, doctors began to record medical information in an increasingly standardized form, as social and physical mobility meant that they might treat patients they had never seen before. This trend continued as health records were established for immigrants to America at the advent of the twentieth century.

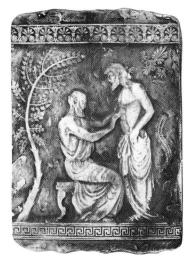

Hippocrates was one of the first health-care practitioners to document diseases.

In 1917, the **American College of Surgeons (ACS)** developed a hospital standardization program that established the **minimum standards**, which identified the elements required for reporting care and treatment. Minimum standards ensured that the health record communicated an accurate account of the healthcare information as well as the status of the patient. Some of the suggested standards for maintaining the patient record included patient identification, personal and family history, reason for encounter, history of current illness, physical examination, diagnosis, treatment, progress notes, and discharge. These standards are still being used almost a century later.

Today, healthcare providers have focused on documenting the patient's past and present care. The health record is an essential part of a patient's healthcare because it helps the provider make an informed treatment decision and is a tool for communication among caregivers.

Beyond traditional shelf filing of handwritten paper records, there have been few advances in medical records storage. Microfilm was used in the 1950s and optical scanning in the 1980s, but no real advancements in actual record keeping were made until the birth of the EHR.

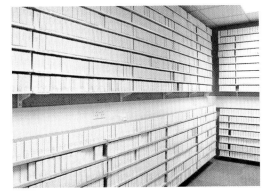

Medical records were often stored on microfilm starting in the 1950s.

Dr. Lawrence L. Weed is considered to be one of the pioneers in the EHR movement. Dr. Weed, a medical doctor specializing in internal medicine, along with Jan Schultz, developed the **Problem-Oriented Medical Record (POMR)**, a systematic approach to the documentation of medical records. In the 1970s, they also developed a software program called **PROMIS (Problem-Oriented Medical Information System)** at the University of Vermont under a federal grant. Healthcare providers did not embrace PROMIS, primarily because too much information was needed to

EXPAND
YOUR LEARNING

Review the following infographic at the HealthIT website to learn more about the history of the electronic health record:

www.paradigmcollege.net /exploringehr/infographic

complete the required fields, so physicians felt that they spent too much time focusing on documentation rather than patient care.

Purposes of the Health Record

The primary purpose of the health record, whether electronically recorded or put on paper, is to document the health history of the patient. The health record is comprised of **data**, which includes the descriptive or numeric attributes of one or more variables. Data collected and analyzed becomes **information**. A **record** is a collection, usually in writing, of an account or an occurrence. The **health record** is an accumulation of information about a patient's past and present health. Typically, the health record begins at the first visit or admission. A patient may have different records with each healthcare provider, such as a primary care physician, cardiologist, dermatologist, or dentist. Each provider must accurately enter the information in the record, such as who provided the health services; what, when, and why the services were provided; and the eventual outcome. The information in the health record is essential when tracking the patient's illnesses along with the treatments, communication, and continuity of care among healthcare providers. In addition, the health record provides information for billing and reimbursement, legal documentation, quality review, research, education, credentialing, and collection of health statistics for government agencies such as the Centers for Disease Control and Prevention (CDC) and the National Committee on Vital and Health Statistics (NCVHS). Health records may also provide crucial information that may indicate food supply contamination or bioterrorism.

Health Record Data

There are four major categories of information in the health record: administrative data, clinical data, legal data, and financial information. **Administrative data** includes demographic information about the patient such as the patient's name, address, date of birth, race, primary language, religion, and marital status. **Clinical data** is information such as admission dates, office visits, laboratory test results, evaluations, or emergency visits. **Legal data** is composed of consents for treatment and authorizations for the release of information. The last category, **financial data**, includes the patient's insurance and payment information for healthcare services. (See Figure 2.1.)

Administrative Data

Administrative data is information that the patient provides or populates in the health record. The administrative information typically found in the health record includes:

- Patient's name
- Address
- Telephone number
- Place of birth
- Date of birth

- Age
- Sex
- Marital status
- Ethnic origin
- Emergency contact information

The healthcare staff collects administrative information to verify the patient's identity and to help create a patient's demographic profile. See Figure 2.2 for an example of a form used to collect administrative information.

Figure 2.1   Types of Health Record Data

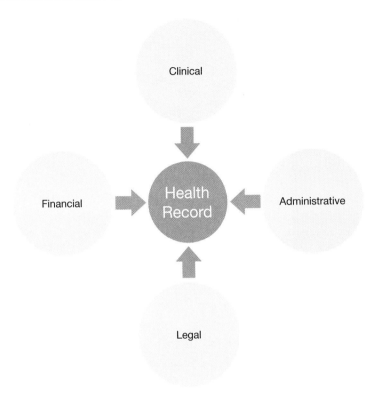

Figure 2.2   Admission Face Sheet

Center City Outpatient Program
ADMISSION FACE SHEET

Patient Name: Last _____ First _____ Middle _____

Are you known by a previous name? ❑ No   ❑ Yes: _____

Patient Address: _____

Home Phone:_____ Work Phone:_____ Cell Phone:_____

Date of Birth: _____

Sex: ❑ M   ❑ F

Occupation: _____

Marital Status: ❑ Single   ❑ Married   ❑ Separated   ❑ Divorced   ❑ Widowed   ❑ Life Partner

Clinical Data

Clinical data includes the medical information taken and recorded by the healthcare provider. It is important that the clinical data is detailed, complete, precise, timely, and accurate because the information plays a large role in the overall health plan of the patient. The clinical data includes documentation such as:

- Pathology and laboratory reports

- History and physical assessments

- Allergies

- X-rays

- List of medications

- Surgeries

- Hospital admissions

- Progress notes

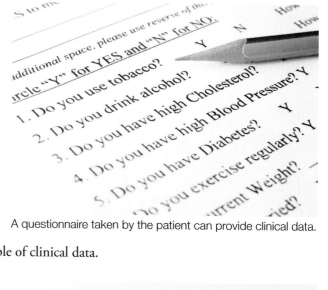

A questionnaire taken by the patient can provide clinical data.

Figure 2.3 provides an example of clinical data.

Legal Data

Legal data in the health record may be found on a variety of forms that are also considered legal documents. Some of these documents include:

- Release of records—written request to release patient's health information to another healthcare provider or other entity in need of the patient's information

- Health Insurance Portability and Accountability Act (HIPAA) forms—HIPAA notice of privacy authorization

- General consent for care—agreement to general treatment and care

- Informed consent—agreement to a procedure

- Advance directives—written statement describing a patient's wishes regarding medical treatment recorded in the event that the individual is no longer able to make such decisions due to illness or incapacity

Figure 2.4 illustrates an example of a form considered to be a legal document. Chapter 6 further explores legal documents in more detail, describing how they are added to and released from the EHR.

Because the health record contains a variety of legal documents, it is considered a legal document. A court of law may use the health record in many different types of legal proceedings. The healthcare facility protects itself by requiring proper documentation and ensuring accurate information where and whenever it is required.

Figure 2.3 Clinical Data Form

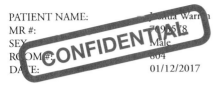

PATIENT NAME: Joshua Warren
MR #:   70935?8
SEX: Male
ROOM #:   804
DATE: 01/12/2017

TREADMILL STRESS TEST

INDICATION
The patient was admitted to Brookfield Medical Center complaining of mild chest pains. He is a 26-year-old white male who is actually quite athletic but has been noted on several occasions to have borderline hypertension. He has a family history of coronary artery disease in the father (who, incidentally, was a smoker), who died at the age of 54 secondary to coronary artery disease.

TECHNIQUE
The patient was exercised according to standard Bruce protocol for a total of 9 minutes and 30 seconds, at which time the test was stopped because he had obtained the target heart rate.

FINDINGS
He has a maximal heart rate of 181, which was approximately 93% of the predicted maximum of 195. He developed some clear up-sloping ST- and T-wave segment changes of 1–2 mm, specifically in leads V3, aVF, and anterior leads V3 through V6, but this resolved in the rest period. He developed only a mild blood pressure rise to a maximum of 146/90 at maximal exercise. Blood pressure returned to his resting normal quickly in recovery.

IMPRESSION
Negative treadmill stress test, with negative hypertensive response.

PLAN
Patient was given signs and symptoms of cardiac chest pain, including pressing substernal chest pain, shortness of breath, sweating, nausea or vomiting, or increase of pain with activity.

ADDENDUM
Patient was given extensive cardiovascular precautions, including the possibility of significant cardiac disease despite a seemingly negative treadmill stress test. The patient voiced understanding of this fact and also the need to seek immediate clinical attention should chest pain or other cardiovascular symptoms appear.

_____
Sondra Southward, MD

SS/XX
D: 01/12/2017
T: 01/13/2017

Financial Data

Financial data consists of insurance and employer information. A copy of the patient's insurance coverage, when available, may also be included. There may be times when a patient pays for healthcare services with a payment plan or another type of financial arrangement. The financial data section of the health record would note this agreement. Figure 2.5 shows a financial data form that a patient may be asked to complete at the time of the visit. Financial data is often combined with administrative data, meaning that both types of data are collected on the same form.

Figure 2.4 Legal Data Form

Authorization to Release Medical Records and Billing Information

Name: _____

Address: _____

City: _____ State: _____ ZIP: _____

Date: _____ (MM/DD/YYYY)

Name of Hospital or Physician: _____

Address: _____

City: _____ State: _____ ZIP: _____

I, _____, hereby authorize _____ (hospital or physican name) to release to _____ (name of person to receive records), any information in my personal medical records, including all X-rays, computed tomography scans, and any other information pertinent to my treatment, along with all billing information while under the care of _____ during the time period from _____. I give my permission for this medical information to be used for insurance claim purposes. I do not, however, give permission for any other use or for any redisclosure of this information.

Signature: _____

Patient Name (Printed): _____

Date: _____

This authorization will expire one year from the date of the signature below. I understand that I can revoke this authorization at any time by writing to the healthcare provider, but that revoking this authorization will not affect disclosures made or actions taken before the revocation is received.

I also understand that:

–I am not required to sign this authorization and that my healthcare or payment for care will not be affected by my refusal.

–Federal privacy regulations will no longer apply to the information disclosed, and that the entity receiving the records may not be subject to patient privacy laws and may redisclose the records.

–I am entitled to receive a copy of this authorization.

–A copy of this authorization may be utilized with the same effectiveness as an original.

Figure 2.5 Financial Data Form

Patient Insurance Information

Primary Policyholder Information

Insurance Plan: _____

Policyholder's Name: _____

Address: _____

_____

Home Phone: _____ Work Phone: _____ Cell Phone: _____

Birth Date: _____

Relationship to Patient: _____

Employer Name: _____

Employer Address: _____

The electronic health record (EHR) must meet the same requirements of a paper health record to be considered a legal document. Healthcare providers must accurately document vital signs, chief complaints, history, orders, plans, and prescriptions. The procedures and tools must also comply with the state's and organization's requirements. Documentation must be original, corrected, clarified, and amended. The EHR must maintain clinical messages, reports, and auditing tools. In addition, healthcare organizations must implement policies to include how unique health records are created and maintained; how content is chosen to be required; how they are authenticated and accessed; how the privacy, confidentiality, and security are maintained; and how amendments and corrections are made. Healthcare organizations must create policies for record retention, archiving, destruction, abstracting, and reporting. Healthcare organizations should work with vendors to ensure that their EHR software adheres to the regulations to maintain a legal health record. What else can healthcare organizations do to maintain the legal health record in an EHR system? What might EHR vendors do to help healthcare organizations maintain a legal health record?

NCVHS Core Data Elements

In 1996, the **National Committee on Vital and Health Statistics (NCVHS)** completed a review of core health data elements and developed a list and definitions of the 42 core elements that can be used in a variety of healthcare settings. The patient provides the patient/enrollment data at the initial visit with the healthcare provider or facility, not at subsequent visits. Table 2.1 provides these core data elements and their definitions.

In addition to the core data elements proposed by NCVHS, other data sets have been proposed as national guidelines to encourage the exchange of information across healthcare providers and settings. The American Health Information Management Association (AHIMA) developed a core data set for the physician practice EHR, with its core elements divided into demographic and administrative information, vital signs, reason for visit, present illness, past medical history, physical examination, problem and medication list, screenings, immunization, summary, referrals, and authentication.

Core Data Element	Definition
Patient/Enrollment Data	
Personal/Unique Identifier	Two options: A. Name—Last, first, middle, suffix B. Numeric identifier Without a universal unique identifier or a set of data items to form a unique identifier, it is impossible to link data across healthcare facilities and providers.
Date of Birth	MM,DD,YYYY
Sex	M/F

Race and Ethnicity	Recommendation to be self-reported
	Race
	  1. American Indian/Eskimo/Aleut
	  2. Asian or Pacific Islander
	  3. Black
	  4. White
	  5. Other
	Ethnicity
	  1. Hispanic origin
	  2. Not of Hispanic origin

Residence	Full address and ZIP code

Marital Status	1. Married—married (currently married; classify common-law marriage as married)
	   a. Living together
	   b. Not living together
	2. Never married—never married or annulled
	3. Widowed—person widowed or not remarried
	4. Divorced—person divorced and not remarried
	5. Separated—person legally separated
	6. Partner—civil unions (some forms now include this option)

Living/Residential Arrangement	Living Arrangement
	  1. Alone
	  2. With spouse (alternate: with spouse or unrelated partner)
	  3. With children
	  4. With parent or guardian
	  5. With relatives other than spouse, children, or parents
	  6. With nonrelatives
	Residential Arrangement
	  1. Private residence/household
	  2. Homeless shelter
	  3. Housing with services or supervision
	  4. Jail/correctional facility
	  5. Healthcare institutional setting
	  6. Homeless
	  7. Other residential setting

Core Data Element	Definition
Self-Reported Health Status	There is no consensus on how to define health status, but a common measure is: Excellent Very good Good Fair Poor
Functional Status	The functional status of a person is an increasingly important health measure shown to be strongly related to medical care utilization rates. Many scales have been developed that include both (a) self-report measures such as limitations of activities of daily living and instrumental activities of daily living, and National Health Interview Survey age-specific summary, and (b) clinical assessments such as the International Classification of Impairments, Disabilities and Handicaps, and the Resident Assessment Instrument. Self-report measures and clinical assessments are both valuable and informative.
Years of Schooling	Years of schooling completed by the enrollee/patient as a proxy for socioeconomic status. This core data element is highly predictive of health status and healthcare use.
Patient's Relationship to Subscriber/Person Eligible for Entitlement	1. Self 2. Spouse 3. Child 4. Other
Current or Most Recent Occupation/Industry	Used to track occupational diseases
Type of Encounter	1. Inpatient 2. Outpatient 3. Emergency department 4. Observation 5. Ambulatory 6. Other
Admission Date (inpatient)	Format MM, DD, YYYY
Encounter Data	
Discharge Date (inpatient)	Format MM, DD, YYYY
Date of Encounter (ambulatory and physician services)	Format MM, DD, YYYY
Facility Identification	Identifier for hospitals, ambulatory surgery centers, nursing homes, hospices, among others
Type of Facility/Place of Encounter	Identifier for type or place of encounter; part of the National Provider Identifier (NPI)
Healthcare Provider Identification (outpatient)	The NPI enables each provider to have a universal unique number across the system
Provider Location or Address of Encounter (outpatient)	Full address and ZIP code for the location of the provider
Attending Physician Identification (inpatient)	The unique national identification assigned to the clinician of record at discharge
Operating Physician Identification (inpatient)	The unique national identification assigned to the clinician who performed the principal procedure
Provider Specialty	Part of NPI system that identifies the provider's specialty
Principal Diagnosis (inpatient)	The condition determined to be chiefly responsible for patient admission

Table 2.1 National Committee on Vital and Health Statistics Core Data Elements *(continued)*

Core Data Element	Definition
Primary Diagnosis (inpatient)	The diagnosis responsible for the majority of the care given to the patient
Other Diagnoses (inpatient)	Conditions should be coded that affect patient care in terms of requiring: 1. Clinical evaluation 2. Therapeutic treatment 3. Diagnostic procedures 4. Extended length of hospital stay 5. Increased nursing care/monitoring
Qualifier for Other Diagnoses (inpatient)	The following should be applied to each diagnosis coded under *other diagnoses* 1. Onset prior to admission 2. Onset not prior to admission 3. Onset uncertain
Patient's Stated Reason for Visit or Chief Complaint (ambulatory)	Reason at the time of the encounter for seeking attention or care
Diagnosis Chiefly Responsible for Services Provided (ambulatory)	Contains the code(s) for the diagnosis, condition, problem, or the reason for encounter/visit chiefly responsible for the services provided
Other Diagnoses (ambulatory)	Additional code(s) that describe any conditions coexisting at the time of the encounter/visit and require management
External Cause of Injury	Code for the external cause of an injury, poisoning, or adverse event; completed whenever there is a diagnosis of an injury, poisoning, or adverse event
Birth Weight of Newborn (inpatient)	Specific birth weight of the newborn recorded in grams or in pounds and ounces
Principal Procedure (inpatient)	The principal procedure is one that was performed for definitive treatment, rather than one performed for diagnostic or exploratory purposes, or necessary to take care of a complication. If there appear to be two procedures that are principal, then the one most related to the principal diagnosis should be selected as the principal procedure. 1. Is surgical in nature 2. Carries a procedural risk 3. Carries an anesthetic risk 4. Requires specialized training
Other Procedures (inpatient)	All other procedures that are considered significant. A significant procedure is one of the following: 1. Is surgical in nature 2. Carries a procedural risk 3. Carries an anesthetic risk 4. Requires specialized training
Dates of Procedures (inpatient)	MM, DD, YYYY
Services (ambulatory)	Describe all diagnostic services of any type, including history and physical examinations, laboratory studies, X-rays, and others performed and are pertinent to the patient's reasons for the encounter; all therapeutic series; all preventive services and procedures at time of encounter
Medications Prescribed	All medications prescribed by the healthcare provider at the time of the encounter. Include dosage, strength, and amount prescribed

Table 2.1 National Committee on Vital and Health Statistics Core Data Elements

Core Data Element	Definition

Disposition of Patient (inpatient)	1. Discharge status
	   a. Discharged alive
	   b. Discharged dead
	   c. Status not stated
	2. Discharge setting
	   a. Discharged to home or self-care
	   b. Discharged to acute care hospital
	   c. Discharged to a nursing facility
	   d. Discharged to other healthcare facility
	   e. Discharged home to be under care of a home health services agency
	   f. Left against medical advice

Disposition (ambulatory)	Provider's statement of the next steps in care of patient. The following are the suggested classifications: 1. No follow-up planned 2. Follow-up planned or scheduled 3. Referred elsewhere
Patient's Expected Sources of Payment	Name of each source of payment including primary and secondary sources
Injury Related to Employment	Yes or No
Total Billed Charges	Co-payment or update payment data when available

CHECKPOINT 2.1

1. Explain the differences among the following terms: *data*, *information*, and *record*.

   _____

   _____

   _____

2. Describe several types of information that may be found within a health record.

   _____

   _____

   _____

Health Record Format

Format is related to the arrangement of a paper health record. There are no specific requirements on how paper health records are formatted, as long as an organization uses the same format throughout its facility. There are three organizational formats used in paper health records: source-oriented record, integrated health record, and problem-oriented record.

Source-Oriented Record

The **source-oriented record (SOR)**, is the most common format used by healthcare facilities. This format organizes the health documents into sections that contain information collected from a specific department or type of service; for example, all progress notes, laboratory reports, and radiology reports are assembled together in their respective sections. Within each section, the health record content is organized in chronologic order. (Most healthcare facilities using the source-oriented format keep the health content in chronologic rather than reverse chronologic order.) SORs allow for the rapid retrieval of health content, although the format can be challenging to view the complete health status of the patient.

Integrated Health Record

The second format type is the **integrated health record**, which is organized either in chronologic or reverse chronologic order. The health content is not separated by department or type of service; therefore, health documentation is viewed by date. Healthcare facilities may use the integrated health record format in several ways. The medical chart may place all forms together or be organized by healthcare setting (for example, all dental forms in one section, all primary care documents in another, etc.). The integrated health record provides a complete view of the health status of the patient, although this format makes it difficult to compare findings from the same type of service, such as comparing two radiology reports completed at the beginning and at the end of a patient's stay.

Problem-Oriented Record

The third format type is the **problem-oriented record (POR)**. As discussed previously, Dr. Lawrence L. Weed developed this type of record because the SOR did not provide a complete view of the patient's health status. The POR focuses on assessment of the clinical documentation by healthcare providers and the creation of a plan that addresses the patient's health concerns. This type of format promotes a team approach to documentation through the use of the SOAP format progress notes.

The **progress notes** in a POR are written in the **SOAP format**:

- S (Subjective)—the reason why the patient is at the healthcare facility for care, as well as comments from the patient or patient's family about the existing condition

- O (Objective)—specific notes such as results from a laboratory test completed during the patient's visit

- A (Assessment)—the healthcare provider's opinion on the condition or diagnosis

- P (Plan)—the healthcare provider's plan to diagnose or treat the patient

The SOAP format is used in both paper and electronic records.

CHECKPOINT 2.2

1. Describe the source-oriented health record format.

_____

_____

_____

_____

2. What are the four components of the SOAP progress note format?

a. _____

b. _____

c. _____

d. _____

Health Record Content

The content of a health record will vary depending on the type of healthcare facility. (Chapter 4 will go into greater detail on the different types of healthcare facilities.) In this chapter, the health record content of patients in acute and ambulatory settings will be discussed. Note the variances in the patient records of these two types of facilities.

Acute Care Setting

Facilities that provide acute care include hospitals and long-term care centers. Patients who are admitted to these facilities are called inpatients. **Inpatients** occupy a hospital bed for at least one night in the course of treatment, examination, or observation.

Record Content

For an inpatient admitted to an acute care setting, a health record usually contains the following content:

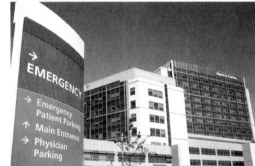

A hospital is an inpatient, acute care facility.

- Admission Record—state of the patient when he or she is admitted to an acute care facility

- History and Physical—information regarding the patient's past and current health condition, assessment, and treatment or diagnostic workup plan

- Progress Notes—entries of the patient's care and progress reported by the healthcare providers

- Laboratory Tests—test and laboratory results ordered by healthcare providers

- Diagnostic Tests—medical tests that assist in the diagnosis of the patient's health issue

- Operative Notes—notes immediately written after surgery that document the procedure and results

- Pathology Reports—detailed information on the review of specimens from tissue or cell biopsy

- Physician Orders—orders given by the physician for medications, fluids, patient testing, etc.

- Consents—authorizations for treatment

- Consultations—reports provided by other healthcare providers that review the patient's health issues

- Emergency Department Encounters—documentation of visits or encounters in the emergency department

- Discharge Summary—summary of the patient's course of care signed by the attending physician

The content in each record may be supplied in different formats but typically contains similar data.

Ambulatory Care Setting

Ambulatory care is an increasingly popular mode of healthcare delivery. Some ambulatory care settings include:

- Physician offices

- Clinics

- Surgery centers

- Dental offices

- Imaging centers

- Occupational health centers

- Oral and maxillofacial offices

- Podiatrists

- Pain management

- Community or college health centers

- Urgent care centers

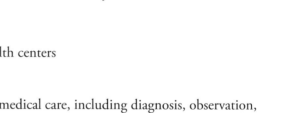

A dental office is an example of an ambulatory care facility.

The term *ambulatory* is used for medical care, including diagnosis, observation, treatment, and rehabilitation services. Patients receiving treatment in an ambulatory setting are called outpatients. **Outpatients** are patients who do not spend more than 24 hours in a healthcare facility.

Record Content

Each facility, unless part of an organization, creates and maintains its own health record for a patient. The ambulatory care record typically contains the following content:

- Demographic Information—patient's name, address, date of birth, and other patient information not medical in nature

- Contact Information—various telephone numbers and email addresses, as well as emergency contacts

- History and Physical—health history, a review of vital signs, and a complete organ-specific physical examination

- Immunization Records—comprehensive list of dates and types of vaccines received as a child, as well as additional vaccines such as flu, tetanus, and hepatitis

- Problem Lists—list of patient's current health issues

- Allergy Lists—list of medications, food, and other items to which a patient is allergic

- Prescription Lists—list of current medications, including dosages

- Progress Notes—updates to the patient's healthcare issues; may be in a SOAP format

- Assessment—summary of the likely causes of the patient's current health issues; provides course of action to address health issues

- Consultations—documentation of a patient's visit to another healthcare provider and what that healthcare provider recommends or concludes

- Referrals—permission or suggestions for the patient to be seen by another healthcare provider

- Treatment Plans—plan for treatment of the patient's health issues

- Patient Instructions—directions and orders to be followed by the patient to help with his or her health issues

- Laboratory Tests and Results—test and laboratory results ordered by the healthcare provider

- Consents—authorizations for treatment

- Communication—letters, emails, telephone messages, or any other documented communication

- External Correspondence—communication between the healthcare provider and any other provider or carrier that provides information about the patient

- Financial Information—payment arrangements and insurance information

Each specialty practice may provide the health information in a slightly different way, but the concept and purpose of each of the contents is the same.

CHECKPOINT 2.3

1. Name five content areas found in an acute care health record.

   a. _____

   b. _____

   c. _____

   d. _____

   e. _____

2. Name five content areas found in an ambulatory care health record.

   a. _____

   b. _____

   c. _____

   d. _____

   e. _____

Documentation in the Health Record

The healthcare facility is responsible for the quality of care provided to its patients. Direct documentation of this care must be provided in a paper record or EHR system and is the responsibility of the healthcare provider. This documentation must be accurate and complete, reflecting all procedures, treatments, medications, tests, assessments, observations, and communications involved with patient care. Remember the saying, "If it's not documented, it didn't happen."

The maintenance and accuracy of the health record are important responsibilities of health information staff, whose duty is to ensure that healthcare records are readily available when patients arrive for care. The staff must also ensure that all forms are in each patient's record, verify that the healthcare provider has documented care, validate the accuracy of the coding of service, and adhere to established healthcare data standards.

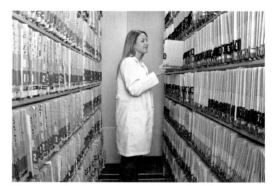

Paper medical records must be pulled from shelves and be readily available when patients arrive at a healthcare facility..

Documentation Guidelines

General guidelines should be followed when documenting within the health record. These guidelines may include:

- Confirming the patient's identity
- Identifying the service provider
- Completing the proper forms in a timely manner
- Ensuring correct and complete documentation

In addition, healthcare personnel must follow specific guidelines when entering health record information, including using black ink for copying, faxing, and imaging; leaving no blank lines; and avoiding backdating of entries.

Lastly, when working with health records, healthcare personnel need to be aware of three areas of concern that affect patient safety: the legibility of the entries, the use of only approved abbreviations and acronyms in the documentation, and the protocol for changing or correcting documented entries. Specifics of these safety concerns are outlined below.

Legibility of Entries

When working with paper record entries, interpreting the handwriting of healthcare providers may be difficult (see Figure 2.6). Consequently, healthcare personnel must query any unclear entries with the appropriate staff members. This verification check protects both the safety of the patient as well as the liability of the healthcare worker and the facility.

The Use of Abbreviations and Acronyms

Abbreviations and acronyms are often used in the health record. Therefore, to ensure clear communication, there are standards for abbreviations and symbols that should be followed when documenting information. Some examples of approved abbreviations are provided in Table 2.2. Healthcare facilities can place additional rules in their bylaws that indicate other acceptable abbreviations per facility preference.

Figure 2.6 Handwritten Progress Note

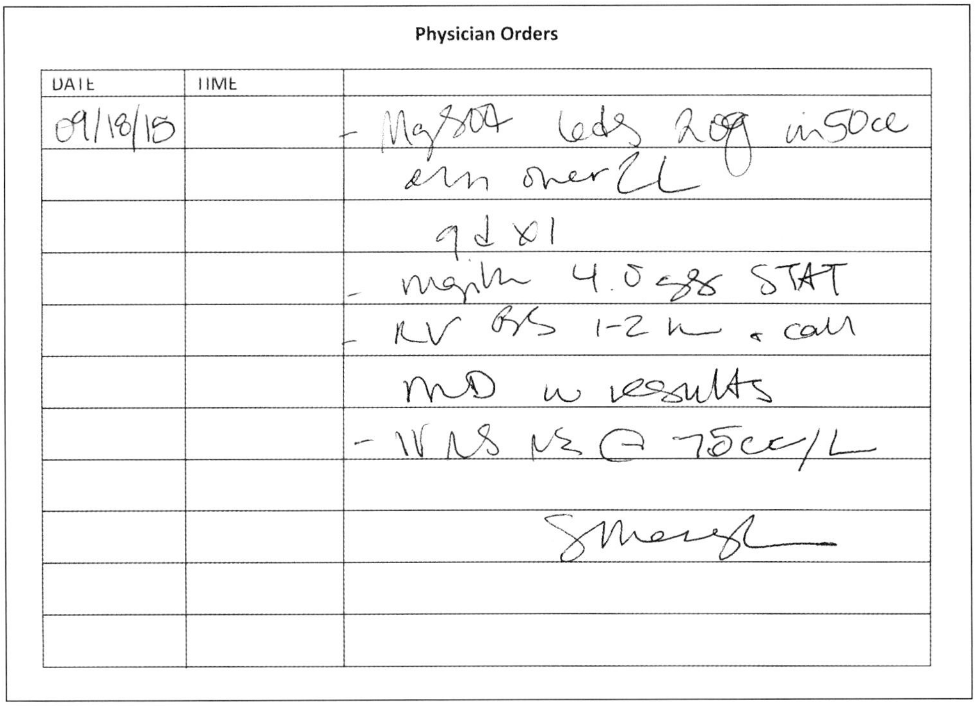

Physician Orders

Table 2.2 Health Record Abbreviations and Acronyms

Abbreviation	Meaning	Abbreviation	Meaning
ABN	Advanced Beneficiary Notice	MMR	Measles, Mumps, and Rubella
BMI	Body Mass Index	MS	Musculoskeletal
BP	Blood Pressure	Neuro	Neurologic
CV	Cardiovascular	NPP	Notice of Privacy Practices
DOB	Date of Birth	02	Oxygen
DPT	Diphtheria, Pertussis, and Tetanus	OR	Operating Room
ENMT	Ears, Nose, Mouth, and Throat	p.o.	By Mouth
ETOH	Alcohol	PCP	Primary Care Provider
GI	Gastrointestinal	PRN	As Needed
GYN	Gynecologic	ROS	Review of Systems
HPI	History of Present Illness	Temp	Temperature
LMP	Last Menstrual Period	VIS	Vaccine Information Sheet
MD	Medical Doctor		

The Joint Commission developed an Official "Do Not Use" List of Abbreviations as part of its information management standards that healthcare organizations must follow. In addition, the commission has proposed a list for possible future inclusion in the Official "Do Not Use" List. The "Do Not Use" list is found in Figure 2.7.

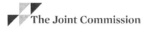
The Joint Commission

Facts about the Official "Do Not Use" List

In 2001, The Joint Commission issued a *Sentinel Event Alert* on the subject of medical abbreviations, and just one year later, its Board of Commissioners approved a National Patient Safety Goal requiring accredited organizations to develop and implement a list of abbreviations not to use. In 2004, The Joint Commission created its "do not use" list of abbreviations (see below) as part of the requirements for meeting that goal. In 2010, NPSG.02.02.01 was integrated into the Information Management standards as elements of performance 2 and 3 under IM.02.02.01.

Currently, this requirement does not apply to preprogrammed health information technology systems (for example, electronic medical records or CPOE systems), but this application remains under consideration for the future. Organizations contemplating introduction or upgrade of such systems should strive to eliminate the use of dangerous abbreviations, acronyms, symbols, and dose designations from the software.

Official "Do Not Use" List[1]

Do Not Use	Potential Problem	Use Instead
U, u (unit)	Mistaken for "0" (zero), the number "4" (four) or "cc"	Write "unit"
IU (International Unit)	Mistaken for IV (intravenous) or the number 10 (ten)	Write "International Unit"
Q.D., QD, q.d., qd (daily)	Mistaken for each other	Write "daily"
Q.O.D., QOD, q.o.d, qod (every other day)	Period after the Q mistaken for "I" and the "O" mistaken for "I	Write "every other day"
Trailing zero (X.0 mg)* Lack of leading zero (.X mg)	Decimal point is missed	Write X mg Write 0.X mg
MS	Can mean morphine sulfate or magnesium sulfate	Write "morphine sulfate" Write "magnesium sulfate"
MSO_4 and $MgSO_4$	Confused for one another	

[1] Applies to all orders and all medication-related documentation that is handwritten (including free-text computer entry) or on pre-printed forms.

*Exception: A "trailing zero" may be used only where required to demonstrate the level of precision of the value being reported, such as for laboratory results, imaging studies that report size of lesions, or catheter/tube sizes. It may not be used in medication orders or other medication-related documentation.

Changing or Correcting Documented Entries

Healthcare personnel need to follow established procedures when changing or correcting documented entries in a paper health record. Information is not allowed to be erased.

When correcting information in an electronic medical record (EMR), providers usually write an addendum to the existing report. Information may not be deleted from an entry.

Health Record Standards

Several accreditation, professional, and regulatory organizations provide guidelines and support on maintaining the integrity of patient health records. By affiliation with these organizations and meeting their professional standards and goals, healthcare facilities can distinguish their services from others as well as reduce the number of state and federal reviews. A focus of all of these organizations is to improve the quality of patient care and health record documentation.

Accreditation Organizations

Four accreditation organizations affiliated with healthcare quality include The Joint Commission, the National Committee for Quality Assurance (NCQA), the Community Health Accreditation Program (CHAP), and the Accreditation Association for Ambulatory Health Care (AAAHC).

The Joint Commission, formerly known as the Joint Commission on Accreditation of Healthcare Organizations (JCAHO), is an independent, not-for-profit organization that accredits and certifies a variety of healthcare organizations, ranging from dentistry to behavioral health to acute care facilities. Health record content standards are addressed in each field of healthcare.

The **National Committee for Quality Assurance (NCQA)** is an independent, nonprofit organization that focuses on healthcare quality. Healthcare organizations such as individual or group healthcare providers and health plans that seek NCQA accreditation do so voluntarily.

The **Community Health Accreditation Program (CHAP)** and the **Accreditation Association for Ambulatory Health Care (AAAHC)** are two examples of specialty accrediting organizations.

EXPAND
YOUR LEARNING
Search for these organizations on the Internet to learn more about how they promote high standards in documenting health information.

Professional Organizations

The American Health Information Management Association (AHIMA) and the Healthcare Information and Management Systems Society (HIMSS) are two professional organizations that support healthcare information personnel in maintaining quality assurance of health records.

The **American Health Information Management Association (AHIMA)** is a professional organization that provides resources, education, and networking with other professionals. AHIMA focuses on the quality of health information used in the delivery of healthcare. Initially, the organization focused on hospital records, but it now supports ambulatory, community health, and many other healthcare delivery (HCD) organizations.

The **Healthcare Information and Management Systems Society (HIMSS)** focuses on using information technology and management systems to improve the quality and delivery of healthcare.

Regulatory Organizations

Lastly, two healthcare organizations actively involved in setting standards for health records are the Association for Healthcare Documentation Integrity (ADHI) and the Centers for Medicare & Medicaid Services (CMS).

The **Association for Healthcare Documentation Integrity (AHDI)** has vowed "to set and uphold standards for education and practice in the field of clinical documentation that ensure the highest level of accuracy, privacy, and security for the U.S. healthcare systems in order to protect public health, increase patient safety, and improve quality of care for healthcare consumers."

Centers for Medicare & Medicaid Services (CMS) is a federal government agency that oversees federal healthcare programs, including Medicare Conditions of Participation (CoPs). In 2009, CMS expanded its role to include the implementation of EHR incentive programs, meaningful use of certified EHR systems, drafting standards for certified EHR technology, and updating privacy and security regulations under HIPAA.

Ownership of the Health Record

Health record ownership is a controversial topic that grows increasingly more complex as healthcare facilities move from paper health records to EHRs. Generally speaking, the healthcare facility that created the record owns the physical health record. A **sole practitioner** (a single, independent healthcare practice) owns the record created in his or her practice. A hospital or long-term care facility owns records for all patients admitted.

Obtaining a Health Record

Patients have the right to access and/or obtain a copy of their health records, depending on federal and/or state laws. To request a copy of the health record from the healthcare provider, a patient typically provides a written request, signs a HIPAA-compliant release of records form, and then pays the necessary fees. The cost of a copy of the health record varies depending on the provider and facility; usually the provider or facility charges a certain number of cents per page, plus a fee for the staff's time to retrieve and copy the record. Some patients requesting a copy of X-rays or scans are required to pay for the actual cost of copying the films. Once any necessary fees are paid, the healthcare provider makes the records available for pick up or mailing. See Figure 2.8 for an example of a release of information form for a patient's health record. As more health records are housed in EHR systems, an increasing number of patients will request to receive an electronic copy of their records. The ability to receive electronic records is discussed in more detail in Chapter 3.

Ownership of Health Information

There are many differing opinions about who owns health information, and the subject remains controversial. Is the patient the owner because he or she is the subject of the record? Or, is the HCD system the owner because it generated the information and physically has possession of the record? It is generally accepted that the HCD system owns paper records and EMRs because these records are the legal records of what took place during patient encounters at HCD systems. The EHR is viewed differently, however. The patient is generally recognized as the owner of an EHR because it is not a legal record but a subset of information from various HCD systems where the patient had encounters.

Many leaders in health information management anticipate that future legislation will address the subject of the ownership of health information, ultimately creating a uniform definition of ownership.

Figure 2.8 Release of Information

EMC Medical Center   MRN/Chart #_____

PATIENT INFORMATION

Name _____ Address _____ City _____ State _____ ZIP _____

Date of Birth _____ Daytime Phone _____ Previous Name (if applicable) _____

AUTHORIZES

Name of Healthcare Provider/Plan _____

Address _____

TO DISCLOSE TO

❏ Self
        Delivery Options: ❏ Pick Up ❏ View on Site ❏ Mail to Address Above

❏ To Be Picked Up By Another Person
        I hereby authorize _____ to pick up my records.

Send to: ❏ _____
        Name of Healthcare Provider/Plan

        _____   _____
        Address   Fax Number

DATE(S) OF INFORMATION TO BE DISCLOSED: From _____ to _____. If left blank, only information from the past two (2) years will be disclosed.

INFORMATION TO BE DISCLOSED:
❏ All medical records related to (specify condition, treatment, etc.): _____
❏ All billing records related to (specify condition, treatment, etc.):_____
❏ Radiology films/images (specify test): _____
❏ Other records: _____
_____

DO NOT DISCLOSE THE FOLLOWING INFORMATION:
❏ Alcohol/drug use   ❏ HIV test results   ❏ Mental health status   ❏ Developmental disabilities

PURPOSE (check all that apply):
❏ Further Medical Care   ❏ Legal   ❏ Insurance   ❏ Personal   ❏ Other:_____

YOUR RIGHTS WITH RESPECT TO THIS AUTHORIZATION
I am aware that I have the right to inspect and receive a copy of the health information I have authorized to be used and/or disclosed by this authorization. I understand that I may be charged a fee for record copies. In addition, I understand that I do not need to sign this authorization in order to receive treatment. I understand that I may revoke this authorization by notifying the disclosing medical records/health information department in writing. However, I understand that my revocation will not be effective as to uses and/or disclosures: (1) already made in reliance upon this Authorization; or (2) needed for an insurer to contest a claim/policy as authorized by law if signing the Authorization was a condition to obtaining insurance coverage. I realize that the information used and/or disclosed pursuant to this Authorization may be subject to redisclosure and no longer protected by federal privacy law.

SIGNATURE OF PATIENT/LEGAL REPRESENTATION
_____ DATE: _____

Importance of EHR Transition

Unfortunately, it took a natural disaster to underscore the importance of transitioning from the paper health record to an EHR.

On Monday, August 29, 2005, Hurricane Katrina made landfall in southeastern Louisiana. The impact of the hurricane caused the levee system in New Orleans to break, and many parts of the city flooded significantly as a consequence. This disaster washed away thousands of paper records, and many residents of the greater New Orleans area lost all of their medical information. In addition, many healthcare providers fled New Orleans, which left many patients adrift in their healthcare needs. These patients had no record of their health history, current health status, or information regarding their medications and had no way to contact their healthcare providers. In response, the U.S. federal government, along with public and private organizations, created the KatrinaHealth website to help healthcare providers and pharmacies obtain access to patients' prescription information. Although this service helped many New Orleans citizens, one segment of the city's population still had access to their medical records: veterans. The U.S. Veterans Health Administration uses VistA, which is an EHR system that was created in the 1970s to assist with the HCD for veterans and their families. Because this information was electronic, displaced veterans were able to access their records no matter where they chose to relocate.

Hurricane Katrina highlighted the necessity for health information to withstand natural disasters, an important lesson that supports the initiative for the development of EHRs.

Many paper health records were destroyed in Hurricane Katrina.

Consider This

St. John's Hospital in Joplin, Missouri, converted its medical records from paper to electronic data on May 1, 2011, three weeks before a devastating tornado hit the area. Because the hospital had an electronic health record (EHR) system, it was able to recover patient information and send it to other healthcare facilities. In addition, St. John's set up mobile surgical and scanning equipment in its parking lot to provide further patient services. The only glitch in accessing the EHR system was a temporary loss of electrical power. However, once power was restored, healthcare providers could continue to care for their patients because the data had not been lost.

Since then, many healthcare facilities using EHRs have addressed the loss of electrical power. What measures could circumvent this issue?

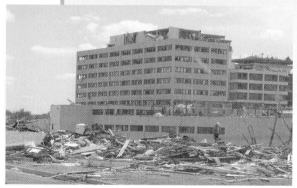

St. John's Hospital in Joplin, Missouri, was back up and running quickly after a 2011 tornado because the facility had recently implemented an EHR system.

Conversion from Paper Health Records to EHRs

The transition from paper health records to EHRs is slowly building momentum as healthcare providers are experiencing the challenges of working with a records management system that cannot keep pace with changing technology.

Limitations of Paper Records

Paper health records have served an important role in patients' healthcare for many decades. However, they also present many challenges to healthcare providers, including:

- Increasing complexity of healthcare delivery
- Single location of records
- Restricted access, allowing only one user to view records at a time
- Inconsistent documentation
- Unsecured storage in the event of a natural disaster or human error

In addition, the paper health record is time-consuming and labor-intensive. Figure 2.9 shows a typical workflow for a paper health record in an ambulatory care setting.

Figure 2.9 Paper Health Record Flowchart

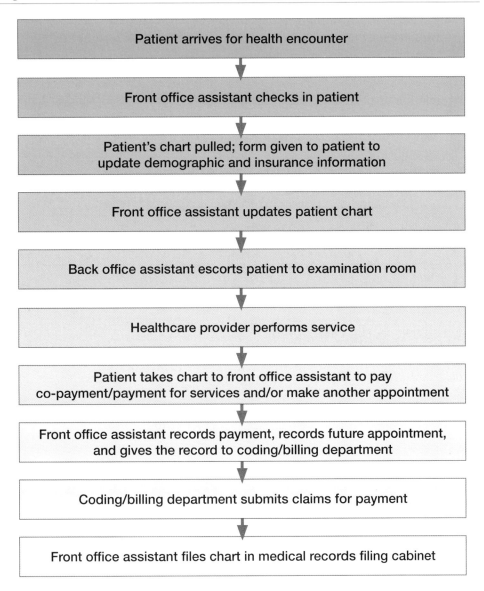

Due to the challenges presented by this time-consuming workflow, and the increasing amount of patient and provider information required to be documented, the concept of using an EHR system became increasingly embraced by healthcare practitioners.

In 1991, the initiative for EHRs expanded, and the **Institute of Medicine of the National Academies (IOM)** developed a committee to explore EHRs, suggesting that "an electronic patient record that resides in a system specifically designed to support users by providing accessibility to complete and accurate data, alerts, reminders, clinical decision support systems, links to medical knowledge, and other aids." The IOM initially called the patient record system a "computer-based patient record," but revised the title to the more widely accepted EHR.

Advantages of EHRs

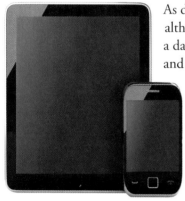

As discussed in Chapter 1, an EHR is not just an electronic version of a paper record, although common data elements exist between the two. Rather, an EHR begins with a database populated with health content from the patient's healthcare encounters and includes demographic information, progress notes, assessments, results, consultations, and many of the other documents found in a paper health record. The database of the patient's healthcare encounters is updated each time the patient seeks medical care. See Figure 2.10 for an example of an EHR database.

Healthcare providers can enter information in an EHR using laptops, desktop machines located in a patient examination room, or wireless devices during patient encounters. This ease of accessibility to a patient's health record is certainly a key advantage over a paper record that must be accessed from one location. The provider can log in to the EHR using a unique username and a secure password. Once the record is accessed by the provider, his or her activities within the record are tracked by the system.

Health information can be entered on laptops, desktop machines, or wireless devices such as tablets or mobile phones.

Figure 2.10 EIHR Chart

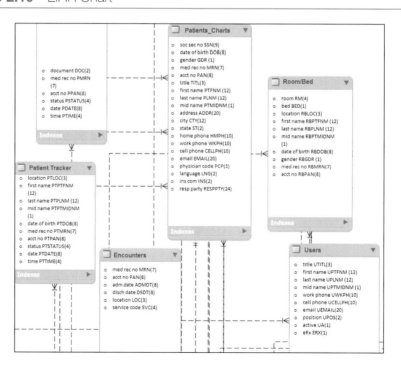

The record itself offers a standardized format containing drop-down menus, lists, icons, and free-text areas for practitioners to enter health information into the database. Because of this standardization, EHRs can be easily searched for specific patient information as well as automatically prompt clinicians to send reminders and follow up with patients. Lastly, the electronic data format provides users with a complete picture of a patient's overall health status.

The workflow of an EHR differs from the pathway of a paper health record. As you can see in Figure 2.11, the process is more streamlined for healthcare personnel.

Figure 2.11 EHR Flowchart

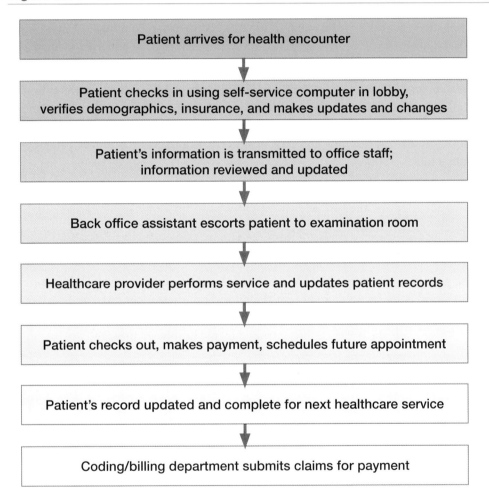

Patient arrives for health encounter

↓

Patient checks in using self-service computer in lobby, verifies demographics, insurance, and makes updates and changes

↓

Patient's information is transmitted to office staff; information reviewed and updated

↓

Back office assistant escorts patient to examination room

↓

Healthcare provider performs service and updates patient records

↓

Patient checks out, makes payment, schedules future appointment

↓

Patient's record updated and complete for next healthcare service

↓

Coding/billing department submits claims for payment

Challenges of EHR Transition

Implementing an EHR system also presents some challenges. Converting the paper records into an electronic format is time-consuming as well as costly. As HCD systems convert from paper to an electronic health format, portions of patient records will be stored electronically as well as on paper, with the end result being a **hybrid health record**. Healthcare providers with small patient populations are likely to be able to convert to EHRs in a shorter time frame than healthcare providers with large patient populations, such as major hospitals. For these larger facilities, the conversion may take several years and, consequently, hybrid health records will need to be implemented.

There may be additional challenges to making the conversion from paper health records to EHRs, such as dealing with duplicate records, establishing the identities of patients/unique patient identifiers, detecting insurance fraud, or identifying questionable identities of patients in various components in the EHR system.

Once all the records have been converted, healthcare workers must review records to ensure accuracy. Even with EMRs, there is room for error during the data entry or data conversion process. Removing erroneous information from an EMR is not allowed, and doing so may be seen as fraud if it is attempted.

Training all users of the EHR system to use EHR content can be difficult. Employees may lack the necessary technologic skills, and some users may be reluctant to learn a new system.

The goal of an EHR system is to improve patient healthcare by providing access to multiple providers across all aspects of healthcare, as well as involving the patient more directly, so that all players have current information of the patient's past and present health status. Having accurate and accessible EHRs will result in improved patient care and outcomes.

Chapter Summary

The purpose of the health record is to document the health history of the patient. The record is an accumulation of information about the patient's past and current health status. Typically, the health record begins with the patient's first visit and continues while the patient is being treated by the healthcare provider.

There are four major categories of information that may be found in the health record: administrative, clinical, legal, and financial information. The data in the health record is based on elements developed by the National Committee on Vital and Health Statistics. The information in the paper health record follows one of three formats: the Source-Oriented Record, the Integrated Health Record, or the Problem-Oriented Medical Record. Different formats of the health record exist depending on the healthcare setting. Documentation guidelines for data entries must be followed by healthcare personnel.

There are several organizations that provide standards for health records, including The Joint Commission, National Committee for Quality Assurance, Community Health Accreditation Program, Accreditation Association for Ambulatory Health Care, American Health Information Management Association, and the Association for Healthcare Documentation Integrity.

The healthcare provider or facility owns the health record, but the patient has the right to a copy of his or her health information. As health records in many facilities make the transition from paper records to electronic health records, both practitioners and patients will benefit from having access to complete health histories.

EHR Review

Check Your Understanding

To check your understanding of this chapter's key concepts, read the following multiple choice and true/false questions and then record your answers on a separate sheet of paper. Write your answers as modeled in these examples: 1a; 2b; 6T; 7F; etc.

1. An ambulatory healthcare facility may be all of the following except a/an

   a. surgery center.

   b. intensive care unit.

   c. dental office.

   d. psychologist office.

2. The four major categories of information in the health record include administrative, clinical, financial, and

   a. demographic.

   b. diagnostic.

   c. procedural.

   d. legal.

3. The acronym POMR means

   a. Problem-Oriented Medical Record.

   b. Progress-Oriented Medical Record.

   c. Patient-Oriented Medical Record.

   d. Patient-Oriented Medication Record.

4. The treatment plan is

   a. an itemized list of the patient's health problem(s).

   b. an organized collection of the patient's health problem(s).

   c. a list of reasons why the patient is at the healthcare facility.

   d. a plan for treatment of the patient's health problem(s).

5. Information standards include an Official "Do Not Use" list of abbreviations. Which organization developed this list?

   a. American College of Surgeons

   b. The Joint Commission

   c. National Committee for Quality Assurance

   d. Association for Healthcare Documentation Integrity

6. True/False: The health record is limited to a patient's acute care health information.

7. True/False: An advantage of an electronic health record (EHR) is accessibility by multiple healthcare providers.

8. True/False: The second step in the workflow of an EHR is that the patient checks in using a self-service computer, verifies demographics and insurance information, and makes updates and changes to his or her record.

9. True/False: Abbreviations and acronyms are often used in the medical record. The abbreviation for "by mouth" is p.o.

10. True/False: An ambulatory care setting is where the patient stays longer than 24 hours.

Learn the Terms

COURSE
NAVIGATOR

Go to the Course Navigator to access flashcards for Chapter 2 of *Exploring Electronic Health Records*.

Acronyms

AAAHC: Accreditation Association for Ambulatory Health Care

ACS: American College of Surgeons

AHDI: Association for Healthcare Documentation Integrity

AHIMA: American Health Information Management Association

ARRA: American Recovery and Reinvestment Act of 2009

CDC: Centers for Disease Control and Prevention

CHAP: Community Health Accreditation Program

CMS: Centers for Medicare & Medicaid Services

CoPs: Medicare Conditions of Participation

CPRS: U.S. Veterans Health Administration's Computerized Patient Record System

DAP format: Data, Assessment, Plan

HCD: healthcare delivery

HIMSS: Healthcare Information and Management Society

HIPAA: Health Insurance Portability and Accountability Act of 1996

IOM: Institute of Medicine of National Academies

NCQA: National Committee for Quality Assurance

NCVHS: National Committee on Vital and Health Statistics

NPI: National Provider Identifier

POMR: Problem-Oriented Medical Record

POR: Problem-Oriented Record

PROMIS: Problem-Oriented Medical Information System

SOAP format: Subjective, Objective, Assessment, Plan

SOR: Source-Oriented Record

VHA: Veterans Health Administration

EHR Application

Go on the Record

To build on your understanding of the topics in this chapter, complete the following short answer questions.

1. Discuss the importance of the workflow of paper health records and EHRs. Include in your discussion what would happen if a paper or electronic record missed a step in the workflow process.

2. Explain the purpose of the health record.

3. Compare and contrast the various accreditation, professional, and regulatory organizations involved in paper health records and EHRs.

4. Identify the four types of data found in the health record. Provide an example of each type of data.

5. Explain the concept of the health record ownership.

Navigate the Field

To gain practice in handling challenging situations in the workplace, consider the following real-world scenarios and then use the guiding questions to help you formulate your responses.

1. You are in charge of the medical records department. Your healthcare facility is preparing for a state department of health review, and you want to ensure that your facility's health records follow the suggested standards. There are several organizations that provide accreditation standards as well as guidance on the content and format of the health record. Select two of the following organizations and prepare a report on the importance of the organization: The Joint Commission, National Committee for Quality Assurance, Community Health Accreditation Program, Accreditation Association for Ambulatory Health Care, American Health Information Management Association, and Association for Healthcare Documentation Integrity. After researching the two organizations, develop a checklist for reviewing your department's medical records based on the guidelines suggested by the two organizations.

2. As Director of Health Information, you are in charge of training the new physicians and nurses on the Official "Do Not Use" List of Abbreviations developed by The Joint Commission. Prepare a summary document that the providers can use after the training session.

EHR Evaluation

Think Critically

Continue to think critically about challenging real-world scenarios and complete the following activities.

1. Match the following description of the Problem-Oriented Medical Record with the SOAP format.

   a. Subjective

   b. Objective

   c Assessment

   d. Plan

   _____ A. X-rays of the right hand will be ordered. If a fracture is seen, the patient will be referred to the orthopedic surgeon. The patient will be given a tetanus booster because he has not had one in the past 10 years. His wounds will be cleaned today, and antibiotic ointment and light bandages will be applied. He will be restricted from using his right hand at work for the next three days with no gripping. He will keep his wounds clean and watch for infection. He will follow up in the clinic in four days to reassess his injury and hopefully return back to full duty.

   _____ B. Mr. Smith is a 35-year-old man who was operating a cherry picker forklift today at work when he backed up and smashed his right hand in between the handle of his lift and a wooden pallet. He complains of pain in his second, third, and fourth fingers. He notes that his fingers are swollen and that they hurt when he tries to bend them. He has not noted any numbness in the fingers but says they are throbbing in pain. He also states that there are several cuts on his hand. He was seen by the company nurse who cleaned his wounds and put bandages on them. He was sent here by his company for evaluation.

   _____ C. VS BP 120/72 P74 Temp 98.7° F

   Right hand: The second, third, and fourth fingers are swollen from the PIP joints to the MCP joints. Bruising is present. ROM of the PIP joints is limited. There is normal ROM of the DIP and MCP joints. Extensor and flexor tendon strength is intact. Distal sensation is intact. Capillary refill is brisk. There are several abrasions noted on each finger. The remainder of the hand and wrist is free of injury.

   _____ D. 1. Right hand contusion

   2. Abrasions right hand

2. A 36-year-old woman with sudden onset upper back pain presents to the emergency department. This is the patient's first visit to Northstar Medical Center. Using the sample medical record located in Appendix B or at www.paradigmcollege.net /exploringehr, identify the following components of the medical record.

    A. Demographic information—include the patient name, address, and date of birth

    B. Contact information—home, work, and cell phone numbers, as well as email address

    C. History and Physical—health history, review of vital signs, and complete organ-specific physical examination

    D. Problem list—list of current health issues

    E. Allergy list—list of medications, food, and other items to which a patient is allergic, if any

    F. Prescription list—list of current medications, including dosages

Make Your Case

Consider the following scenario and create a presentation on the following topic.

This chapter illustrated how Hurricane Katrina affected medical records. Dig deeper into this topic by locating five reputable Internet sites that discuss the impact of the hurricane on the medical records of local citizens. Read and consider the information carefully. Then create a preparedness plan that would prevent a loss of medical information in a future catastrophe.

Explore the Technology

To expand your mastery of EHRs, explore the following online activities.

1. Conduct an Internet search for patient registration/admission forms at two acute and two ambulatory care facilities. Identify and explain the registration/ admission process at each type of facility. Is the patient required to complete the forms before admission/visit? If so, are there forms the patient downloads and completes? Does the patient register online? If so, how does the patient do that? Is there a patient portal that requires the patient to create an account? If so, are the instructions clear? What are the advantages and disadvantages of the system the care facility is using?

2. Research the three different formats of the health record. Explain the advantages and disadvantages of each type of format.

3. Locate three websites that provide information and resources on proper health record documentation. Do the three sources provide different guidelines for proper health record documentation? How are they similar and different?

4. Research why the NCVHS list of 42 core elements is important. How will the core elements affect the EHR?

Are You Ready?

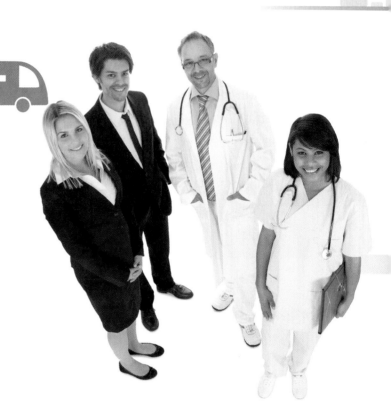

As you begin your studies in health information technology, you probably do not know where your career will take you. One thing is for certain, though: no matter what aspect of healthcare you plan to pursue, you will come into contact with an electronic health record (EHR). With that in mind, the simulated EHR software accompanying this textbook will teach you the basic skills necessary to master the real-world EHR system that is a future certainty for all healthcare facilities.

Beyond the Record

- In 2011 there were more than 300 different EHR software vendors, and many more are expected to appear on the market in the coming years.

- A 2010 study showed that 50% of physicians use smartphones or tablets to help aid medical decisions.

- A six-letter password takes a hacker about 10 minutes to crack, and the most common password is 123456. To ensure security, passwords in an EHR system need to be strong.

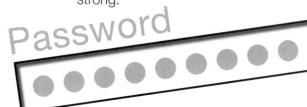

Password

Chapter 3

Introduction to Electronic Health Record Software

This textbook uses a comprehensive, realistic electronic health records (EHR) system called EHR Navigator. EHR Navigator is designed to introduce and practice the key functions found in EHR systems (e.g., patient admission, registration, scheduling, communication, privacy, security, coding, billing, reimbursement, clinical decision support, and patient portals). Using the EHR Navigator throughout this textbook will help you experience how an EHR system works in the field.

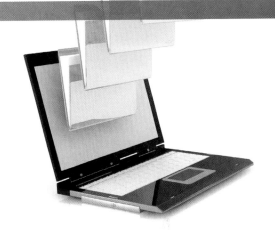

Field Notes

Electronic health records (EHRs) have improved quality of care with regard to medical records, helping to standardize processes throughout our hospitals at a regional level. We can now quickly and effectively analyze patient information to prevent any issues that may arise. Physicians complete charts timely and accurately with fewer medical errors (e.g., poor legibility, unapproved abbreviations). Maintaining an EHR saves money and time by eliminating the cost of storing, retrieving, transporting, and printing records. An EHR also allows practitioners to quickly view records from other hospitals and hospital affiliates, thus improving patient care.

– Misty A. Glasgow, MBA
HIM/Privacy Officer

- Define the terms *input*, *output*, *processing*, *storage*, and *local area network*.

- Identify the role of the health information professional in the electronic health record (EHR).

- Explain the certification of EHR systems by the Certification Commission for Health Information Technology (CCHIT).

- Demonstrate how to set up and navigate an EHR system.

- Describe the password and security measures of the EHR system.

- Identify menu options in an EHR system.

- Examine charting features in an EHR system.

- Review the various scheduling features of an EHR system.

- Examine secure messaging, document management, laboratory integration, and e-prescribing features of an EHR system.

- Examine mobile features in an EHR system.

An electronic health record (EHR) system manages all aspects of a patient visit, from the time a patient contacts the healthcare facility to the time the insurance and billing are both processed. This system can be accessed by healthcare personnel who work in an acute care setting as well as those individuals who work in an ambulatory care facility. As defined in Chapter 2, an acute care facility treats patients who have acute health issues that require inpatient care. An ambulatory care setting services outpatients, or patients who do not require admission to acute care facilities. There are many types of ambulatory care facilities such as a physician's office, a hospital emergency department, a dental office, a surgery center, or a health clinic. An EHR system provides interoperability among various healthcare facilities, which allows the facilities to communicate with each other and view the patient's health record. To help you understand how an EHR system operates, you must become familiar with the system's features and have plenty of opportunities for practice. The EHR Navigator will help you do just that.

Introduction to the EHR Navigator

The EHR Navigator is a comprehensive EHR and practice management system that provides you with hands-on experience within a realistic EHR system. This practice software, accessed through the Course Navigator learning management system, provides you with the necessary skills to work in any EHR system you might encounter in either an acute care or ambulatory care setting. You will become familiar with patient management, scheduling, medical charting, laboratory integrations, medical documents, e-prescribing, clinical collaboration, reporting, referral letters, and billing. You will also practice patient portal activities.

In addition to instruction on the features of an EHR system, the text examines the security settings and requirements of a typical EHR system; discusses the importance of having a backup system; and explains how to evaluate and implement an EHR system. Lastly, this chapter discusses the current and future role of digital devices as healthcare providers embrace the adoption of EHR systems. Together, the text and the EHR Navigator activities will guide you through the concepts and applications of EHR systems.

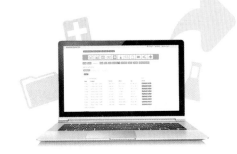

Information Processing Cycle

The **information processing cycle** provides the building blocks for the EHR system and includes four components: input, processing, output, and storage (see Figure 3.1). The information processing cycle converts data entered into the computer into valuable information for healthcare personnel.

The **input** component is the data entered by the user of an EHR system (e.g., the patient's first name, last name, identification number).

The **processing** component takes that data and makes the information usable within the system. In an EHR, the processing component determines whether entered test results are values within a critical or normal range.

Figure 3.1 Information Processing Cycle

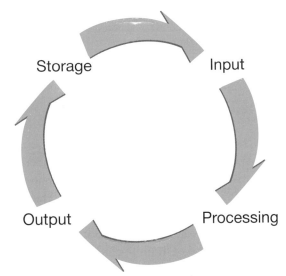

The **output** component is the data produced that provides meaningful information for the user. A report on a patient's laboratory test results is an example of an output in an EHR system. A healthcare provider may use the report to guide treatment decisions.

Storage is the fourth component of the information processing cycle. Patient information is stored so that it can be retrieved, added to, or modified for later use. Data are processed once they are entered into an EHR. There are various types of **storage devices** that an EHR system uses. EHR systems may be stored on a dedicated server at the healthcare facility or on a server provided by a vendor. If an EHR system is networked, then the storage may exist on the healthcare system's server. **Cloud storage** is data stored on virtual servers.

As technology continues to develop, EHR systems become easier to use. Internet and intranet technologies may allow you to access and share an EHR system in one building as well as in remote locations. This accessibility can be a liability, which is why an EHR system must be secure and accessed based on necessary functions to perform a specific job. As an additional security measure, the data entered and extracted from the EHR system is encrypted to maintain security and protect patient privacy.

Hardware Support

An EHR system is most commonly accessed through a computer workstation. A typical **workstation** includes a computer and input and output devices. Healthcare providers may also be supplied with digital mobile devices not wired to a workstation. Both computer workstations and digital devices can be found in healthcare facilities

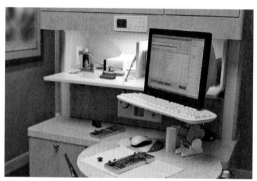

EHR systems are most commonly accessed through a computer workstation.

today. An **input device**—such as a keyboard, mouse, scanner, microphone, camera, stylus, or touchscreen—is used to enter data into an EHR system. An **output device**—such as a computer monitor, digital device screen, or printer—displays the results from EHRs. Because the printing functionality of an EHR is a security issue, healthcare staff members must adhere to their facilities' Policy and Procedure manual for the permissible circumstances for printing a patient's health record.

Network Systems

The workstation also includes access to the Internet and intranet system. Computer workstations are networked through a **local area network (LAN)**. LAN is a group of computers connected through a network confined to a single area or small geographic area such as a building or hospital campus. The network is secure and reliable, enabling safe mobility of the data among the workstations. The networked computer system allows computer workstations to work and communicate together. The network should provide a great deal of flexibility and should be adaptable to new technologies, such as fiber-optic cables, new software, wireless communication, etc. The LAN utilizes a dedicated server for the workstations. The network is connected either through wired or wireless connections. The advantage of a wireless connection is that the healthcare provider may be anywhere and have access to an EHR system. Figure 3.2 shows a visual representation of a network system.

A **wide area network (WAN)** is a network that covers a broader area than a LAN. It is a computer network that spans regions, countries, or the world. As healthcare becomes more global and interoperable, more WANs will be used to connect the LANs of separate healthcare facilities.

Figure 3.2 Network System

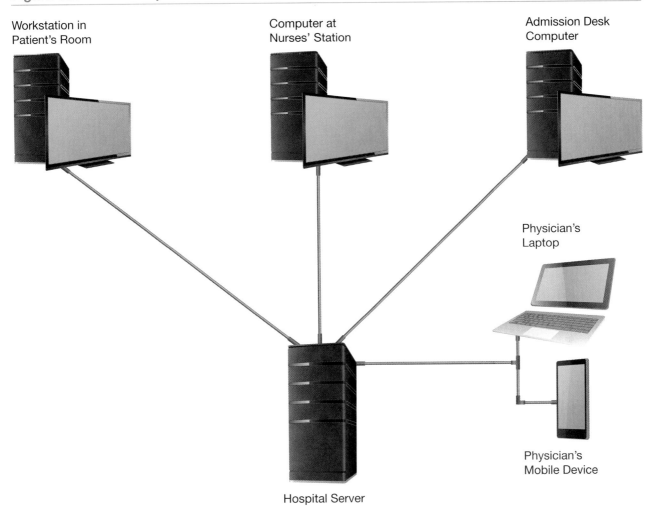

Workstation in Patient's Room

Computer at Nurses' Station

Admission Desk Computer

Physician's Laptop

Physician's Mobile Device

Hospital Server

EHR Accessibility

The expense of having a computer workstation in every service room may prevent providers from expanding an EHR system as widely as necessary for maximum efficiency. However, not having access to a workstation may cause a delay in updating and adding information to an EHR for other healthcare providers to view. One solution for this accessibility issue is the use of mobile and digital devices, which some healthcare providers are beginning to utilize. Mobile and digital devices will be explored later in this chapter.

Data may be entered into EHRs via a keyboard. Some EHR systems have voice recognition software that will adapt to your voice and speech patterns and input data into the system. Electronic handwriting or touch screen input may also be available, depending on the EHR system design. Some EHR systems have templates that allow you to select text options from a drop-down menu, allowing standard data to be quickly added to the patient's record.

EXPAND
YOUR LEARNING

The use of EHR software can be instrumental in the training of healthcare providers. Because healthcare providers may be exposed to different types of EHR systems, the providers are able to recognize the benefits. Watch a video testimonial about the benefits of EHRs at www.paradigmcollege .net/exploringehr/ testimonial.

CHECKPOINT 3.1

1. Name the four components of the information processing cycle.

   a. _____

   b. _____

   c. _____

   d. _____

2. Explain how a LAN affects the use of an EHR system.

   _____

   _____

   _____

Privacy and Security in the EHR System

The privacy and security settings of an EHR system must conform to Health Insurance Portability and Accountability (HIPAA) regulations. (For more information on HIPAA regulations, refer to Chapter 6.) These settings include the use of passwords and user permissions.

Password Protection

An EHR system must allow acute and ambulatory care facilities to create, change, and safeguard passwords. Facilities must have policies and procedures in place for managing passwords. Typically, passwords are six to eight characters long, with a combination of alpha and numeric characters, and typically contain at least one uppercase letter. When you enter your password, characters appear as dots, asterisks, or other symbols, thus preventing other users from seeing the password. Generally, you must change your password every 90–120 days. In addition to using a password to enter the system, specific areas of an EHR system may also be password-protected to maintain the privacy and security of patient health records. The password is encrypted in the transmittal process between your workstation and an EHR system. An audit manager or administrator records the user log-ins and log-outs to monitor use of the EHR system. EHR systems allow for back-end auditing so there is an objective record available that indicates all users who have accessed a patient's chart. Audit records can be reproduced to address access issues or HIPAA noncompliance.

When you first log in to an EHR system, you will key in a default password, then follow the prompts to change your password. Typically, you can attempt to log in three times before being locked out and requiring the password to be reset by the administrator or information technology (IT) manager at the facility.

User Permissions

An EHR contains a patient's **protected health information (PHI)**. If you are an employee of an acute care or ambulatory care facility, you must have a unique user name that registers your identity and tracks your activity in an EHR system. Each user's access to information is based on the type of information he or she will need to view or modify. Therefore, users are assigned access according to their job functions (e.g., healthcare provider, nurse, health information professional, registrar). For example, a registration or admission clerk may not have access to a patient's X-rays but would have access to the patient's insurance information. This assigned access ensures the security and confidentiality of patient records. Figure 3.3 illustrates how an administrator can assign you permission to access various areas of an EHR system based on your job position. These permissions define the areas of the software a user may view, add, edit, or delete information. For example, a front desk clerk at an outpatient facility may see a screen similar to the one shown in Figure 3.4 when accessing the EHR Navigator. When admitting a patient, an admission clerk would view a screen similar to the one shown in Figure 3.5.

Figure 3.3 Assign User Permissions

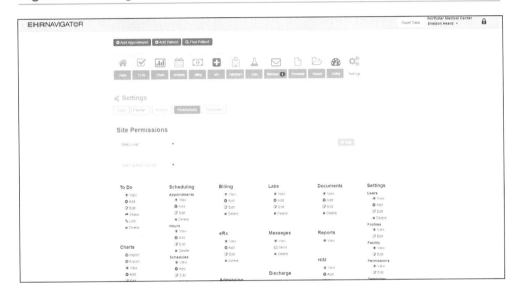

Figure 3.4 Home Screen – Outpatient

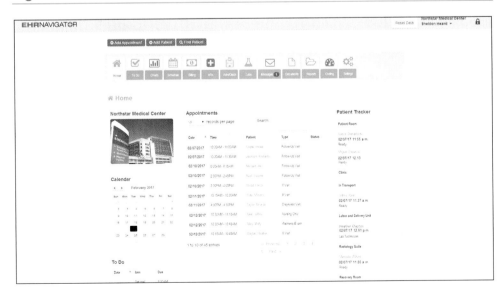

Figure 3.5 Patient Admission - Inpatient

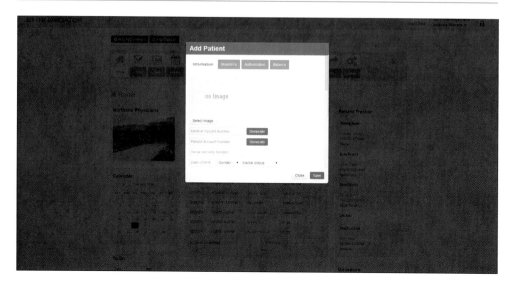

Hibernation Mode

When you must step away from your workstation, an EHR system should be set to **hibernation mode**, a privacy feature that prevents disclosure of PHI. Patients and healthcare providers alike may be able to see a workstation as they pass by, so the information on the screen must be protected. When you are not actively using the EHR system, or if you must step away for a few minutes, an EHR system must be in the hibernation mode. If you do not set the hibernation mode manually, it will automatically go into hibernation mode after a period of inactivity. To escape the hibernation mode and reaccess a patient's health record, you must reenter your username and password. Figure 3.6 shows these precautions.

Patients have the right to receive their health records. Some healthcare facilities provide patients with their health records on a type of portable device such as a flash drive. Other patients create PHRs they can access anywhere that has Internet connectivity (see Figure 3.7). Still, some patients prefer to have their health record in a hard copy format, which is also an option. Chapter 11 explores these types of records in more detail.

Flash Drive

Figure 3.6 Log-in Due to Hibernation

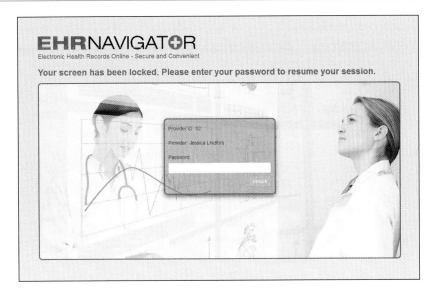

Figure 3.7 Personal Health Record

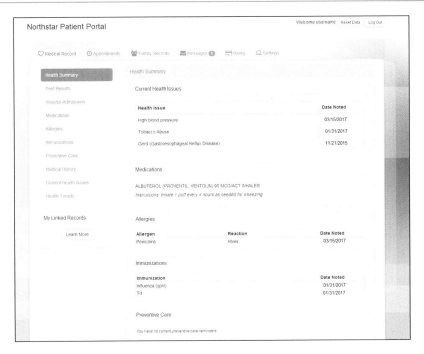

Accessing the EHR Navigator

In this chapter, as well as throughout *Exploring Electronic Health Records*, hands-on activities using the Web-based EHR Navigator will provide you with practical experience. Each activity is an interactive tutorial that is designed to demonstrate an EHR concept. These activities are based on a review of many inpatient and outpatient EHR systems and, therefore, are transferable to a variety of healthcare settings. When you log in to the Course Navigator learning management system to launch the tutorials and complete the activities, you will be guided by an audio recording through each step of the tutorial. The activities will begin by reviewing various features and capabilities of the software. Once you have mastered the software, you will begin to apply the EHR concepts presented in the text. As a final check, there are additional activities at the end of each chapter that assess your understanding of the chapter concepts and their applications.

Capabilities of EHR Systems

The Certification Commission for Health Information Technology (CCHIT) has defined the capabilities that are necessary for the meaningful use of EHR technology. These capabilities include functionality, interoperability, and security. **Functionality** is the ability to create and manage EHRs for all patients in a healthcare facility. In addition, functionality includes the ability to automate workflow in a healthcare facility. **Interoperability** is the ability of an EHR system to exchange data with other sources of health information, including pharmacies, laboratories, and other healthcare providers. Interoperability is achieved through standards such as Health Level Seven International (HL7), which aims to facilitate sharing and passage of clinical information from one system to another. **Security** is the standard that prevents data loss and ensures that patient health information is private. Therefore, each component of the EHR system will be explained based on the four CCHIT capabilities.

EHR Software Features

This text addresses the software features that improve efficiency in the administrative and clinical components of a healthcare facility. Some of the administrative features examined in this text include messaging, to do list, scheduling, patient management, billing, and coding. Several features that are used in a clinical setting are also discussed, including medical charting, clinical collaboration, results reporting, clinical decision support, and PHRs.

Using the EHR Navigator

The EHR Navigator encompasses an inpatient and outpatient EHR system. Within each menu are submenu options. Figure 3.8 illustrates the inpatient system, Northstar Medical Center. The outpatient system, Northstar Physicians, is shown in Figure 3.9. Examples of the inpatient and outpatient menus are shown in Figures 3.10 and 3.11.

Figure 3.8 EHR Overview – Inpatient

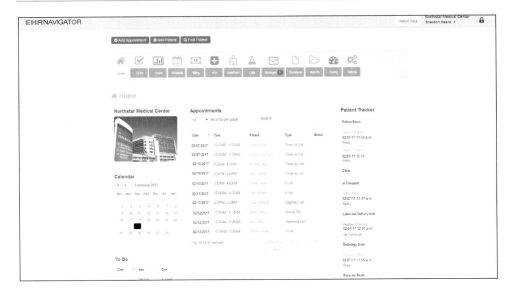

Figure 3.9 EHR Overview – Outpatient

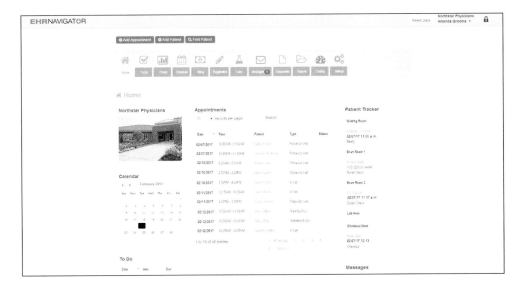

Menus

The menu bar is at the top of the screen. The options on the Northstar Medical Center menu bar are Home, To Do, Charts, Schedule, Billing, eRx, Admission/Discharge, Labs, Messages, Documents, Reports, Coding, ROI, and Settings (see Figure 3.10).

Figure 3.10 Menus – Inpatient

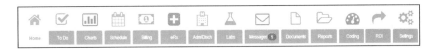

The options on the Northstar Physicians menu bar are Home, To Do, Charts, Schedule, Billing, eRx, Registration, Labs, Messages, Documents, Reports, Coding, ROI (Release of Information), and Settings (see Figure 3.11).

Figure 3.11   Menus – Outpatient

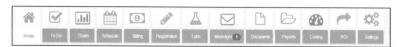

When you click on each of the menu options, a list of functions will appear below the menu option.

Settings

The EHR Navigator has a *Settings* feature that allows the healthcare facility to add users, edit facility information, grant user permissions, and customize features to meet the needs of the healthcare facility. Figure 3.12 illustrates the Settings feature for both inpatient and outpatient facilities.

Figure 3.12   Settings

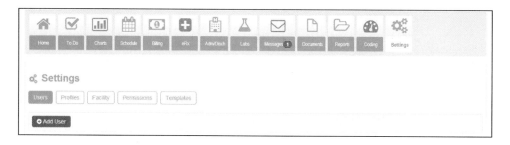

Users

In the *Users* submenu option, all users are listed along with their respective roles (e.g., physician, HIM professional, unit clerk, pharmacist). This site is also where the EHR administrator or office manager can add or edit users (see Figure 3.13).

Figure 3.13 Users Submenu

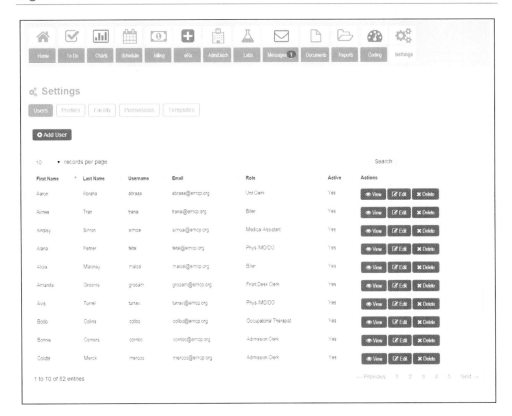

Profiles

By selecting *Profiles*, you may update your basic information (see Figure 3.14).

Practice

In the *Facility* submenu of the EHR Navigator (see Figures 3.15 and 3.16), the *Facility* menu option allows you to view basic information about the facility, including:

- Identifiers such as a National Provider Identifier (NPI), Employer Identification Number (EIN), Medicare, Medicaid, and the Tricare provider number

- Healthcare organizations list (details a list of related healthcare organizations)

- Payer list (details a list of payers)

Figure 3.14 Profiles Submenu

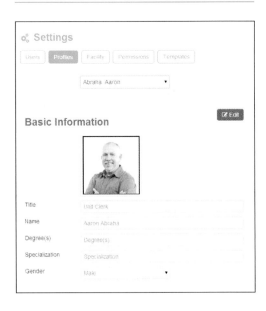

Figure 3.15 Facility Submenu

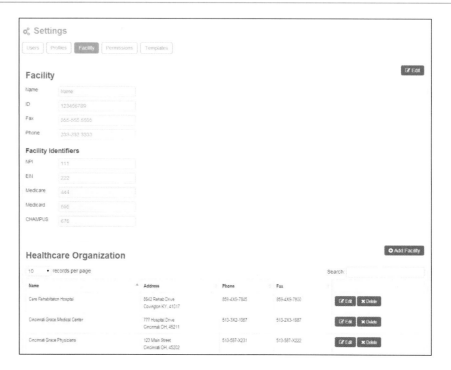

Figure 3.16 Facility Submenu Continued

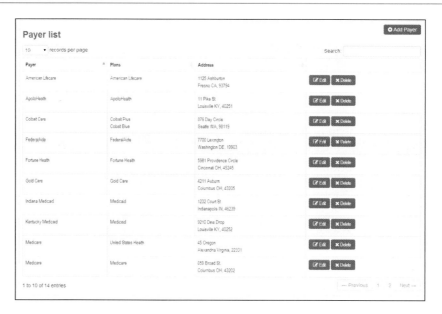

Permissions

The *Permissions* submenu in the EHR Navigator is where employee access to EHR functions is managed. Options to view, add, edit, and delete permissions are selected for each user. For example, all users are granted access to the *To Do* option on the Users menu, but only certain healthcare personnel that can order medications (such as physicians, physician assistants, nurse practitioners, and pharmacists) can override drug allergies. Figure 3.17 provides an example of how adjustments for permissions may be made to drug-drug and drug-allergy alerts.

Figure 3.17   Permissions for Drug Alerts

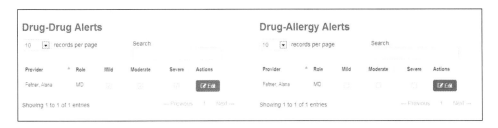

Templates

The *Settings* menu allows you to manage charting templates. When you select *Templates*, facility templates appear on the left panel, and a list of templates you may like to use in a patient's chart appears on the right panel. You may create custom templates by selecting *Add Templates*. Figure 3.18 provides a list of templates.

Figure 3.18   Facility and User Templates

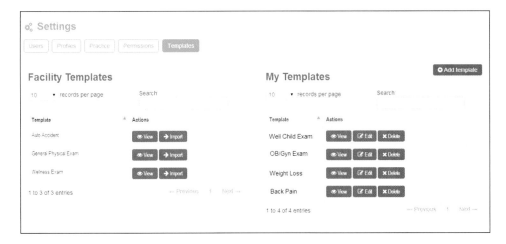

Administrative Features

The administrative features in the EHR Navigator include reports, messages, scheduling, billing, some charting information, and documents.

Home

On the Home menu there are six submenus: *Calendar*, *To Do*, *Appointments*, *Patient Tracker*, and *Messages* (see Figure 3.19). The *Calendar* provides quick access to specific dates, and the *To Do* section allows you to create reminders, prioritize activities, and organize lists to be more efficient and effective on the job. *Appointments* displays your appointments for the current week, and *Patient Tracker* identifies a patient's physical location while he or she is in the facility. *Messages* is an internal communication tool for all users of the EHR Navigator.

Figure 3.19   Home Menu

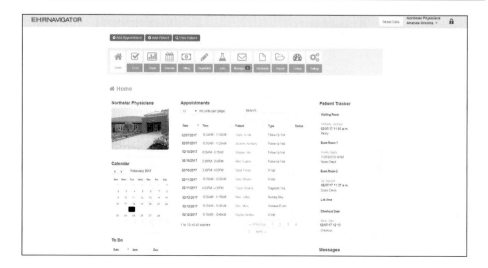

Patient Tracker

In the *Home* menu, a *Status* feature allows you to change the status of the patient. For instance, the patient status may change from *Scheduled* to *Arrived*, *No Show*, or *Canceled*. This allows the administrative staff to easily track patients. Once a patient's status is changed to *Arrived*, the patient is displayed in the *Patient Tracker*. Then the administrative staff or healthcare provider may change the status to *Waiting*, *Patient Room*, *Checkout Desk*, etc., in the system. Figure 3.20 shows the Patient Tracker status.

Figure 3.20 Patient Tracker Status

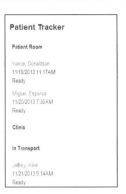

 ## Reports

As you learned in Chapter 1, the HITECH Act provides incentives for implementing an EHR system based on meaningful use criteria, and many of these systems have a dashboard to track this use. Typically, an administrator of an EHR system monitors the progress the healthcare facility has made toward completing each criterion. In the EHR Navigator, the meaningful use information can be accessed under the *Reports* tab. Figure 3.21 illustrates an example of a typical *Meaningful Use* report. Criteria may be calculated based on provider, year, attestation duration, and start and end dates.

Figure 3.21 Meaningful Use Report

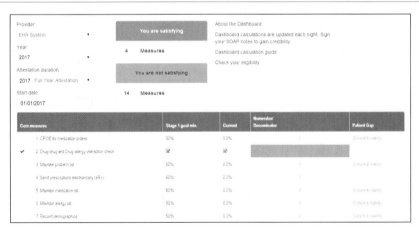

You can also access the Activity Feed feature on the Reports tab. The *User Activity Feed* feature in the EHR Navigator tracks your access to various components in the system and provides two views, either a user's activities within the EHR system. Each time you log in or out, or each time you make updates or add data to a patient's chart, the activity is tracked. If you create an appointment or submit a prescription to the pharmacy, that activity will also appear in the *User Activity Feed*. This feed, seen in Figure 3.22, enables the administrator to get a longitudinal view of actions occurring in the healthcare facility.

Figure 3.22 User Activity Feed

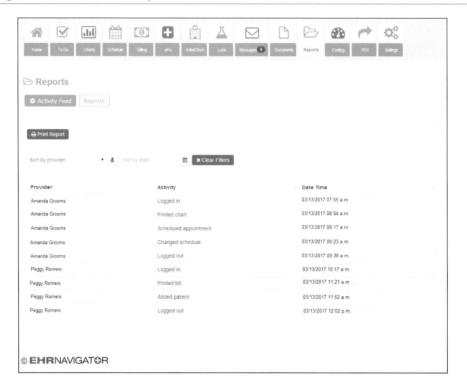

The *Reports* feature in the EHR Navigator allows users of Northstar Medical Center and Northstar Physicians to convert the facility's data into information that can be analyzed. Reports may be run on clinical data or administrative information, or by provider and date range. Figure 3.23 lists the various reports and descriptions available in the EHR Navigator.

Figure 3.23 List of Reports

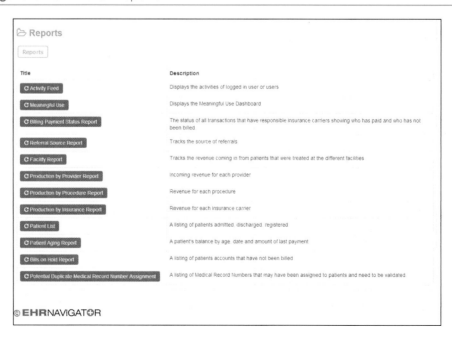

The EHR Navigator *Reports* feature queries special reports based on particular criteria. An example of a query report might include generating a list of women age 50 and older who have not yet scheduled mammography in the past year.

✉ Messages

The EHR Navigator messaging system allows you to communicate with other system users in your organization. Some EHR systems contain a HIPAA-compliant messaging feature that permits physicians, nurses, and other healthcare providers to communicate with medical colleagues outside their healthcare facility. This feature is similar to a social media–type messaging system used to improve the collaboration and continuity of patient care.

The *Message* function allows you to send messages to patients, providers, and employees of the healthcare facilities using the EHR Navigator. The menu provides three options: *Inbox*, *Sent Messages*, and *Archived Messages*.

The *Inbox* lists messages received by the user or healthcare facility. Figure 3.24 illustrates the EHR Navigator Inbox. You may reply, forward, save, or delete messages. You may also send a new message, as illustrated in Figure 3.25. As shown in Figure 3.26, messages may be saved to a patient's chart to allow you to document communication among healthcare providers, facilities, pharmacies, and the patient.

Figure 3.24   Messages – Inbox

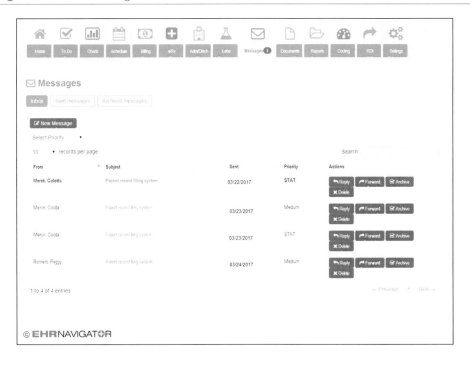

Figure 3.25 Messages – New Message

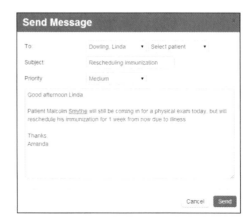

Figure 3.26 Messages – Archived Messages

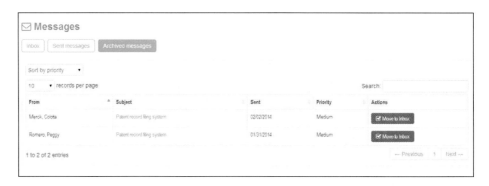

Schedule

The *Schedule* feature in the EHR Navigator gives you access to the calendar in monthly, weekly, and daily views. The calendar overview allows you to quickly access the schedules of providers, departments, or both. For example, a nurse may view the operating room schedule for a particular day, at Northstar Medical Center. At Northstar Physicians, for example, the front desk clerk can view a doctor's schedule for an entire month (see Figure 3.27).

In addition to the calendar overview, Northstar Medical Center and Northstar Physicians can use the *Hours* feature to customize the availability of appointments by setting parameters for the days and times that Northstar is able to schedule patients. Figures 3.28 and 3.29 illustrate how Northstar may select days and hourly times, respectively, when appointments are available.

Figure 3.27 Calendar Overview – Northstar Physicians

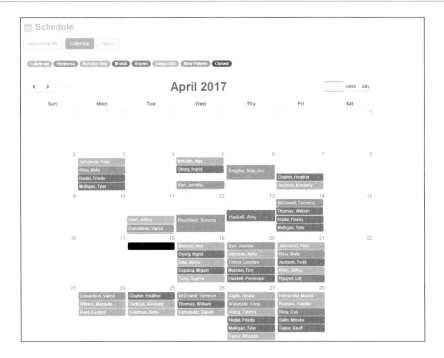

Figure 3.28 Facility Days and Hours

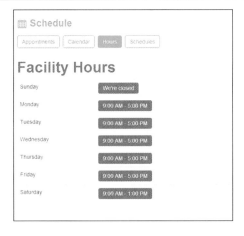

Figure 3.29 Customize Hours

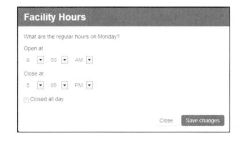

Weekly Calendar

Appointment times are defaulted to 15 minutes and may be scheduled in the *Weekly Calendar* view, although the healthcare facility may customize standard appointment times when necessary. If the patient requires additional time, you can select multiple time slots for longer appointments. A healthcare provider or facility may also filter the *Weekly Calendar* view to see appointments. Figures 3.30 and 3.31 show the weekly calendar for Northstar Medical Center Radiology Department and the weekly calendar for Northstar Physicians, respectively.

Figure 3.30   Northstar Medical Center Radiology Department Weekly Calendar

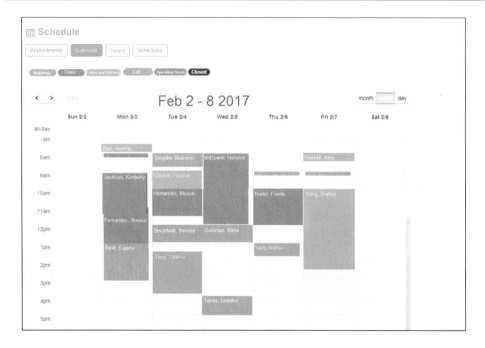

Figure 3.31   Northstar Physicians Weekly Calendar

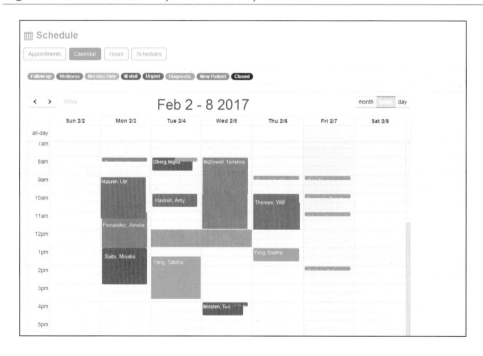

Daily Calendar

The administrative and clinical staff are likely to use the *Daily Calendar* feature in a variety of ways. The *Daily Calendar* allows you to see the appointments scheduled for the healthcare facility on a given day, as well as individual providers' scheduled appointments. Figures 3.32 and 3.33 illustrate the daily calendar views for Northstar Medical Center and Northstar Physicians, respectively.

Figure 3.32   Daily Calendar for Northstar Medical Center

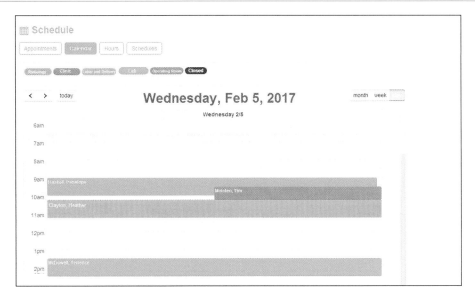

Figure 3.33   Daily Calendar for Northstar Physicians

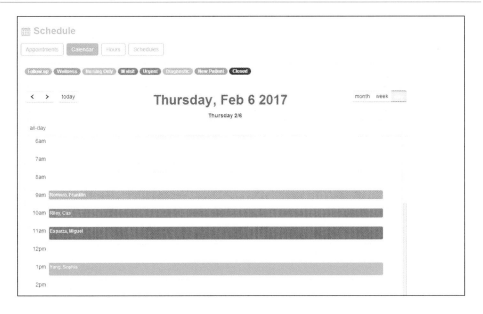

$ Billing

Billing for treatment and services rendered is a main function of any healthcare organization. Figure 3.34 shows the main billing screen found in the EHR Navigator. You will experience the *Billing* functions of the EHR Navigator in Chapter 9.

Figure 3.34 Billing

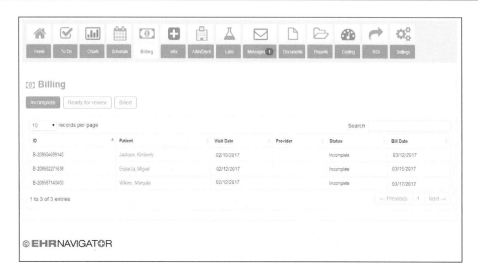

Charts

The *Charts* feature in the EHR Navigator contains both administrative *and* clinical information. This section addresses only the administrative information, and the clinical information will be discussed in the Clinical Features section on page 83. In the *Charts* feature, a list of patients treated at the healthcare facility appears. The user is able to find, filter, and add patients. The administrative features in the EHR Navigator contain patient demographics, insurance information, setting, clinical information, and a list of appointments. Within the patient chart, the healthcare facility can enroll a patient in a PHR, print a patient chart, send a referral or response letter, export a patient record, export an immunization registry, and provide public health surveillance information. Figures 3.35 and 3.36 provide examples of the patient list and patient chart found in the *Charts* feature.

Figure 3.35   Charts – List of Patients

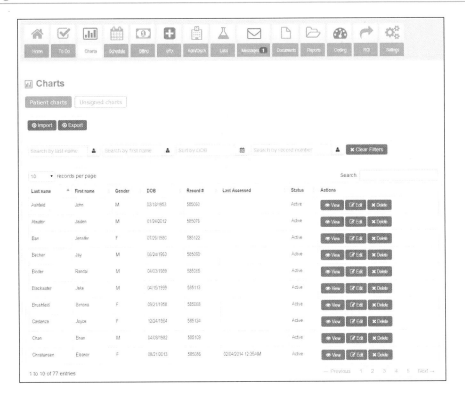

Figure 3.36   Charts – Patient Chart

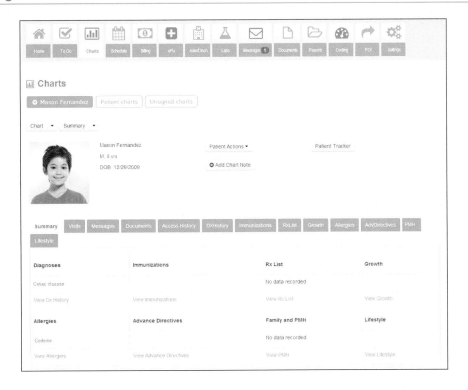

Documents

The EHR Navigator allows you to upload and save scanned or digital files—such as a scanned insurance card, a patient photo, an X-ray, or a dictation—to a patient's chart. The system also allows you to make notations on a document before assigning the file to a patient's chart and to digitally sign documents. Figure 3.37 shows how to upload a document.

Figure 3.37   Uploading Documents

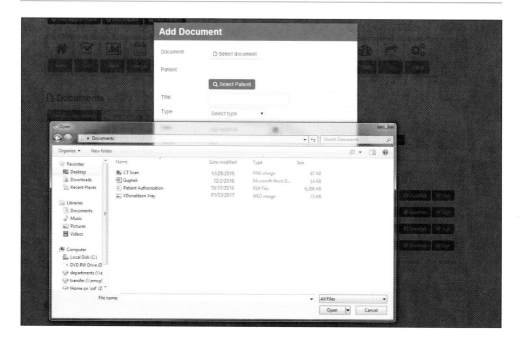

Documents can be viewed either as pending or signed, and they may be filtered by provider and document type. Figure 3.38 illustrates pending documents. For example, a pending document may be a physician order waiting for a doctor to authenticate.

Figure 3.38   Pending Documents

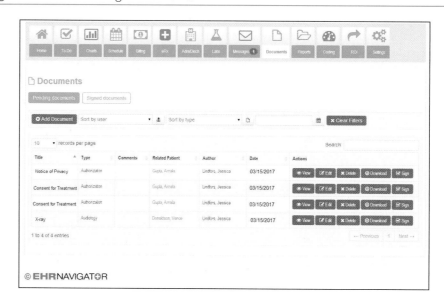

CHECKPOINT 3.2

1. Name three different ways to view appointments in the Schedule tab.

    a. _____

    b. _____

    c. _____

2. Explain why *Messages* is an important feature in an EHR system.

    _____

    _____

    _____

Activity 3.3 — EHRNAVIGATOR

EHR Administrative

Go to the Course Navigator to launch Activity 3.2. As a physician, practice the administrative features using the EHR Navigator

Clinical Features

In addition to the administrative features, there are a number of clinical features available to an EHR user. The clinical features of the EHR Navigator include patient chart information, e-prescriptions (eRx), managing physician orders, and viewing laboratory and diagnostic test results.

Charts

The EHR Navigator *Charts* feature is the source for the patient's clinical data, including medical diagnoses, treatments, procedures, allergies, medical history, medications, test results, and reports. *Charts* provides you with a unique view of the entire record at a glance, without having to navigate to other areas of the EHR system to view patient information. The EHR Navigator allows multiple users to have access to a patient's chart. Figure 3.39 illustrates the past medical history component of the patient chart.

The EHR Navigator *Charts* feature also allows you to add a chart note, as shown in Figure 3.40.

Figure 3.39 Charts – Patient History

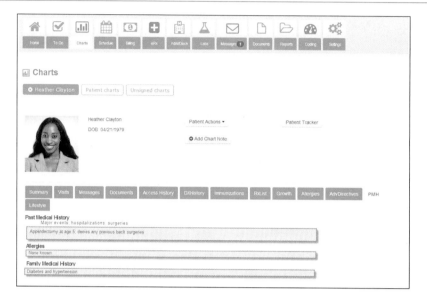

Figure 3.40 Add Chart Note

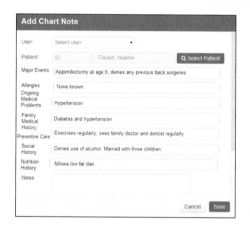

 eRx

A typical EHR system has an eRx (electronic prescription) feature that enables the system to electronically submit prescriptions to pharmacies all across the United States. The use of e-prescribing helps to reduce medication errors, thus improving patient safety and increasing practice efficiency. An EHR system that integrates an e-prescribing function increases facility productivity and efficiency by allowing a healthcare provider to view the patient's medication history in the EHR rather than pulling a chart and writing a prescription by hand. Figure 3.41 shows the *eRx* screen in the EHR Navigator.

Figure 3.41 eRx

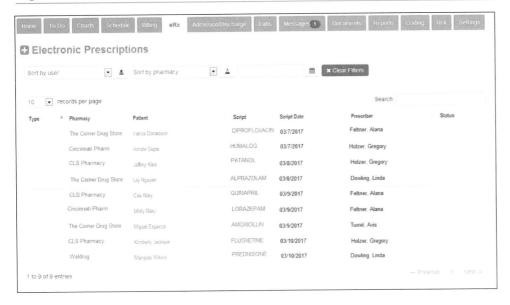

Labs

EHR systems include an integrated laboratory feature, which enables healthcare facilities and providers to connect with national and regional laboratories or maintain an existing laboratory partner. The EHR Navigator *Labs* feature allows you to view *Pending Labs* and *Signed Labs*. Pending labs are those awaiting test processing and results reporting. Signed labs are those that have been viewed and signed by a physician, physician assistant, or nurse practitioner. Integrating laboratories into an EHR system gives you the ability to create laboratory orders and view results from any computer at any time, with abnormal results flagged and organized for easy review. Figure 3.42 illustrates the *Labs* feature in the EHR Navigator.

Figure 3.42 Labs – Views

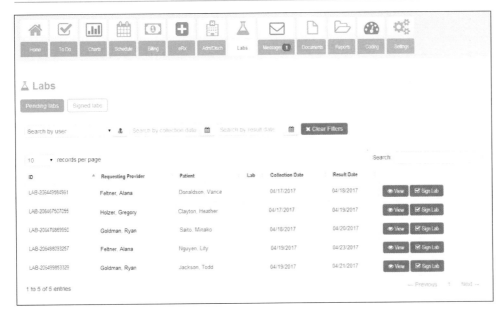

Manage Orders

Every EHR system contains a computerized physician order entry (CPOE) component. In the EHR Navigator, the CPOE component is located under *Manage Orders*. Depending on their level of access, users add, view, and cancel physician orders for treatment and care—for example, laboratory orders, dietary orders, and therapy orders—by using *Manage Orders*. The EHR Navigator *Manage Orders* feature allows you to view *Pending Orders* and *Signed Orders*. Pending orders are those awaiting response. Signed labs are those that have been viewed and signed by a physician, physician assistant, or nurse practitioner. Figure 3.43 illustrates the *Manage Order* screen in EHR Navigator. You will learn about CPOE, in detail, in Chapter 8 of this text.

Figure 3.43 Manage Orders

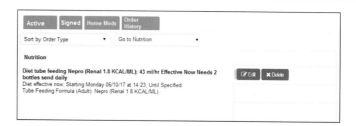

Diagnostic Test Results

Patients undergo many different diagnostic tests during the course of treatment, particularly patients in the acute care setting. Upon the completion of these tests, physicians and other healthcare providers can immediately access the results in an EHR system. In the EHR Navigator, test results are available for review under the *Diagnostic Test Results* tab (see Figure 3.44). You will learn about this function in more detail in Chapter 8 of this textbook.

Figure 3.44 Diagnostic Test Results

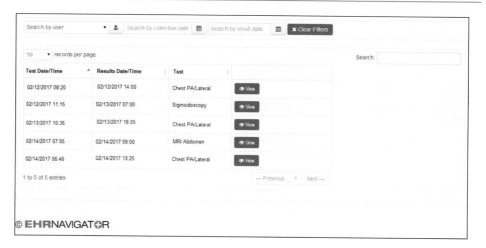

CHECKPOINT 3.3

1. Name four types of clinical information found in a patient's chart.

   a. _____

   b. _____

   c. _____

   d. _____

2. Explain the importance of an integrated laboratory feature.

   _____

   _____

   _____

Activity 3.4   EHR NAVIGATOR

EHR Clinical

Go to the Course Navigator to launch Activity 3.4. As a physician, practice reviewing patient clinical information using the EHR Navigator.

Backup System

EHR systems can be Web-based or locally installed. Regardless, the EHR system data belongs to the healthcare facility. If the healthcare facility decides to switch from a Web-based to a locally installed EHR system, the data may be exported from a cloud-based server and imported into the local EHR system.

No matter what type of server is used, the EHR system must have a secure backup plan. This contingency plan is critical in the event of a disaster that destroys the health records.

EHR systems, whether Web-based or locally installed, should have a secure backup system. A healthcare facility that has a locally installed EHR system should have its backup plan recorded in the facility's Policy and Procedure manual. The backup system must provide an exact copy of patient health records. Depending on the backup system—be it on-site, magnetic storage, cloud-based, or off-site—the same security measures must be followed to prevent the unauthorized access or release of patient PHI. Policies and procedures must include controlled access, password protection, and a secure location. Web-based EHR system is stored on a secure server utilizing the highest levels of encryption software.

EXPAND
YOUR LEARNING

According to a study published in the U.S. National Library of Medicine's online research journal, approximately 50% of healthcare providers are using some type of mobile device for clinical decision making. Review the study at www.paradigmcollege.net/exploringehr/smartphones to learn more about the advantages and challenges healthcare providers face while using mobile devices when caring for patients.

Mobile Devices

An EHR system may be accessible through a mobile device such as a smartphone or tablet with computer capabilities. Mobile devices allows you to remotely access the EHR system, which will help improve your productivity and quality of patient care. Healthcare providers may choose to use a mobile device because they can bring the device with them when caring for patients. These easy-to-use devices help inform and show patients images such as the location of an injury. However, digital devices in a healthcare facility are not without their challenges; you must ensure that they comply with the security requirements of HIPAA. There can also be difficulty with the ability of a device to easily integrate within the EHR system. Figure 3.45 illustrates the use of an EHR system, Practice Fusion, on an iPad.

Figure 3.45   Practice Fusion for the iPad.

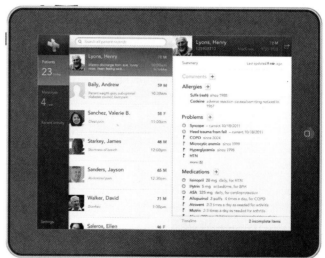

Source: Practice Fusion. Used with permission.

Chapter Summary

There are two primary healthcare settings—inpatient and outpatient—and each setting requires its own features within an electronic health record (EHR) system. Rather than learning one specific EHR system, mastering the knowledge behind an EHR system allows you the flexibility of working with a variety of EHR systems that you may encounter in the workplace. CCHIT-certified EHRs possess similar capabilities and functions as a result of standardized requirements for compliant EHRs.

With that in mind, the EHR Navigator provides you with the hands-on activities to help you master this basic knowledge. Assigning rights and permissions, managing and scheduling patients, reviewing medical documents, charting, reviewing laboratory results, filling e-prescriptions, and sending secure messages are all important features to understand, no matter what EHR system you use. The structure of an EHR system, such as the information processing cycle, is also crucial background knowledge to learn.

Data security and accessibility are important features of an EHR system. EHRs should always have a backup system and a secure server location. Accessing this server via mobile devices is becoming more commonplace as mobile technology becomes more affordable, secure, and adaptable to various EHR systems.

EHR Review

Check Your Understanding

To check your understanding of this chapter's key concepts, read the following true/false and multiple-choice questions and then record your answers on a separate sheet of paper. Write your answers as modeled in these examples: 1a; 2b; 6T; 7F; etc.

1. Data storage in an electronic health record (EHR) may be handled by all of the following methods *except* a

   a. cloud server.

   b. vendor server.

   c. facility server.

   d. flash drive.

2. The four components of the information processing cycle are

    a. input, print, output, and save.

    b. input, output, print, and storage.

    c. input, processing, output, and storage.

    d. enter, print, save, and storage.

3. CCHIT is the acronym for

    a. Certified Committee for Health Information Technology.

    b. Certification Committee for Health Information.

    c. Certified Commission for Health Information Technology.

    d. Certification Commission for Health Information Technology.

4. Meaningful use provides

    a. incentives for a healthcare facility that meets established criteria for an EHR system.

    b. a report to the patient on his or her healthcare information.

    c. a measurement of the functionality of the EHR system.

    d. incentives for patients who use a personal health record.

5. Mobile devices include

    a. iPads.

    b. iPhones.

    c. Androids.

    d. all of the above.

6. True/False: Interoperability allows various healthcare facilities to communicate with each other.

7. True/False: A microphone is a type of input device.

8. True/False: A local area network is a computer connected to the Internet.

9. True/False: All users of an EHR system have the right to access all components of the EHR.

10. True/False: EHR systems may be customized to meet the needs of the facility.

Learn the Terms

Go to the Course Navigator to access flashcards for Chapter 3 of *Exploring Electronic Health Records.*

COURSE NAVIGATOR

Acronyms

CCHIT: Certification Commission for Health Information Technology

CPOE: computerized physician order entry

EIN: employer identification number

HIPAA: Health Insurance Portability and Accountability Act

HITECH Act: Health Information Technology for Economic and Clinical Health Act

HL7: Health Level Seven International

IT: information technology

LAN: local area network

NPI: National Provider Identifier

PHI: protected health information

PHR: personal health record

WAN: wide area network

EHR Application

Go on the Record

To build on your understanding of the topics in this chapter, complete the following short answer questions.

1. Discuss the importance of assigning passwords and rights to users of an electronic health record (EHR) system.

2. Explain why it is important to lock an EHR system when not actively working with it.

3. Compare and contrast the advantages and challenges of using mobile devices with an EHR system.

4. Explain the advantage of using the e-prescribing feature of an EHR system.

Navigate the Field

To gain practice in handling challenging situations in the workplace, consider the following real-world scenarios and then use the guiding questions to help you formulate your responses.

1. You are the health information technology (HIT) training specialist at Northstar Medical Center, and you have been tasked with training new employees on the EHR Navigator. Prepare an outline you will follow for training employees.

2. After completing an overview of the EHR Navigator in this chapter, prepare a list of features that are most important to your job as the HIT training specialist at Northstar Medical Center. Explain why each feature is important and how each will help you complete your job more effectively and efficiently.

EHR Evaluation

Think Critically

Continue to think critically about challenging real-world scenarios and complete the following activities.

1. Tabitha Iris Wang calls to schedule an appointment with Dr. Alana Feltner. List the steps of an EHR system that you must take to schedule this patient.

2. You are the information technology (IT) manager for your healthcare facility. A new employee will begin in the Health Information Management (HIM) department. Prepare a list of the steps you would take to add a new user and assign permissions to this new HIM employee.

Make Your Case

Consider the following scenario and create a presentation on the following topic.

You are chairing a committee on selecting the EHR system for Cincinnati Grace Medical Center. The committee has decided to select a Web-based EHR system because the facility does not have a large IT staff. You are in charge of researching Practice Fusion, a free Web-based EHR system. Create a presentation based on the instructions provided to you by your instructor.

Explore the Technology

To expand your mastery of EHRs, explore the following online activities and complete the EHR Navigator assessments.

COURSE NAVIGATOR

Ensure you are comfortable with the functionality presented in the EHR Navigator activities, such as exploring the system, adding a new employee and assigning rights, exploring the administrative screens, and exploring the clinical screens. Then, complete the EHR Navigator assessments for Chapter 3 located on the Course Navigator.

1. Research the EHR certification criteria established by the Certification Commission for Health Information Technology (CCHIT). Prepare a table that lists the criteria and another table that lists the names and Web addresses of the CCHIT-certified EHR systems.

> " I believe we are seeing the tide turn toward widespread and accelerating adoption and use of health IT. "
>
> —David Blumenthal, MD, MPP
> National Coordinator for Health Information Technology
> Department of Health and Human Services

Are You Ready?

By choosing to pursue a career in health information technology (HIT), you are at the start of something monumental. Healthcare jobs are increasing, and it is estimated that 10 of the 20 fastest-growing occupations over the next 10 years will be in healthcare. Additionally, an estimated 50,000 new jobs will need to be filled to implement electronic health record (EHR) systems.

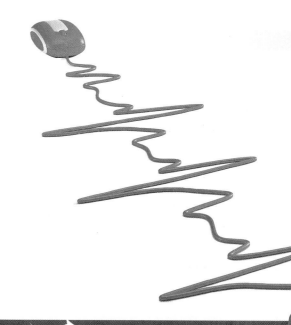

Beyond the Record

- Healthcare is the second most searched topic on Google.

- 66% of users are looking for information on diseases.

- 56% of users are searching for information on medical treatments.

- 44% of users are searching for doctors.

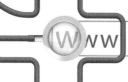

Administrative Management

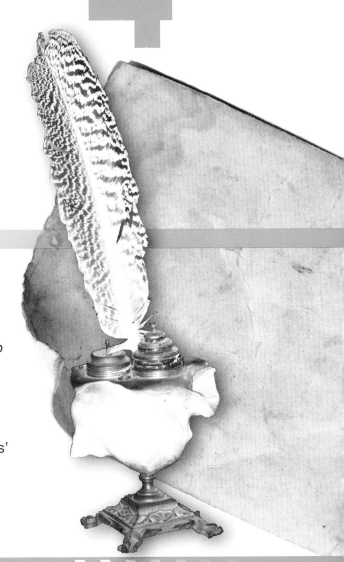

EHR Historical Context

Did you know that the roots of informed consent date back to the Middle Ages? Early medical practitioners would ask their patients to sign a *pro corpore mortuoto* ("hold harmless document"), absolving them of responsibility for any adverse effects from medical procedures or treatments. Ironically, the vast majority of patients at this time could not read or write and, consequently, had to place their trust in their caregivers' verbal communication about their treatment plan and possible complications.

Advance Directives 〉〉〉

National Healthcare Decisions Day is April 16. This annual initiative, which started in 2007, was established to educate adults about the importance of advanced care planning and to encourage them to document their wishes for end-of-life care. To find out more about this initiative, visit www.paradigmcollege.net/exploringehr /nhdd. This website provides a wealth of information on advance directives, including a list of sites that individuals can visit to download documents for completion.

- Identify various healthcare settings.

- Understand the difference between an established patient and a new patient for admission and registration purposes.

- Identify various documents found in an acute care or ambulatory care record.

- Define the term master patient index.

- Explain the registration process for a patient requiring ambulatory care.

- Explain the admission process for a patient requiring acute care.

- Understand the distinction between a subscriber and a guarantor.

- Examine the birthday rule.

Healthcare providers create and maintain an individual health record for every patient. Each health record contains the reason for the visit, the services rendered, diagnoses, and recommended treatments. Regardless of whether a patient is treated in a clinic, hospital, physical therapy facility, or imaging clinic, his or her health records require administrative management. As more healthcare facilities implement electronic health record (EHR) systems, more administrative functions will be electronically performed. This technology will change the daily tasks of healthcare personnel, streamline the workflow of health records, and improve the accuracy of documentation. For example, front-desk personnel will input patient appointments into the EHR system rather than enter the data on a physical calendar, thus reducing the chance of error. Staff will directly input patient demographic data into the EHR instead of pulling it from a paper form. Billing specialists will enter insurance data into the system and update the electronic record if the patient's insurance changes, thus ensuring accurate billing. These administrative functions will also allow healthcare providers and other staff members easy access to a patient's medical record, providing them with a complete picture of the patient's health history.

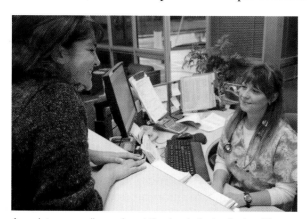

A registrar usually works at the front desk of a healthcare facility.

Generally, the initial contact for a patient is the healthcare personnel at the admission or registration desk. This person, called a **registrar**, is often required to collect information prior to and at the time the patient is seen. Increasingly, healthcare facilities may refer to professionals performing the registration or admission process as *patient access specialists*.

At the initial visit, the patient provides **demographic information** that connects the registrar to the correct EHR. If no record exists for the patient, the registrar must create a new record and add it to the **master patient index (MPI)**.

Depending on the nature of the appointment, patient information may be new or may require editing such as updating insurance coverage, contact information, or demographic data. The Health Insurance Portability and Accountability Act (HIPAA) Notice of Privacy Practices for Protected Health Information and the advance directives notice are also given at registration. Collecting accurate information from the patient is a critical job requirement for the registrar who completes the admission/registration process for the patient. Accurate data entry is also crucial to ensuring patient safety and avoiding communication problems among providers.

Different Types of Healthcare Settings

As you learned in Chapter 2, patient care is divided into two main categories: acute care and ambulatory care.

An acute care facility's goal is to care for patients who have short-term illnesses and require an overnight stay in a hospital. Acute care facilities provide round-the-clock diagnostic, surgical, or therapeutic care to patients.

An ambulatory care facility provides care to patients who do not require an overnight stay. Ambulatory care centers have grown within the past 30 years as technology has improved and fewer medical procedures require patients to stay overnight. In addition, health insurance has changed how patients pay for services and procedures, and many policies will not cover extended overnight care in a hospital if it is not medically necessary. There are times when a patient may go to an ambulatory care facility for a procedure and complications occur, requiring the patient to be admitted to an acute care facility. The patient would then be an acute care patient, rather than an ambulatory care patient.

Patient care in the acute and ambulatory settings is different. The following sections examine the differences in these two care settings.

Patient Care in an Acute Care Setting

Hospital personnel provide acute care to patients who experience sudden health issues or illnesses and cannot be treated in an outpatient care facility. Patients requiring acute care are either admitted to a hospital through the emergency department or sent from an outpatient clinic or a physician.

Acute care can range from a minimum stay of 24 hours to a maximum stay of 30 days, although exceptions to this guideline may occur. For example, if a patient dies before treatment, this patient is still considered as acute care because the physician planned for the patient to be admitted.

The day and time the patient is admitted to the acute care facility is the **admission date**. The admission registrar is the initial contact with the patient, which is, in part, why this interaction is

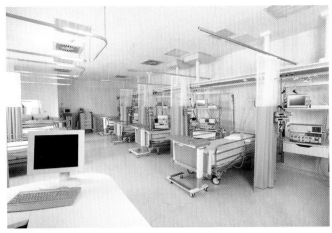

A hospital is an acute care facility.

increasingly referred to as patient access. In the acute care setting, the patient will receive room, board, and care from the hospital. The day and time the patient leaves the facility are included in the **discharge date**. A patient is admitted to the hospital by the physician who must document the admission order in the patient record. The physician must also document a discharge order to officially discharge the patient from the hospital.

Patient Care in an Ambulatory Care Setting

Ambulatory care includes services provided to the patient that do not require hospitalization or institutionalization. In most cases, the patient is discharged from the ambulatory care center in less than 24 hours. However, there are some exceptions to this rule such as a patient who is placed on observation status.

Ambulatory care settings are numerous and include (but are not limited to):

- Surgery centers
- Physician offices
- Clinics
- Group practices
- Emergency departments
- Therapeutic services

- Dialysis clinics
- Birthing centers
- Cancer treatment centers
- Home care
- Correctional facilities
- Dentist offices

Although gathering patient data is similar within an acute care or ambulatory care setting, there are some differences. Table 4.1 compares the two healthcare delivery systems.

Table 4.1 Management of Patient Data in Acute and Ambulatory Care Settings

	Acute	Ambulatory
Patient Contact	Admit a patient	Schedule an appointment
Health Record Content	History and physical exam, diagnostic records, treatment records, and discharge summary	SOAP, progress, or chart note
Patient Care	Admission	Visit
Length of Stay	More than 24 hours	Length of appointment, or less than 24 hours
List of Patients	MPI	Patient list
Completion of Patient Care	Discharge	Checks out
MPI = master patient index; SOAP = subjective, objective, assessment, plan		

Other Healthcare Settings

Other types of healthcare settings are identified either by length of stay or by specialty of care:

- A **long-term care facility** typically has patients who reside more than 30 days.

- A **behavioral health setting** provides care to patients with psychiatric diagnoses. The facility may offer a combination of acute care and ambulatory care for patients.

- A **rehabilitation facility** may also offer acute care and ambulatory care, typically serving patients recovering from accidents, injuries, or surgeries.

- **Hospice care** is palliative, or short-term, care provided to terminal patients within acute care or home care settings. The purpose of hospice care is to make patients comfortable until death and to support their families during this difficult time.

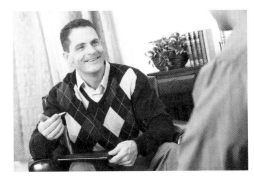

Behavioral health therapists may provide both acute care and ambulatory care.

CHECKPOINT 4.1

1. Name four types of healthcare settings.

   a. _____

   b. _____

   c. _____

   d. _____

2. When may a patient transition from an ambulatory care to an acute care setting?

   _____

   _____

   _____

Initial Patient Contact

The admission or registration begins when the patient or healthcare provider contacts the acute care or ambulatory care facility to make an appointment or schedule an admission in person or by telephone, email, or secure patient portal. If the facility uses an EHR system, then the patient may begin the registration process on the patient portal. If the healthcare facility uses a combination of electronic and paper forms for registration, then a patient may download forms from a healthcare facility website, or the forms may be provided by mail, email, or in person when the patient arrives. In addition to demographic information, these forms also collect payer information. This information is used to determine patient benefits and any required approvals from the third-party payer. Figure 4.1 shows a sample of a patient registration form.

When the patient arrives at the healthcare facility, a staff member must verify the patient's identity by copying or scanning the patient's insurance card and checking a driver's license or other proof of identification.

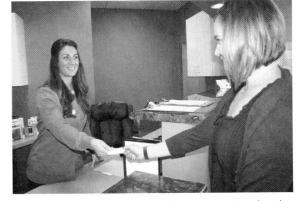

A patient provides insurance and co-payments when he or she checks in for an appointment.

Figure 4.1 Patient Registration Form

EMC MEDICAL CENTER

EMC Medical Center

Patient Registration Form

For Office Use Only:

MRUN: _____

Registrar: _____

PATIENT INFORMATION

Patient's Last Name		First	Middle Initial	Type of Care: ❑ Inpatient ❑ Same-Day Surgery ❑ Maternity ❑ Surgery ❑ Outpatient

| Race | Marital Status | Religion | Primary Language | Date of Birth (mm/dd/yyyy) | Date of Scheduled Visit |

| Physician's Last Name | First Name | ❑ Female ❑ Male | Social Security No. |

| Patient's Street Address | Apt. No. | City | State | ZIP |

| Home Phone ( ) | Work Phone ( ) | Cell Phone ( ) | Visit Reason or Diagnosis | Admission Date |

| Temporary Address | Apt. No. | City | State | ZIP |

| Patient's Current Employer Name | Employer Address | City | State | ZIP |

| Employer Phone ( ) | Patient's Occupation | Employment Status: ❑ Not Employed ❑ Full Time ❑ Part Time ❑ Student ❑ Retired and Date: |

| Full Name of Emergency Contact | Relationship | Home Phone ( ) | Work Phone ( ) |

Have you ever been a patient at EMC Medical Center? ❑ Yes ❑ No | If yes, when was your last visit? | Under what name?

Guarantor

| Last Name | First | Middle Initial | Relationship | Date of Birth (mm/dd/yyyy) |

| Street Address | Apt. No. | ❑ Female ❑ Male | Marital Status | Social Security No. |

| City | State | ZIP | Home Phone ( ) | Work Phone ( ) | Cell Phone ( ) |

| Employer Name | Employer Address | City | State | ZIP |

| Employer Phone ( ) | Occupation | Employment Status: ❑ Not Employed ❑ Full Time ❑ Part Time ❑ Student ❑ Retired and Date: |

Insurance Information

Primary Insurance Name | Name of Insured (exactly as it appears on card)

| Insurance Billing Address | City | State | ZIP | Phone No. ( ) |

| Policy No. | Group No. | Plan Code | State | Effective Date | Expiration Date |

| Subscriber's Full Name | Subscriber's Soc. Sec. No. | Subscriber's Date of Birth (mm/dd/yyyy) | ❑ Female ❑ Male |

| Subscriber's Employer Name (if self-employed, company name) | Relation to Insured | Subscriber's Employment Status: ❑ Not Employed ❑ Full Time ❑ Part Time ❑ Student ❑ Retired and Date: |

| Subscriber's Employer Address | City | State | ZIP | Phone No. ( ) |

Effective Date (mm/dd/yyyy)

_____ ❑ Part A (Hospital Benefit)

_____ ❑ Part B (Medical Benefit)

| Effective Date | State |

Name of Insured (exactly as it appears on card)

| State | ZIP | Phone No. ( ) |

| State | Effective Date | Expiration Date |

| Subscriber's Date of Birth (mm/dd/yyyy) | ❑ Female ❑ Male |

Subscriber's Employment Status: ❑ Not Employed ❑ Full Time ❑ Part Time ❑ Student ❑ Retired and Date:

| State | ZIP | Phone No. ( ) |

| Date of Accident: (mm/dd/yyyy) | Claim No. |

| Phone No. ( ) | Insurance Name |

| State | ZIP | Phone No. ( ) |

Advance Directive

Do you have an Advance Directive, such as a Living Will or Durable Power of Attorney for Healthcare? ❑ Yes ❑ No

Please specify the type: _____

*** If yes, please bring a copy at the time of your admission. ***

Self-Pay

* If insured but your procedure is not covered or verified by your plan, a deposit is required at the time of admission.

* If you do not have insurance, please call our *EMC Financial Services at (XXX)-XXX-XXXX* before your scheduled arrival date to discuss financial terms.

Additional Information

Do you need special accommodations, such as Translation, Visual Aid, etc.? ❑ Yes ❑ No

*** If yes, please specify so that prior arrangements can be made for the day of your visit. ***

❑ Language Interpreter _____ ❑ Sign Language Interpreter ❑ Visual Aid ❑ Other: _____

Master Patient Index

Most acute care facilities that use an EHR system call their list of patients a **master patient index (MPI)** or **patient list**. The MPI is a database created by a healthcare organization to assign a unique medical record number to each patient served, thus allowing easy retrieval and maintenance of patient information.

Patient Identifiers

Typically, the EHR system automatically generates and assigns a unique patient or medical record number, also known as a patient identifier. Figure 4.2 illustrates the button used to generate the patient number through the EHR Navigator.

HIPAA proposes the implementation of a unique patient identification system. The patient identifier would be similar to a Social Security number and consist of a set of numbers that seamlessly connects a person to his or her healthcare information.

It is crucial that healthcare providers use the MPI to verify that a patient has only one patient identifier (i.e., medical record number). If a patient has multiple identifiers, then providers may not see the true picture of a patient's health status because important healthcare information may be misplaced, lost, or duplicated.

Figure 4.2 Generating a Patient Number

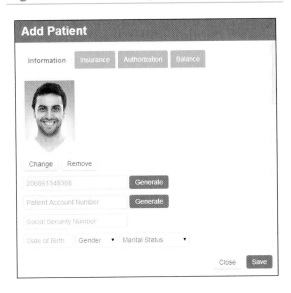

EXPAND YOUR LEARNING

There has been debate over the implementation of a unique patient identification system. To learn more on this controversy, read the following articles:

www.paradigmcollege.net/exploringehr/patient_ID_1

www.paradigmcollege.net/exploringehr/patient_ID_2

Purpose and Goals of the MPI

The EHR system stores the master patient index permanently (see Figure 4.3).

The goals of the MPI are to:

- match the patient with his or her MPI record.
- minimize duplication.
- merge and enterprise the MPI.
- retain lifelong health records.

Meeting these goals allows the efficient and effective use of the MPI.

The MPI contains the patient record number, with each information field containing data about a patient. These data fields produce a unique record. Healthcare providers

Figure 4.3 Master Patient Index

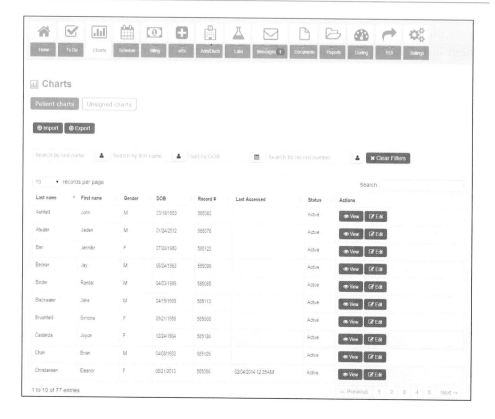

use the MPI to determine whether a patient record exists in the EHR system. If such a record exists, that same patient identifier is used each time a healthcare provider or facility sees the patient. In doing so, the patient identifier can be used to track all of the patient's encounters at the healthcare facility.

Core Data Elements

The American Health Information Management Association (AHIMA) recommends searching for a patient based on **core data elements** for indexing. In an MPI, the core data elements of a patient record are:

- Patient identification number
- Patient name
- Date of birth
- Sex
- Race
- Ethnicity
- Address
- Previous name

- Social Security number
- Facility identifier
- Account number
- Admission date
- Discharge date
- Service type

Optional Data Elements

AHIMA has identified the following **optional data elements** for the MPI:

- Marital status
- Telephone number
- Mother's maiden name
- Place of birth
- Advance directive decision making

- Organ donor status
- Emergency contact
- Allergies
- Problem list

Enterprise Master Patient Index

As healthcare continues to incorporate acute care and ambulatory care practices, there is a need to maintain patient identifier information across an EHR system for all healthcare settings. This systemwide database is called the **enterprise master patient index (EMPI)**. The EMPI allows the healthcare organization to compile the patient's information into one index using registration, scheduling, financial, and clinical information.

Two key data elements differentiate the MPI from the EMPI: the **enterprise identification number (EIN)** and the **facility identifier**. The enterprise identification number (EIN) in the EMPI is an identifier used by the organization to identify the patient across the various healthcare settings, whereas the facility identifier is used to indicate the healthcare setting where the patient is seeking care. Healthcare providers have created a system in the EHRs that automates the data elements in the patient record. Recommended EMPI data elements include:

- EIN
- Facility identifier
- Internal patient identification
- Patient name
- Date of birth
- Sex
- Race

- Ethnicity
- Address
- Social Security number
- Telephone number

Activity 4.1	EHRNAVIGAT✚R

EHR Master Patient Index/Patient List

Go to the Course Navigator to launch Activity 4.1. As an admission clerk, practice the various ways to search for a patient using the EHR Navigator.

Patient Registration/Admission

The patient registration/admission process may be slightly different for acute care and ambulatory care settings, but personnel in both settings focus on collecting accurate patient information.

Acute Care Registration

As mentioned earlier, the registrar is typically the first person the patient approaches upon arrival at the care facility. The registrar collects demographic and administrative information from the patient. If the patient is already in the EHR system, then the registrar will verify the accuracy of that information. Although similar to the registration process for ambulatory care, acute care personnel must follow the **Uniform Hospital Discharge Data Set (UHDDS)** for inpatient care. Developed by a committee in 1969, the UHDDS outlined a set of patient-specific data elements. This protocol, revised by the National Committee on Vital and Health Statistics (NCVHS) in 1984, was adopted by federal health programs in 1986. Since then, the UHDDS has been revised several times.

The recommended **UHDDS core data elements** are:

- Patient identifier
- Date of birth
- Sex
- Ethnicity
- Address
- Healthcare setting identification
- Admission date
- Type of admission
- Discharge date
- Attending physician identification

- Surgeon identification
- Principal diagnosis
- Other diagnoses
- Qualifier for other diagnoses
- External cause of injury code
- Birth weight of neonate
- Significant procedures and dates
- Disposition of patient
- Expected source of payment
- Total charges

Ambulatory Care Registration

In an outpatient or a physician office setting, the front office staff usually handles the registration process. The information gathered in the outpatient setting should follow the **Uniform Ambulatory Care Data Set (UACDS)** for outpatient services. The primary purpose of using this data set is to ensure that all healthcare settings and providers are gathering identical types of information on each patient, and that the data collected is defined consistently across all healthcare settings.

The NCVHS approved this data set in 1989. The UACDS is used in surgery centers, physician offices, and outpatient clinics, as well as emergency departments. The UACDS is not required but highly recommended.

Some of the recommended UACDS data elements include:

- Patient identification
- Address
- Date of birth
- Sex
- Ethnicity
- Provider identification
- Provider address
- Provider specialty
- Place of encounter
- Reason for encounter
- Diagnostic services
- Problem, diagnosis, assessment
- Therapeutic services

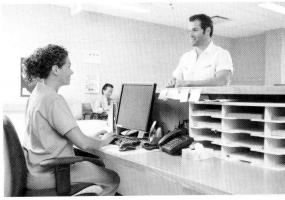

The registrar verifies the patient's information.

- Preventive services
- Disposition
- Source of payment
- Total charges

New vs. Established Patients

After identifying the patient, you must determine if he or she is an established patient or a new patient. To make this determination, it is important to understand the differences between these types of patients.

New Patient

For the purposes of admission and registration, a **new patient** is defined as a patient who has not received any services from a provider or a provider in the group in the same specialty within the past three years. For instance, if the patient was seen two years and eleven months ago, then he or she is likely to have an existing record; however, if the patient was seen three years and one day ago, then he or she is considered a new patient.

Consider This

When a patient arrives at an emergency department (ED), he or she is neither a new patient nor an established patient. The patient may have a record in the EHR system, but patients in the ED are not identified as being new or established. The terms *new* and *established* are primarily used for patients in an ambulatory care setting. Patients may have been to the ED for a previous visit, but they would not be classified as *established*.

How would you handle a situation in which a patient states that he has been to Shoreview Emergency Department before and, consequently, should not have to provide his information again?

To add a new patient to the system, the registrar must collect administrative information, including demographics used to identify the patient, report statistics, conduct research, and allocate resources.

The demographic information gathered includes:

- First, middle, and last names
- Medical record number (if known by the patient)
- Address
- Telephone numbers: home, work, and cell
- Sex
- Date of birth
- Place of birth
- Marital status
- Ethnicity
- Social Security number
- Emergency contact
- Date of service
- Physician
- Dentist

Activity 4.2 — EHRNAVIGATOR

Preadmission of a Patient

Go to the Course Navigator to launch Activity 4.2. As an admission clerk, practice preadmitting a patient using the EHR Navigator.

Established Patient

An **established patient** has received professional services from a healthcare provider or a provider in the same group and/or specialty within the past three years.

Begin by searching for the patient to determine whether the patient record is entered in the EHR Navigator. There are multiple ways to search for a patient using a variety of criteria such as:

- the patient's full or partial name in the *Last Name* and *First Name* fields.
- the patient's medical record or patient number in the *Patient Record* field.
- the patient's date of birth in the *Date of Birth (DOB)* field.

Healthcare staff members can also use of combination of the above criteria to find an established patient.

When searching for an established patient, search by different core data elements, e.g., patient name, patient record number, DOB, Social Security number, or admission date, to ensure the patient record exists in the EHR system.

Figure 4.4 shows the search screen for determining whether the patient is registered in the EHR Navigator.

If the patient is registered in the EHR system, confirm the information with the patient. If the patient needs to edit or update any demographic information, select the patient record and click on Edit Patient, as shown in Figure 4.5, and then update any patient demographic information required. To edit patient information, select the field and key in the appropriate data.

Figure 4.4 Search Screen

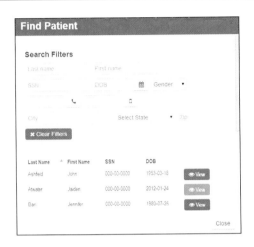

Figure 4.5 Update Patient Demographic Information

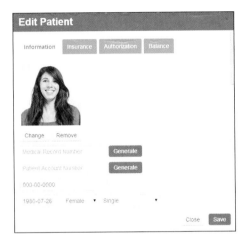

Activity 4.3 **EHRNAVIGAT⊕R**

Editing a Record for an Established Patient

Go to the Course Navigator to launch Activity 4.3. As a front desk clerk, practice editing a record for an existing patient using the EHR Navigator.

Insurance Information

Insurance information includes details about the patient's insurance coverage such as the insurance company, co-pay, and identification numbers to assist with processing claims. Some patients may not have insurance or may not wish to use insurance and are considered cash payers. Figure 4.6 on the following page is an example of a typical insurance card a patient may provide to the healthcare facility. A staff member will scan the insurance card into the EHR system and enter the insurance coverage information.

The insurance card contains the member name, member identification number, group number, and contact numbers for member services and claims/inquiries.

Figure 4.6 Insurance Card

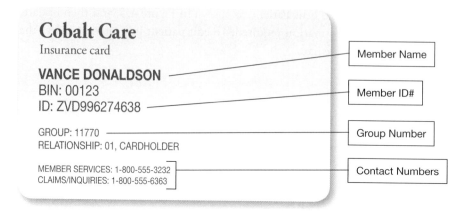

Insurance Subscriber and Guarantor

Two other key components of health insurance coverage are the subscriber and the guarantor. The **subscriber** is the person whose insurance coverage is used for acute or ambulatory care. The **guarantor** is the person or financial entity that guarantees payment on any unpaid balances on the account. The guarantor will be discussed in detail in the next section.

When a patient provides the healthcare facility with his or her insurance information, the coverage of treatment is based on the primary reason for the visit and a list of established insurance rules, which are addressed below.

- If a patient is injured, the healthcare setting must determine how the injury occurred. If there was an accident, primary coverage may be provided by the company, property insurance, or accident insurance.

- If a service at an acute care or ambulatory care setting is not accident-related, and each adult on the policy has his or her own insurance, then the patient's own insurance is primary.

- If a child is seen at an acute care or ambulatory care setting, and there are two insurance plans that cover the child, then the **birthday rule** is applied. The birthday rule specifies that the insurance of the parent whose birthday falls first in a calendar year will be the primary insurance. The ages of the separate cardholders have no bearing on this rule.

- If a patient has Medicare coverage and the services meet Medicare coverage guidelines, primary coverage is provided by Medicare.

- If a patient is older than age 65, is being seen for something other than an injury, has two insurances (Medicare and a supplemental plan), is unemployed, and is not covered by a spouse's insurance, the primary insurance would be Medicare and the supplemental plan would be the secondary insurance. Typically, a supplemental plan pays the deductible, co-pay, and any other charges not paid by Medicare.

- If a patient has Medicaid and a private insurance plan, the private insurance would be primary and Medicaid would be secondary.

For patients with insurance coverage through more than one provider, the primary coverage is determined by industry rules adopted by state insurance commissioners. The patient or the insured is responsible for informing the healthcare facility whether he or she has more than one insurance coverage.

New Insurance

When entering the patient's insurance and financial information into the EHR, you must also enter the patient's guarantor and guarantor account information. Subsequently, if an acute or ambulatory healthcare facility sends a bill for a balance of a service or services not covered by insurance, the bill will go to the patient's guarantor.

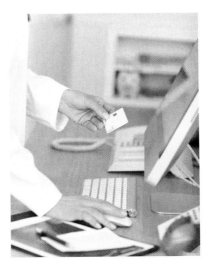

The registrar verifies the patient's insurance information.

A guarantor is the person or financial entity financially responsible for the patient. The guarantor may be the patient, another person, or a financial entity. Most patients older than age 18 are their own guarantors. Minors usually have their parents or legal guardians as their guarantors. Any patient with decreased mental capacity typically has a guarantor.

Every patient must have at least one guarantor account prior to being admitted or checked in to a healthcare facility. The **guarantor account** is a record that saves the information about the guarantor, including the guarantor's name and address.

There are several types of guarantor accounts, as seen in Table 4.2.

Table 4.2 Guarantor Account Types

Personal/Family	For general healthcare services, the guarantor is typically the subscriber of the primary insurance.
Workers' Compensation	The employer's workers' compensation insurance carrier is billed and then if there are remaining charges, or injuries are deemed not work-related, the patient is responsible for the charges.
Third-Party Liability	A third party, such as an insurance company, is responsible for payment.
Corporate	Company requires patient to receive services from healthcare facility or provider.
Research	Patient is involved in research or is a provider at the healthcare facility.

EHRNAVIGAT⊕R

Adding Insurance

Go to the Course Navigator to launch Activity 4.4. As a biller, practice adding insurance information using the EHR Navigator.

Update Insurance Information

Figure 4.7 Patient's Insurance Information

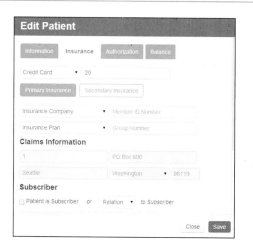

If a patient no longer has the original health insurance in his or her EHR, then the EHR will need to be updated, which is done by finding the patient's EHR and selecting the Insurance menu option on the left panel. You can make changes to existing coverage or add new coverage. It is important to key in the end date of the old insurance coverage to ensure that claims are submitted to the correct insurance provider.

The patient's current and previous health insurance coverages will appear on the Patient Insurance tab of the EHR, as shown in Figure 4.7.

Once you have entered the patient information and updated any administrative information, the patient may be scheduled for appointments.

CHECKP⊕INT 4.2

1. Name the five different types of guarantors.

   a. _____

   b. _____

   c. _____

   d. _____

   e. _____

2. Explain the birthday rule. Why is it important?

   _____

   _____

   _____

Adding Documents to a Patient Record

The EHR system gives you the ability to add scanned or uploaded documents to the patient's chart. The types of documents depend on the type of facility but may include documents such as privacy notices, financial agreements, consent forms, and advance directives.

Privacy Notices

An ambulatory care facility may scan or upload a Notice of Privacy Practices for Protected Health Information, which is a document based on a Department of Health and Human Services (HHS) document that informs patients about the use and disclosure of information by the healthcare facility. The document informs patients of their rights and responsibilities and provides contact information for any questions they may have.

The patient or the patient's representative must review and approve the Notice of Privacy Practices. An example of a Notice of Privacy Practices is shown in Figure 4.8. After you supply the patient with a copy, you must discuss the privacy notice with him or her. When the patient signs the document, you may upload the completed form into the individual's EHR. Some facilities use electronic patient signatures for these documents.

Figure 4.8 Notice of Privacy Practices

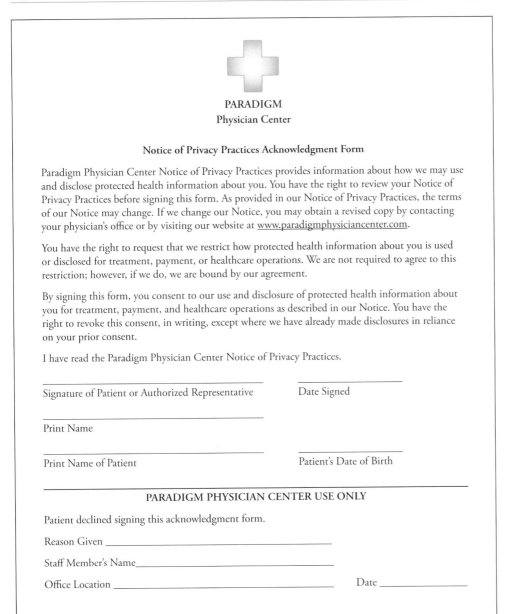

PARADIGM
Physician Center

Notice of Privacy Practices Acknowledgment Form

Paradigm Physician Center Notice of Privacy Practices provides information about how we may use and disclose protected health information about you. You have the right to review your Notice of Privacy Practices before signing this form. As provided in our Notice of Privacy Practices, the terms of our Notice may change. If we change our Notice, you may obtain a revised copy by contacting your physician's office or by visiting our website at www.paradigmphysiciancenter.com.

You have the right to request that we restrict how protected health information about you is used or disclosed for treatment, payment, or healthcare operations. We are not required to agree to this restriction; however, if we do, we are bound by our agreement.

By signing this form, you consent to our use and disclosure of protected health information about you for treatment, payment, and healthcare operations as described in our Notice. You have the right to revoke this consent, in writing, except where we have already made disclosures in reliance on your prior consent.

I have read the Paradigm Physician Center Notice of Privacy Practices.

_____   _____
Signature of Patient or Authorized Representative   Date Signed

_____
Print Name

_____   _____
Print Name of Patient   Patient's Date of Birth

PARADIGM PHYSICIAN CENTER USE ONLY

Patient declined signing this acknowledgment form.

Reason Given _____

Staff Member's Name_____

Office Location _____   Date _____

Financial Agreements

An example of a financial agreement that may be attached to a patient's EHR is the Assignment of Benefits form. The **Assignment of Benefits** form is an authorization by the patient to allow his or her health insurance or third-party provider to reimburse the healthcare provider or facility directly. A sample financial agreement is shown in Figure 4.9. If a healthcare facility requires patients to have a financial agreement on file, a staff member may ask for the patient's signature and then upload the signed document into the patient's EHR.

Figure 4.9   Assignment of Benefits

PARADIGM
Physician Center

Assignment of Benefits

In consideration of the patient receiving services from Paradigm Physician Center, I agree that:

- I am responsible for all expenses for treating the patient.
- Payment of charges is due at the time of the appointment.
- If Paradigm Physician Center files my insurance for me, I agree to pay for noncovered insurance benefits, coinsurance, co-pays, and deductibles.

Patient Signature

Printed Name

Date

Responsible Party's Signature (Parent/Guardian of Minor)

Printed Name

Date

AUTHORIZATION TO RELEASE INFORMATION AND TO PAY BENEFITS

I authorize Paradigm Physician Center to release any of my medical information, including drug, alcohol, and HIV-positive test results, to my insurance company(s), as needed to process my insurance claim.

I authorize my insurance company to make payments directly to Paradigm Physician Center for covered medical and/or surgical services.

Patient's Signature

Printed Name

Date

Responsible Party's Signature (Parent/Guardian of Minor)

Printed Name

Date

Consent Forms

A **general consent for treatment** form is used in acute care facilities. The patient signs the general consent for treatment, giving the healthcare provider the right to treat him or her. The provider may require an informed consent form if the patient is having a specialty procedure. A sample consent form is provided in Figure 4.10. This consent may also request permission to bill the patient and/or the patient's insurance for services rendered.

Figure 4.10 Consent Form

EMC
Medical Center

Informed Consent for Invasive, Diagnostic, Medical, and Surgical Procedures

Patient's Name_____

Date of Birth_____

Medical Record #_____

I hereby authorize _____ and/or _____ and/or such assistants and associates as may be selected by him/her/they to perform the following procedure(s)/treatment(s) upon myself/the patient.

Procedure(s)/Treatment(s) _____

_____

The procedure has been explained to me, and I have been told the reasons why I need the procedure. The risks of the procedure have also been explained to me. In addition, I have been told that the procedure may not have the results that I expect. I have also been told about other possible treatments for my condition and what might happen if no treatment is received.

I understand that, in addition to the risks described to me about this procedure, there are risks that may occur with any surgical or medical procedure. I am aware that the practice of medicine and surgery is not an exact science and that I have not been given any guarantees about the results of this procedure.

I have had enough time to discuss my condition and treatment with my healthcare providers, and all of my questions have been answered to my satisfaction. I believe I have enough information to make an informed decision, and I agree to have the procedure performed. If something unexpected happens and I require additional or different treatment(s) from the treatment I expect, I agree to accept any treatment necessary.

I agree to have transfusion of blood and other blood products that may be necessary in addition to the procedure I am having. The risks, benefits, and alternatives have been explained to me, and all of my questions have been answered to my satisfaction. If I refuse to have transfusions, I will cross out and initial this section and sign a Refusal of Treatment form.

I agree to allow this facility to keep, use, or properly dispose of tissue and parts of organs removed during this procedure.

_____   _____
Signature of Patient or Parent/Legal Guardian of Minor Patient   Date

If the patient cannot consent for himself or herself, the signature of either the healthcare agent or legal guardian acting on behalf of the patient, or the patient's next of kin who is asserting to the treatment for the patient, must be obtained.

_____   _____
Signature of Patient or Parent/Legal Guardian of Minor Patient   Date

_____   _____
Signature and Relationship of Next of Kin   Date

Witness:

I, _____, am a facility employee who is not the patient's physician or authorized healthcare provider named above, and I have witnessed the patient or other appropriate person voluntarily sign this form.

_____
Signature and Title of Witness

Interpreter/Translator (to be signed by the interpreter/translator if the patient required such assistance)

To the best of my knowledge, the patient understood what was interpreted/translated and voluntarily signed this form.

_____
Signature of Interpreter/Translator

Advance Directives

An **advance directive** is a document that provides information about how the patient would like to be treated if he or she is no longer able to make his or her own medical decisions. There are several types of advance directives. Figure 4.11 provides a sample of one type of document that may be attached to a patient's chart in the EHR system.

Figure 4.11   Advance Directives

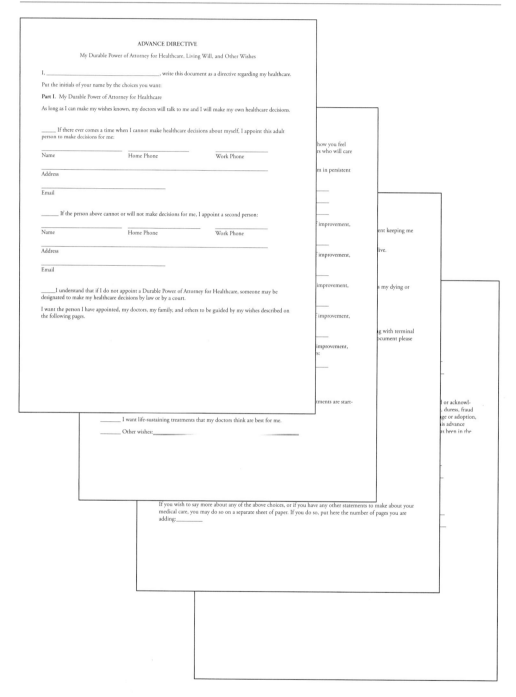

Figure 4.12 illustrates the list of documents that have been uploaded in the EHR system and may be attached to a patient's chart.

Figure 4.12 List of Documents

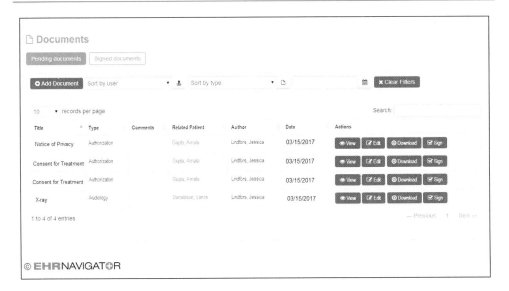

Activity 4.5 — EHR NAVIGATOR

Attaching Documents to a Patient's Chart

Go to the Course Navigator to launch Activity 4.5. As an admission clerk, practice attaching documents to a patient's chart using the EHR Navigator.

Consider This

The Documents feature of an EHR system offers many benefits for healthcare personnel. For providers, this feature allows them to scan or upload documents, such as test results or handwritten notes, and attach them to a patient's chart. This feature also allows providers to sign the notes. For all healthcare staff members, the Documents feature allows them access to view the documents and helps prevent misplaced or misfiled paperwork. In short, the ability to attach documents in an EHR system increases efficiency, productivity, and quality of patient care. With all these benefits, do you think there are still opportunities for documentation errors? What types of errors may occur?

Chapter Summary

Patients seek healthcare at acute care and ambulatory care facilities. Acute care services are provided by hospitals, long-term care facilities, inpatient behavioral units, inpatient rehabilitation units, and hospice care facilities. Ambulatory care services are delivered by clinics, group practices, home care, dentist offices, and many other types of facilities. In fact, ambulatory care facilities represent a growing segment of healthcare as more procedures and services are completed on an outpatient basis.

Depending on the type of care facility, patient visits are managed differently. An important factor of the patient visit in an acute care facility is the master patient index (MPI), which keeps track of the patient encounters and services at the facility. The design of the MPI is based on the core data elements proposed NCVHS. The American Health Information Management Association (AHIMA) recommends using the core data elements when searching the database. The data collected by an acute care facility is based on the Uniform Hospital Discharge Data Set (UHDDS), whereas the data collected by an ambulatory care facility is based on the Uniform Ambulatory Care Data Set (UACDS). Care for a patient in the ambulatory setting is based on the "new versus established" patient rule.

No matter the healthcare setting or whether the patient is new or established, healthcare staff members must collect insurance information. They also are required to gather and complete many documents during the patient's initial visit, including the Notice of Privacy Practices, Assignment of Benefits, Consents, and Advance Directives. In an EHR system, these documents may be electronically signed and attached to the patient's record.

EHR Review

Check Your Understanding

To check your understanding of this chapter's key concepts, read the following multiple-choice and true/false questions and then record your answers on a separate sheet of paper. Write your answers as modeled in these examples: 1a; 2b; 6T; 7F; etc.

1. Demographic information includes
   a. date of birth.
   b. laboratory results.
   c. diagnostic history.
   d. immunizations.

2. The master patient index is a/an
   a. spreadsheet of patient invoices.
   b. database of patients seen at the healthcare facility.
   c. index of patient telephone numbers.
   d. index of patient insurance coverage.

3. AHIMA recommends using which core data element when searching for a patient record in an EHR?
   a. Marital status
   b. Mother's maiden name
   c. Telephone number
   d. Patient record number

4. The Uniform Hospital Discharge Data Set includes all of the following *except*
   a. date of birth.
   b. sex.
   c. reason for encounter.
   d. admission date.

5. If a child is covered by two insurance plans, the primary coverage is the insurance of the
   a. parent who is older.
   b. parent who is younger.
   c. parent whose birth date occurs first in a calendar year.
   d. parent who has the best coverage.

6. True/False: Long-term care facilities have patients who reside more than 30 days.

7. True/False: There is only one type of ambulatory care facility.

8. True/False: Workers' Compensation is a type of guarantor account.

9. True/False: Most EHR systems allow documents to be uploaded to a patient's chart.

10. True/False: EHR systems do not have the capability for a healthcare provider to electronically sign documents.

Learn the Terms

COURSE NAVIGATOR

Go to the Course Navigator to access flashcards for Chapter 4 of *Exploring Electronic Health Records*.

Acronyms

AHIMA: American Health Information Management Association	**MPI:** Master Patient Index
EIN: Enterprise Identification Number	**NCVHS:** National Committee on Vital and Health Statistics
EMPI: Enterprise Master Patient Index	**UACDS:** Uniform Ambulatory Care Data Set
HIPAA: Health Insurance Portability and Accountability Act of 1996	**UHDDS:** Uniform Hospital Discharge Data Set
	UPI: Universal Patient Identifier

EHR Application

Go on the Record

To build on your understanding of the topics in this chapter, complete the following short answer questions.

1. Compare the registration processes in acute care vs. ambulatory care settings.

2. Describe the different types of ambulatory care settings.

3. Explain the differences between the Uniform Hospital Discharge Data Set (UHDDS) and the Uniform Ambulatory Care Data Set (UACDS).

4. Review the image of Vance Donaldson's Cobalt Care insurance card. Identify the different parts of the insurance card.

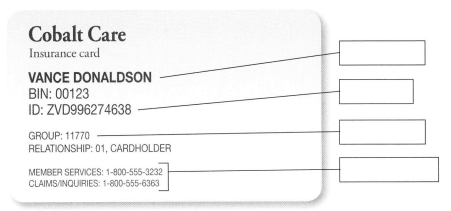

5. Discuss how a patient is identified as either a new patient or an established patient.

Navigate the Field

To gain practice in handling challenging situations in the workplace, consider the following real-world scenarios and then use the guiding questions to help you formulate your responses.

1. You are part of the team from Lincoln County Hospital working with the EHR Savvy company on the design of the master patient index (MPI). What elements are required for the MPI? Create a table with the elements that must be included in the MPI.

2. You are the EHR training specialist with Lincoln County Hospital. You are meeting with the registration staff to review the appropriate procedures for searching for patients. Create a checklist for the registrars to follow when determining whether a patient is new or established.

EHR Evaluation

Think Critically

Continue to think critically about challenging real-world scenarios and complete the following activities.

1. A new patient calls the admissions desk at Northstar Medical Center to preregister for a surgery. Prepare a list of steps that you would take to add the new patient to the EHR system.

2. Identify common errors made in the registration process. How could these errors be avoided/minimized? What is the impact of these errors on patient care?

Make Your Case

Consider the following scenario and create a presentation on the following topic.

You are a member of the Medical Records Department at Lincoln County Hospital. You are training the registration staff on the admission process. Prepare a presentation for your class that provides detailed guidelines to follow when collecting patient information.

Explore the Technology

To expand your mastery of EHRs, explore the following online activities and complete the EHR Navigator assessments.

COURSE
NAVIGATOR

Ensure you are comfortable with the functionality presented in the EHR Navigator activities, such as exploring the Master Patient Index, preadmitting a patient, editing a patient record for an established patient, adding insurance, and attaching documents to a patient's chart. Then, complete the EHR Navigator assessments for Chapter 4 located on the Course Navigator.

Are You Ready?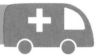

Not sure where to begin your career in health information management (HIM)? Volunteering and job shadowing are worthwhile ways to learn about different HIM disciplines. Choose a hospital, physician's office, or other type of facility where you might like to work to get a good idea of the profession's day-to-day responsibilities and gain insight into the type of atmosphere that will be a good fit for your personality and skill set. Plus, you will be able to add valuable experience to your résumé!

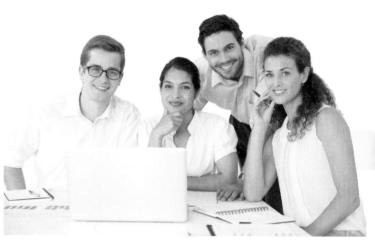

Beyond the Record

- The average wait time in a doctor's office is 24 minutes.

- The average wait time in an emergency department is 4 hours.

- Electronic health records can reduce wait time by streamlining the registration process.

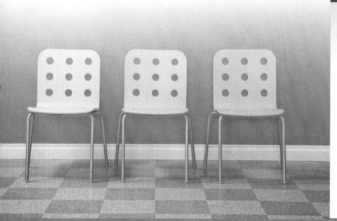

Room for Improvement

Approximately 35% of dentistry practices report sending email reminders of appointments, whereas only 14% of solo physician practices do. On average, 42% of clinical appointments are no-shows, for reasons ranging from issues with work and transportation to just plain forgetfulness. Could email reminders reduce no-shows in physician practices?

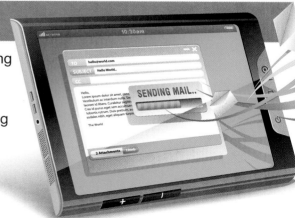

Chapter 5

Scheduling and Patient Management

EHRs in the News

The U.S. Department of Defense is expected to deploy a new electronic health record (EHR) system in 2017. The project has been delayed nine years due to rising costs, but the new EHR system will include 9.7 million active duty and retired armed forces personnel.

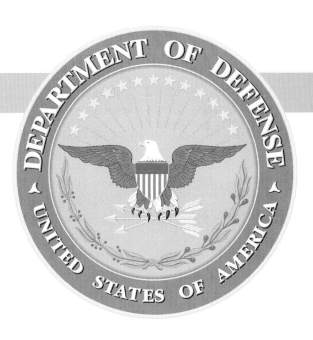

- Apply procedures to customize the schedule.

- Demonstrate how to schedule a patient in an acute care setting.

- Demonstrate how to schedule, cancel, and reschedule an established patient in an outpatient setting.

- Illustrate how to generate a provider schedule.

- Apply procedures to check out or discharge a patient.

- Demonstrate how to transfer a patient in an acute care setting.

- Use the Patient Tracker feature of the EHR Navigator to follow the patient from arrival to checkout.

Scheduling appointments is a common task among healthcare staff members, particularly in an ambulatory care setting. An electronic health record (EHR) system that includes a scheduling feature helps simplify the scheduling—and billing—process in a healthcare facility. The 2011 Certification Commission for Health Information Technology (CCHIT) standards state that an EHR system must "provide the ability to display a schedule of patient appointments, populated either through data entry in the system itself or through an external application interoperating with the system." EHR vendors must meet the CCHIT requirements so that providers using their software programs can show evidence of meaningful use to the federal government. To be compliant with such standards, an EHR system should provide the healthcare facility with a way to schedule patient appointments directly in the system, as you will learn how to do within the EHR Navigator. Some systems will use a separate electronic program to handle scheduling and communicate with the EHR system via a Health Level Seven International (HL7) interface. The system's scheduling component also includes a messaging system for the healthcare facility, provider, and patient to communicate with each other.

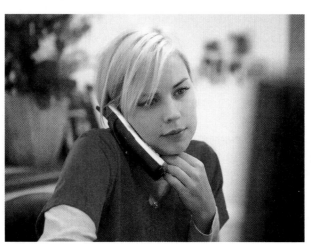

Patients make contact with a healthcare facility to make an appointment.

Before scheduling any patient visits, however, the facility must set up a facility template showing its overall schedule of operations. Once these scheduling parameters have been set, healthcare staff members can schedule patient appointments in the Scheduling tab of the EHR system (see Figure 5.1).

Figure 5.1 Scheduling Tab on the EHR Navigator

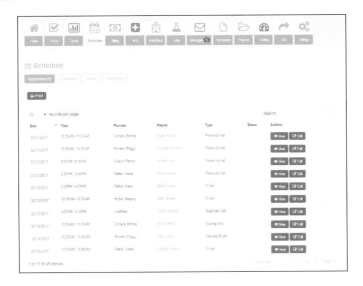

Healthcare Facility Schedule

A healthcare facility should create a matrix that shows available and unavailable appointment times. Unavailable times may include meetings, holidays, lunch hours, surgical schedules, physician rounds, or emergencies. The schedule may be viewed as daily, weekly, or monthly calendars, or may be viewed by patient, provider, or facility. The scheduling tools are used to insert, edit, cancel, or clear an appointment from the schedule. When setting up the EHR system, the acute care or ambulatory care facility enters the parameters for scheduling patients. Typically, a practice administrator or a representative from the healthcare facility works with the EHR vendor to create available days, times, and types of appointments. Such parameters typically include available providers, available scheduling days and hours, and types of visits. A typical EHR schedule for an ambulatory care facility displays a calendar; lists of available providers such as physicians, nurse practitioners, and physician assistants; and a list of open appointments, currently scheduled patients, contact information, types of appointments, and notes (see Figure 5.2).

Figure 5.2 EHR Schedule for Ambulatory Care

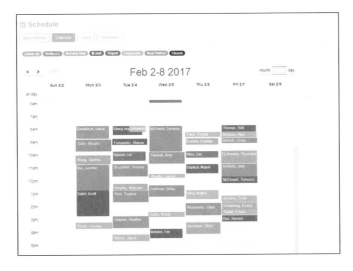

As mentioned earlier, the EHR scheduling system must block off time for holidays, lunch hours, vacations, personal time, and meetings, as necessary. These unavailable hours should be blocked off as soon as possible so patients are not scheduled during those times. These unavailable hours should be blocked off as soon as possible so patients are not scheduled during those times (see Figure 5.3).

Figure 5.3 Blocked Off Time in a Facility Schedule

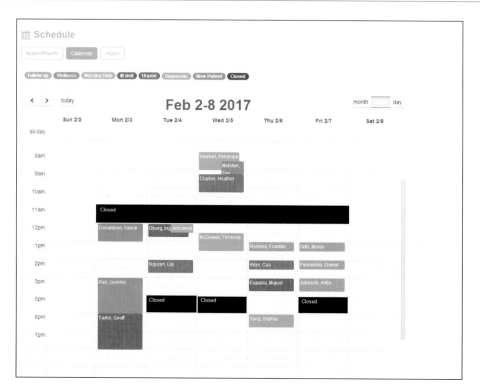

Activity 5.1 EHRNAVIGAT⊕R

Blocking Time in the EHR Schedule

Go to the Course Navigator to launch Activity 5.1. As an office manager, practice closing the office and adjusting the hours for Northstar Physicians using the EHR Navigator.

Patients who desire to be seen by a healthcare provider or receive care at a facility typically make an appointment for a specific date and time. Most healthcare facilities use a fixed schedule, whereas others, such as urgent care clinics or after-hours clinics, take walk-in appointments. Depending on the appointment type (e.g., office visit, surgery), the length of time will vary, with an office visit usually ranging from 10 minutes to as long as one hour. The healthcare facility typically has each type of appointment set up in the EHR scheduling parameters; therefore, when an appointment type is selected, the system will automatically populate the length of the appointment. However, the system also allows staff members to customize the length of an appointment if needed. Figure 5.4 illustrates a typical flowchart for scheduling an appointment for an outpatient.

Figure 5.4 Flowchart of Scheduling an Outpatient Appointment

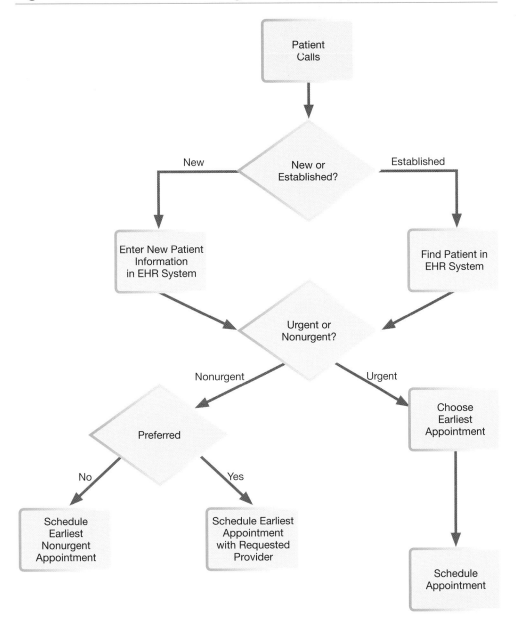

Types of Schedules

There are several different ways healthcare facilities choose to schedule appointments. No matter the type of scheduling method selected by the healthcare facility, the schedule must meet the needs of the facility and its patients. The different scheduling methods are designated as *open hours*, *time-specified*, *wave*, *modified wave*, and *cluster* and are discussed below.

- **Open Hours**: Patients are seen throughout certain time frames or on a first-come, first-served basis. This type of scheduling is typically used in an urgent care setting.

- **Time Specified**: Patients are given a specific date and time to arrive at a facility. A time-specified schedule may be used in an acute care setting where the patient has a specific date and time for surgery.

- **Wave**: Patients are scheduled to arrive at the beginning of the hour (hence, the term "wave"), and the number of appointments is determined by dividing the hour by the length of an average visit or procedure. The expectation is that patient visits will average out the time usage during that hour. This type of scheduling may be used in a primary care office where a group of patients arrive at the top of the hour, and then no appointments are scheduled at the bottom of the hour.

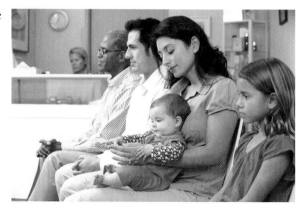

In wave scheduling, all patients arrive at the beginning of the hour.

- **Modified Wave**: Patients arrive at planned intervals in the first half hour; then, in the second half hour, the healthcare provider catches up. This type of scheduling may be used in an internal medicine office where the provider does not have to be in the room with the patient for the entire appointment.

- **Cluster**: Similar appointments are scheduled together at specific times of the day. For example, in a pediatrician's office, well-child visits may be scheduled in the morning and ill-child appointments may be scheduled after lunch.

CHECKPOINT 5.1

1. List the five types of schedules:

   a. _____

   b. _____

   c. _____

   d. _____

   e. _____

2. What types of events are placed on the schedule as blocked off time?

   _____

   _____

   _____

Patient Appointment Scheduling

Once the facility schedule includes the necessary parameters, patient appointments may be scheduled. There are a few ways to schedule an appointment in the EHR scheduling system. Traditionally, patients contact the healthcare facility to schedule his or her appointment. A patient can also schedule an appointment through a patient portal, which gives the patient the opportunity to schedule his or her own appointment.

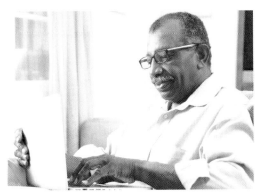

A patient can make an appointment from a home computer using a patient portal.

Information Needed to Schedule an Appointment

When a new inpatient or outpatient contacts the healthcare facility to schedule an admission or appointment, the healthcare staff must collect specific information. For a new patient, this information includes:

- Patient's full name
- Telephone number
- Date of birth
- Chief complaint or reason for appointment
- Type of insurance
- Insurance identification number

- Referring physician
- Social Security number
- Sex
- Address
- Emergency contact
- Responsible party information
- Employer information

Using the master patient index, the healthcare facility may populate the admission or appointment for an existing patient by collecting the following information to schedule an appointment:

- Patient's full name
- Date of birth
- Telephone number
- Chief complaint or reason for appointment

The patient information that already exists in the EHR must be verified and updated at the time of scheduling.

Patient Portal

Many EHR systems contain either a patient portal or a personal health record (PHR) component. The **patient portal** provides a secure communication tool between patients and healthcare providers that is compliant with the Health Insurance Portability and

Accountability Act of 1996 (HIPAA). Patient portals can also provide patients with information for their PHRs. Some patient portals are similar to the EHR Navigator and provide 24-hour, self-service components for patients to use. For example, the patient portal allows the patient to view a provider's calendar of available dates and times and schedule an appointment. This type of portal also allows the patient to enter demographic, insurance, medical history, and current health information prior to the first appointment. Patients who use the patient portal reduce the resources necessary from the healthcare facility.

Scheduling Component

The patient portal scheduling component is used for existing patients of an acute care or ambulatory care facility. The healthcare provider gives an existing patient an access code that allows him or her to schedule an appointment, send a message, update information, view laboratory appointments, request prescription refills, and view his or her health record. See Figures 5.5 and 5.6 for examples of a patient portal.

The patient accesses the patient portal by entering his or her username and password. Once logged in, the patient can view upcoming appointments, schedule appointments, view past appointments, and request referrals.

To begin, the patient would select *Schedule an Appointment.* The patient is able to select a provider and appointment type. The patient is then able to see the available appointments based on the criteria he or she has selected. Once a patient selects an appointment, the information is sent to the healthcare facility, and then the healthcare facility sends an email message to the patient with a confirmation. Figure 5.7 illustrates the Messages component of the patient portal.

Figure 5.5 Main Screen of a Patient Portal

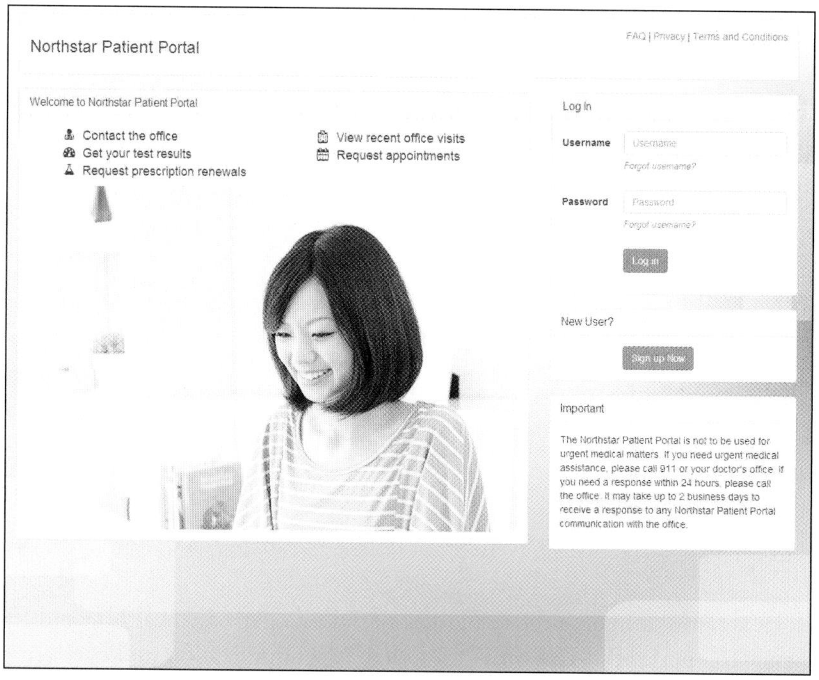

Figure 5.6 Schedule Appointment Screen of a Patient Portal

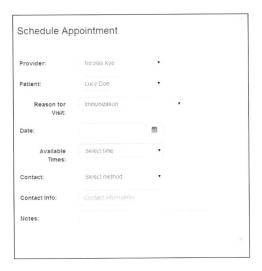

Figure 5.7 Messages in a Patient Portal

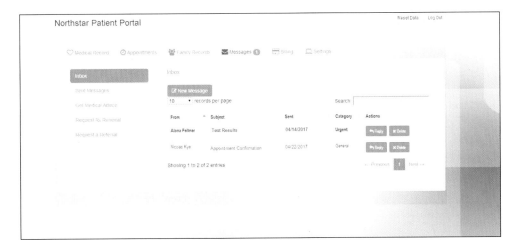

The patient portal makes scheduling convenient for the patient and the healthcare facility. Practices that implement a patient portal provide value to the patient by increasing patient access, enhancing the relationship between patients and providers, improving quality of care, and securing information. The patient portal also meets these four meaningful use criteria:

- Patient engagement criteria 1: electronic copy of health information

- Patient engagement criteria 2: clinical summaries

- Patient engagement criteria 3: appointment recalls

- Patient engagement criteria 4: timely access to health information

Scheduling in the EHR System

EXPAND
YOUR LEARNING

Patient portals are an integral part of EHRs. Read the following articles on how patient portals are improving healthcare and be prepared to discuss the articles' chief arguments.

www.paradigmcollege.net/exploringehr/patient_portal_1

www.paradigmcollege.net/exploringehr/patient_portal_2

www.paradigmcollege.net/exploringehr/patient_portal_3

When a patient telephones the healthcare facility or is present to schedule an appointment, there are three ways to initiate an appointment within the EHR Navigator scheduling feature.

- Select the patient: This method is the easiest way to schedule an appointment because the user is selecting the appointment directly from the appointment grid.

- Select Add Appointment: This method allows the user to make modifications to the traditional appointment times. Figure 5.8 illustrates the Add Appointment method.

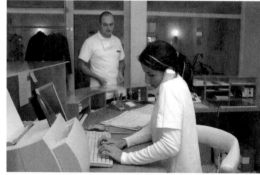

The healthcare worker will search for available appointments when a patient calls the facility.

- Select Calendar: This button allows the user to enter a date and time range to view available appointments. The search button also shows the provider's schedule and what percentage is already filled.

All three methods produce the same result: an appointment. The difference in the various ways to schedule comes down to user needs and preferences. The scheduling feature shows various colors that define the visit type or scheduled department. Staff members are able to accommodate patient preferences by adding sort criteria.

Figure 5.8 Add Appointment

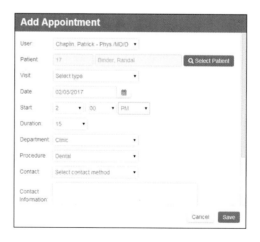

CHECKP⊕INT 5.2

1. Describe the benefits to scheduling using a patient portal.

   _____

   _____

2. What are the three methods for scheduling an appointment in the EHR?

   a. _____

   b. _____

   c. _____

Activity 5.2	**EHR**NAVIGAT⊕R

Scheduling an Inpatient Procedure

Go to the Course Navigator to launch Activity 5.2. As a unit clerk, practice scheduling an inpatient procedure using the EHR Navigator.

Activity 5.3	**EHR**NAVIGAT⊕R

Scheduling an Outpatient Appointment

Go to the Course Navigator to launch Activity 5.3. As a front desk clerk, practice scheduling an outpatient appointment using the EHR Navigator.

There are several other scheduling functions a healthcare staff member will need to use in his or her day-to-day practice, such as canceling a scheduled appointment, rescheduling an appointment, or printing a schedule. Each type of scheduling function will be reviewed below.

Canceling and Rescheduling Appointments

Many facilities struggle with patients who cancel appointments or those who do not show for their scheduled appointments (called **no-shows**). Patients cancel their appointments for a variety of reasons, including scheduling conflicts, emotional issues, financial concerns, and—for no-shows—forgetfulness. Regardless of the reason, each facility must set its own policy on cancellation fees, and each canceled appointment or no show should be documented in the EHR system. Tracking these types of appointments will enable the healthcare facility to run reports and determine its rate of no shows.

Confirming appointments decreases the incidences of no-shows, which in turn increases practice productivity and revenue. Healthcare staff can decrease the number of no-shows by setting up automated confirmation of appointments in the EHR system. To maximize the results of confirming appointments, patients can be given an option to receive a phone call or secure email reminder based on personal preference. Rescheduling may be the outcome of a canceled or no-show appointment.

Canceling and Rescheduling an Appointment

Go to the Course Navigator to launch Activity 5.4. As a medical assistant, practice canceling and rescheduling an appointment using the EHR Navigator.

Printing a Schedule

To meet the CCHIT Certified 2011 Ambulatory EHR criteria, EHR systems must display a schedule of patient appointments. In addition, CCHIT criteria state that the EHR must generate reports of clinical or administrative information. One example is to print the provider's schedule.

| Activity 5.5 | **EHR**NAVIGAT⊕R |

Printing a Provider's Schedule

Go to the Course Navigator to launch Activity 5.5. As a medical assistant, practice printing a provider's schedule using the EHR Navigator.

Transfers in the EHR System

EXPAND YOUR LEARNING

The use of medical scribes to assist providers in more efficient and personal interactions with patients is on the rise. Read the following article to learn how scribes may provide greater efficiency in an EHR environment.

www.paradigmcollege
.net/exploringehr/
scribes

During the time a patient is in a hospital, the need to be transferred from one unit or room to another may arise. Some of the reasons for a patient transfer include a change in patient condition, change in isolation status, or patient preference. All intra-facility transfers must be documented within the EHR system to ensure accuracy in patients' locations and hospital census data.

Change in Patient Condition

During an inpatient stay, a patient's condition may improve or deteriorate to the point that he or she must be transferred to a nursing unit in the hospital that can more adequately address his or her needs. For example, a patient in a room on a postoperative hospital unit who experiences cardiac arrest will likely be transferred to a more intensive nursing unit such as a cardiac intensive care unit. As the patient stabilizes and improves, he or she may be moved to a less intensive care unit.

Change in Isolation Status

Isolation status refers to the precautions that must be taken by healthcare staff and visitors to avoid the spread of bacterial or viral infections. Many hospital rooms are semi-private, meaning there are two patients occupying a room. Patients can only be admitted to the same room if they have the same isolation status. For example, a patient infected with methicillin-resistant *Staphylococcus aureus* (MRSA) cannot be admitted to the same room as a patient without the same infection, as there is a substantial risk that the other patient may also become infected with MRSA.

Patient Preference

Patients may ask to be transferred to another hospital room for many reasons, such as noise levels or roommate issues.

All EHR systems should have a transfer patient function. In the EHR Navigator, this function is accessed through the *Admission/Discharge Tab*.

Activity 5.6   **EHRNAVIGAT⊕R**

Transferring a Patient

Go to the Course Navigator to launch Activity 5.6. As a unit clerk, practice transferring a patient using the EHR Navigator.

Checkout/Discharge Procedures

The procedure for a patient leaving a medical facility varies depending on whether he or she is **checking out** at an outpatient facility, or whether he or she is being **discharged** from an inpatient facility.

Outpatient Checkout

Following an outpatient visit, the patient will check out. The checkout procedure may include collecting payments, ordering tests, making referrals, or scheduling a future appointment for the patient. During the checkout process, all the necessary prescriptions and completed forms must be verified.

Inpatient Discharge

The discharge of an inpatient from an acute care hospital is entered into the EHR Navigator via the *Admission/Discharge* tab. The date and time of the patient's discharge are automatically captured when the nurse or staff member enters the discharge into the EHR system. The **discharge disposition**, or the patient's destination following a stay in the hospital, is also entered. Examples of discharge dispositions include home, skilled nursing facility, rehabilitation hospital, and long-term acute care hospital. If an inpatient dies, the discharge disposition entered is "expired."

Discharge documents may be generated from the EHR system. These documents may include discharge instructions for the patient specific to the patient's diagnoses and the procedures performed. Discharge

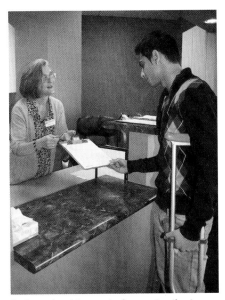

Before checking out of an outpatient facility, a patient may be asked to schedule a follow-up appointment.

documents may also include information regarding recommended follow-up with the patient's surgeon or primary care physician. In addition, to comply with accreditation requirements, a current medication list should be provided from the EHR system to the patient at the time of discharge.

Activity 5.7 — EHR NAVIGATOR

Discharging a Patient

Go to the Course Navigator to launch Activity 5.7. As a unit clerk, practice discharging a patient using the EHR Navigator.

EXPAND YOUR LEARNING

As healthcare facilities implement EHRs, many researchers find that wait time will increase for patients. Other factors, including a shortage of physicians and the demand for specialty areas within facilities, may be a contributing factor to increasing wait times for patients. To learn more about the future of patient wait times, read the following articles: www.paradigmcollege.net/exploringehr/wait_time_1 and www.paradigmcollege.net/exploringehr/wait_time_2

Patient Tracker

An EHR system has the ability to track a patient's location from admission to discharge (for inpatients) or from check-in to checkout (for outpatients). This feature offers a real-time, at-a-glance view of a patient's current status and location. For example, when a patient checks in at Northstar Physicians, the patient-tracking feature would be activated and would follow the patient until checkout. The use of patient tracking by providers improves the healthcare facility's work flow and increases patient satisfaction. The EHR Navigator's Patient Tracker feature is illustrated in Figures 5.9 and 5.10.

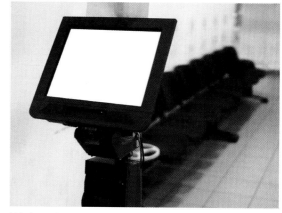

Workstations in the waiting room can be used to check in a patient and begin tracking his or her location.

Figure 5.9 Patient Tracker Feature — Updating Patient's Location

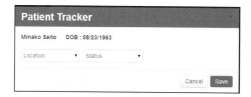

Figure 5.10   Patient Tracker Feature — Patient Status Summary

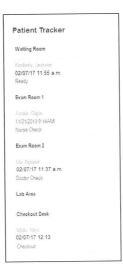

CHECKP◍INT 5.3

1. List the three reasons a patient might be transferred.

   a. _____

   b. _____

   c. _____

2. Describe the purpose of a patient tracker system.

   _____

   _____

   _____

Activity 5.8   **EHR**NAVIGAT◍R

Using the Patient Tracker

Go to the Course Navigator to launch Activity 5.8. In this activity, practice using the EHR Navigator Patient Tracker to follow the patient from arrival to checkout. You will log in as several different staff members of Northstar Physicians.

Chapter Summary

Scheduling patients in an acute care or ambulatory care facility is a key factor in the delivery of healthcare. Scheduling depends on the type of facility and type of appointment. In an acute care facility, the appointment depends on resources, such as the availability of the healthcare provider, the equipment, and the type of procedure ordered. Ambulatory care patients are typically labeled as new or existing. When scheduling a new patient, healthcare staff must gather demographic and financial information.

There are several types of schedules, all of which are dependent on the needs of the facility. The schedule types include *open hours*, *time specified*, *wave*, *modified wave*, and *cluster*. The electronic health record (EHR) system provides features for scheduling, canceling, and rescheduling appointments.

The Certification Commission for Health Information Technology (CCHIT) states that an EHR system must display a schedule of patient appointments and generate reports of clinical or administrative information.

Transferring patients may be necessary due to a change in the patient's condition or isolation status or because he or she is dissatisfied with the room.

Tracking patients allows facilities to know immediately the location and status of a patient, increasing work flow efficiency and patient satisfaction.

EHR Review

Check Your Understanding

To check your understanding of this chapter's key concepts, read the following multiple-choice and true/false questions and then record your answers on a separate sheet of paper. Write your answers as modeled in these examples: 1a; 2b; 6T; 7F; etc.

1. Scheduling an appointment requires that the scheduler collect all of the following pieces of information except

   a. health insurance information.

   b. patient demographics.

   c. reason for the visit.

   d. means of arrival.

2. An electronic health record (EHR) contains unavailable times for scheduling appointments. Unavailable times may include all of the following *except*

   a. holidays.

   b. hospital rounds.

   c. lunch.

   d. pharmaceutical sales visits.

3. A healthcare facility may choose one of the following scheduling methods to create its appointment schedule:

   a. Modified cluster

   b. Wave

   c. Modified wave

   d. Cluster

4. A patient portal is

   a. owned and controlled by a patient, may contain additional information not in the medical record, and is used for managing health information.

   b. generated by a healthcare provider to document a patient's medical and health information and is not directly accessed by a patient.

   c. a secure website that allows patients to access a personal health record (PHR) to communicate with healthcare providers, request prescription refills, review laboratory test results, or schedule appointments.

   d. a nonsecure website that allows patients to access a PHR to communicate with healthcare providers, request prescription refills, review laboratory test results, or schedule appointments.

5. Which of the following is *not* an appropriate reason for a patient transfer?

   a. The patient's condition has changed.

   b. The patient does not like his or her roommate.

   c. The patient is in isolation status.

   d. A nurse does not like the patient.

6. True/False: Scheduling is used to insert, edit, delete, or remove an appointment.

7. True/False: The patient tracker feature in an EHR follows the patient from admission or check-in to discharge or checkout.

8. True/False: Time-specified appointment scheduling requires the patient to be seen on a first-come, first-served basis.

9. True/False: A patient may request a transfer because he or she finds the room too noisy.

10. True/False: A patient portal provides the patient with an opportunity to schedule his or her own appointments.

Learn the Terms

COURSE NAVIGATOR

Go to the Course Navigator to access flashcards for Chapter 5 of *Exploring Electronic Health Records*.

Acronyms

CCHIT: Certification Commission for Health Information Technology

PHR: personal health record

EHR Application

Go on the Record

To build on your understanding of the topics in this chapter, complete the following short answer questions.

1. Why would a healthcare facility choose to use a specific type of scheduling?

2. There are times when a schedule should be blocked from appointments. Explain the different types of activities of a healthcare facility or provider that would necessitate blocked schedule time.

3. What are the different reasons that a patient's appointment may need to be adjusted?

4. Why is it important to track a patient during his or her stay at a healthcare facility?

5. Describe how the patient tracker feature may improve the healthcare facility's work flow and patient satisfaction.

Navigate the Field

To gain practice in handling challenging situations in the workplace, consider the following real-world scenarios and then use the guiding questions to help you formulate your responses.

1. You receive an appointment request from Ms. Ying through the patient portal. She is requesting an appointment time already filled by another patient. You contact Ms. Ying, and she informs you that when she requested the appointment, the time was available and she needs to be seen right away. How should you handle this situation?

2. You are preparing the 2018 calendar for Northstar Physicians. You are working with the physicians, staff, and IT manager to create the schedule in the EHR Navigator. What are the steps you would take to prepare the calendar to be customized for the EHR Navigator? What would be the best way to communicate this to the IT manager so that the EHR Navigator calendar may be customized?

EHR Evaluation

Think Critically

Continue to think critically about challenging real-world scenarios and complete the following activities.

1. A new patient calls to schedule an appointment. Prepare a list of steps you would follow to schedule the appointment.

2. Dr. Nelson's office contacts the Scheduling Department at St. Francis Hospital to schedule Mr. Yadav's double bypass surgery. Mr. Yadav will have to stay a minimum of three days in the hospital. Prepare a list of steps you would follow to schedule the surgery for Dr. Nelson's patient.

Make Your Case

Consider the following scenario and create a presentation on the following topic.

You work for Pleasant Valley Urgent Care, which is implementing a new electronic health record (EHR) system. You are responsible for working with the EHR vendor to determine the scheduling parameters of the system and must provide the vendor with a presentation on the type of scheduling Pleasant Valley Urgent Care will use. Include in the presentation the urgent care days, times, a list of healthcare providers, number of examination rooms, equipment necessary, any nonpatient times, and any additional resources that will be used for scheduling. You will be presenting to the vendor and the director of Pleasant Valley Urgent Care.

Explore the Technology

To expand your mastery of EHRs, explore the following online activities and complete the EHR Navigator assessments.

COURSE NAVIGATOR

Ensure you are comfortable with the functionality presented in the EHR Navigator activities, such as scheduling an inpatient procedure, scheduling an outpatient appointment, canceling and rescheduling an appointment, printing a provider's schedule, transferring a patient, discharging a patient, and using the patient tracker. Then, complete the EHR Navigator assessments for Chapter 5 located on the Course Navigator.

Are You Ready?

Have you found a job that sounds perfect for you? If so, you will want to spend some time perfecting your résumé and cover letter to make a good first impression on a potential employer. Research how to craft an interesting and effective cover letter, and consider meeting with your school's career services office for tips on writing an effective résumé.

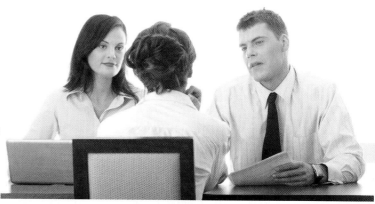

Beyond the Record

- The penalties for criminal violations of the Health Insurance Portability and Accountability Act of 1996 (HIPAA) are steep.

- Knowingly obtaining or disclosing identifiable patient information can result in one year of imprisonment and a $50,000 fine per violation.

- Obtaining patient information for personal or commercial gain or with malicious intent can result in 10 years' imprisonment and a $250,000 fine.

HIPAA Time Line

- **1996**–HIPAA signed into law.

- **1999**–United States Department of Health & Human Services (HHS) becomes responsible for developing privacy standards.

- **1999**–HHS proposes privacy standards and receives more than 50,000 comments on the proposed standards.

- **December 2000**–HHS publishes the Final Rule for Standards for Privacy of Individually Identifiable Health Information, or the Final HIPAA Privacy Rule

- **April 2003**–Deadline for covered entities to comply with the Privacy Rule.

- **April 2005**—Deadline for covered entities to comply with the Security Rule.

Privacy and Security of Health Information

Case Study

On July 27, 2010, Rite Aid Corporation and its 40 affiliated entities agreed to pay $1 million to settle potential violations of the HIPAA Privacy Rule. It also agreed to take corrective action to improve policies and procedures that safeguard the privacy of its customers when disposing of identifying information on pill bottle labels and other health information. The settlements followed an extensive investigation of Rite Aid after television media videotaped pharmacy employees disposing of prescriptions and labeled pill bottles containing individuals' identifiable information in the trash.

- **January 25, 2013**–HHS publishes modifications to the HIPAA Privacy, Security, and Enforcement Rules to comply with the provisions of the Health Information Technology for Economic and Clinical Health (HITECH) Act. This is known as the HIPAA Omnibus Final Rule.

- **September 23, 2013**–HIPAA Omnibus Final Rule compliance is mandatory for covered entities, business associates, and subcontractors.

Learning Objectives

- Define Health Insurance Portability and Accountability Act of 1996 (HIPAA), specifically the Administrative Simplification Provision and the date enacted.

- Define the term *covered entity*.

- Discuss the main components of the Privacy Rule.

- Define the term *protected health information*.

- Discuss the concept of "minimum necessary" as it relates to the release of health information.

- Explain the enforcement and penalty process for violations of HIPAA Privacy and Security regulations.

- Demonstrate competency in the use of electronic health record software as it relates to the release of health information.

- Discuss the Breach Notification Rule.

- State the two primary purposes for the development of the Security Standards of HIPAA.

- Discuss the major sections of the standards of the Security Rule.

- Discuss the difference between required and addressable implementation specifications.

As you have already learned, privacy and confidentiality of health information is a major focus when implementing an electronic health record (EHR) system. As a user of an EHR system, you must understand and follow the laws and regulations regarding privacy, safety, and security of health information. In addition, there are procedures for safeguarding health information that are not mandated by law but should be considered when implementing and using EHRs.

A challenging topic to address is patients' access to their health information and their rights regarding its release to others. Federal legislation that revolutionized the release and security of health information includes the HIPAA Privacy and Security Rules published in 2000, which were subsequently updated in 2010. These rules provide guidance with regard to the release and security of paper health records, as well as the release and security of EHR data.

EXPAND YOUR LEARNING

Locate a website sponsored by the U.S. government that provides information and resources regarding HIPAA.

HIPAA

The **Health Insurance Portability and Accountability Act of 1996 (HIPAA)** was enacted on August 21, 1996. HIPAA includes many provisions that affect all health-care facilities. For example, HIPAA allowed for health insurance to be "portable—in other words, the insurance could be moved from one employer to another without denial or restrictions. HIPAA mainly addresses the confidentiality of patients' medical records, including the safeguards that need to be implemented by a healthcare facility to protect the privacy and security of its patients. In addition to setting standards for health information privacy and security, HIPAA also addresses standards to improve the efficiency and effectiveness of healthcare systems. For example, Sections 261-264, known as the Administrative Simplification Provisions, required the U.S. department of Health & Human Services (HHS) to adopt national standards for electronic health care transactions and code sets, unique health identifiers, and security. To gain a broad picture of the tenets of HIPAA, see Figure 6.1. This chapter will specifically focus on the provisions for the electronic exchange, privacy, and security of health information.

Figure 6.1 HIPAA Administrative Simplification Provisions

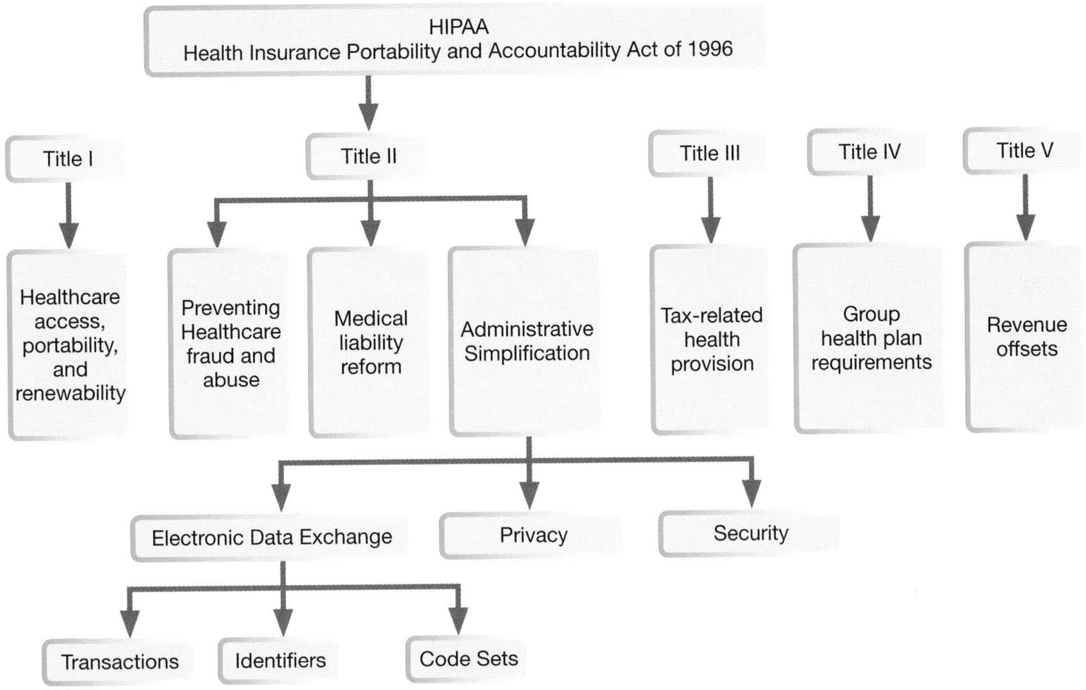

HIPAA Privacy Rule

In response to the HIPAA legislation, the HHS Secretary published the Privacy Rule on December 28, 2000, and later modified the HIPAA Privacy, Security, and Enforcement Rules on January 25, 2013, to comply with the provisions of the Health Information Technology for Economic and Clinical Health (HITECH) Act, particularly with regard to EHRs.

Covered Entities

The Privacy and Security Rules apply to healthcare providers, health plans, and healthcare clearinghouses transmitting health information in an electronic format. These entities are called **covered entities** (see Table 6.1). Individuals, organizations, and agencies meeting the definition of a covered entity under HIPAA must comply with the Rules' requirements to protect the privacy and security of health information, and they must provide individuals with certain access rights with respect to his or her health information.

EXPAND YOUR LEARNING

The Final HIPAA Privacy Rule published December 28, 2000, can be viewed at the following website: www.paradigmcoll ege.net/exploringehr/ privacy_rule.

Modifications made to HIPAA on January 25, 2013, can be viewed at the following website:

www.paradigmcoll ege.net/exploringehr/ HIPAA_Modifications.

Business associates of a covered entity must also follow the Privacy Rule if they perform services to the covered entity involving the use or disclosure of individually identifiable health information.

Table 6.1 Covered Entities

Healthcare Provider	Health Plan	Healthcare Clearinghouse
The term healthcare provider refers to a provider who transmits health information in an electronic format, such as: • Doctors • Clinics • Psychologists • Dentists • Chiropractors • Nursing Homes • Pharmacies • Hospitals	The term health plan refers to the following entities: • Health insurance companies • Health maintenance organizations • Company health plans (some self-administered company health plans with fewer than 50 participants are not covered) • Government programs that pay for healthcare, such as Medicare, Medicaid, and military and veterans' healthcare programs	The term healthcare clearinghouse refers to a public or private entity, including billing services, repricing companies, community health management information systems, community health information systems, or "value-added" networks and switches, that does either of the following functions: (1) Processes, or facilitates the processing of, health information received from another entity in a nonstandard format or containing nonstandard data content into standard data elements or a standard transaction. (2) Receives a standard transaction from another entity and processes or facilitates the processing of health information into nonstandard format or nonstandard data content for the receiving entity.

Noncovered Entities

If an entity is not considered a covered entity, it does not have to comply with HIPAA Privacy and Security Rules. Some examples of **noncovered entities** include workers' compensation carriers, employers, marketing firms, life insurance companies, pharmaceutical manufacturers, casualty insurance carriers, pharmacy benefit management companies, and crime victim compensation programs.

Health Information and the Privacy Rule

Certain types of health information are classified under the HIPAA Privacy Rule. These types include protected health information, individually identifiable health information, and de-identified health information.

Protected Health Information

The Privacy Rule defines **protected health information (PHI)** as all individually identifiable health information held or transmitted by a covered entity or its business associate, in any form or media, whether electronic, paper, or oral.

Individually Identifiable Health Information

Individually identifiable health information is information, including demographic data, that identifies the individual, or for which there is a reasonable basis to believe that the information can be used to identify the individual, and that it relates to at least one of the following:

- the individual's past, present, or future physical or mental health condition.

- the provision of healthcare to the individual.

- the past, present, or future payment for the provision of healthcare to the individual.

Individually identifiable health information includes many common identifiers, such as name, address, birth date, or Social Security number.

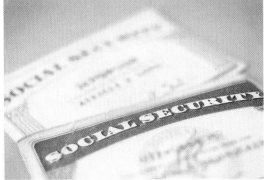

Your Social Security number is a type of common identifier.

De-identified Health Information

The term **de-identified health information** was coined by the Privacy Rule and is health information that neither identifies an individual nor provides a reasonable basis to identify an individual. Therefore, the Privacy Rule does not restrict the use of de-identified health information. Healthcare staff primarily use de-identified health information for summary purposes, as illustrated by the following scenarios:

- the marketing department of a healthcare provider wants to know how many patients are from each ZIP code.

- a dentist office wants to know the number of patients who recently had a cavity filled to determine if the office's use of dental supplies is appropriate.

- a home care agency wants to know the number of physical therapy home care visits made last year to determine whether additional physical therapists should be hired.

Basic Principles of the Privacy Rule

A major purpose of the Privacy Rule is to define and limit the circumstances in which an individual's protected health information may be used or disclosed by covered entities.

A covered entity may not use or disclose PHI except either (1) as the Privacy Rule permits or requires, or (2) as the individual who is the subject of the information (or the individual's personal representative) authorizes in writing.

Required Disclosures

A covered entity *must* disclose PHI in only two situations:

1. To an individual (or his or her personal representative), specifically when he or she requests access to, or an accounting of disclosures of, his or her PHI

2. To HHS, specifically during a compliance investigation, review, or enforcement action

Permitted Disclosures

HIPAA regulations permit health information to be used and/or disclosed in the following scenarios without a prior authorization signed by the patient:

- to the individual patient

- for treatment purposes

- for payment purposes

- for healthcare operations

- incidental to an otherwise permitted use or disclosure

- for public interest and benefit activities

- as a limited data set for purposes of research, public health, or healthcare operations

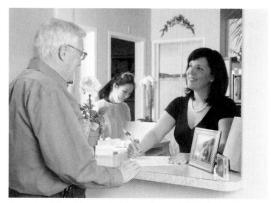

A patient is often asked to sign a HIPAA disclosure asking if it is acceptable to release his or her health information in certain situations.

To learn more about these specific situations for permitted disclosure of health information, refer to the following sections.

Individual Patient A patient has the right to view and receive a copy of his or her health information. The covered entity must release the health information in the format requested by the patient (e.g., paper, CD, or another electronic format). As a result of the HIPAA Omnibus Final Rule, a patient also now has the right to download and transmit his or her health information electronically.

Three types of permitted disclosures are commonly known in the healthcare industry collectively as **treatment, payment, healthcare operations (TPO)**. When health information managers, compliance officers, or administrators are asked questions related to the appropriate release of healthcare information and reply with, "Yes, you can release the health information under the TPO clause," they are referring to these permitted disclosures.

Treatment Purposes **Treatment** is defined as the provision, coordination, or management of healthcare and related services for an individual by one or more healthcare providers, including consultation among providers regarding a patient, and referral of a patient by one provider to another.

HIPAA has made it easier and faster for providers to release information for patient care purposes because written patient authorization is not necessary. This HIPAA provision is particularly important for EHRs, allowing healthcare practitioners to obtain health information within minutes or seconds. In comparison, a written authorization could take hours or days.

A teenage patient brought to the emergency department (ED) of a hospital drifts in and out of consciousness. The ED physician suspects an adverse event from a medication the patient is taking or a possible drug overdose. The physician learns that the patient takes medications that have been prescribed by her primary care physician. Because the patient's EHR is interoperable with the hospital's EHR, the ED physician is able to access the medications prescribed for the patient. How does permitted disclosure of health information in HIPAA's Privacy Rule allow the patient to receive the care she needs? What could happen if the patient needs to wait while the hospital seeks authorization to release her information?

Payment Purposes **Payment** is defined as the activities of a health plan to obtain premiums, to determine or fulfill responsibilities for coverage and provision of benefits, and to furnish or obtain reimbursement for healthcare delivered to an individual.

Under this provision, healthcare providers are allowed to release health information to receive payment for services rendered. In addition, health insurance companies can obtain health information to identify a subscriber's coverage and provision of benefits, as well as to offer reimbursement for healthcare services provided. For example, a nursing home is allowed to provide health information to an ambulance transportation company so that the ambulance company can be reimbursed for the transfer of a nursing home resident to the hospital.

Healthcare Operations **Healthcare operations** are defined as any of the following activities:

- quality assessment and improvement, including case management and care coordination.

- competency assurance activities, including providers of health plan performance evaluation, credentialing, and accreditation.

- conducting or arranging for medical reviews, audits, or legal services, including fraud and abuse detection and compliance programs.

- specified insurance functions, such as underwriting, risk rating, and reinsuring risk

- business planning, development, management, and administration.

- business management and general administrative activities of the entity, including—but not limited to—de-identifying PHI, creating a limited data set, and certain fundraising for the benefit of the covered entity.

Covered entities are allowed to use health information for their own facility or their company's internal operations. The specific activities allowed by HIPAA are listed in the definition of healthcare operations above. Some specific examples of permitted use and disclosures of health information under this provision are as follows:

- health insurance companies only want to contract for healthcare services from the best providers, i.e., those providing the highest quality of care and services for the lowest cost. To select these high-quality, low-cost providers, the insurance company reviews specific health information, and HIPAA permits the use and disclosure of health information for this purpose.

- healthcare providers conduct internal quality assessments to identify policies and procedures to be changed to provide higher quality care. The HIPAA healthcare operations clause allows providers to use health information for these assessments.

It is important to note that covered entities may choose to require a signed patient authorization for any and all disclosures of patient health information, even in circumstances in which the HIPAA law does not require a patient's written authorization. For example, most healthcare providers request that patients sign an authorization to release healthcare information to insurance companies or other payers prior to rendering healthcare services. A good rule for a healthcare provider to follow is to obtain a written patient authorization prior to the release, disclosure, or use of an individual's health information. The authorization form should be HIPAA-compliant and depict certain elements required by law.

Incidental to a Permitted Use or Disclosure The Privacy Rule does not require that every risk of an incidental use or disclosure of PHI be eliminated. A use or disclosure of this information that occurs as a result of, or as "incident to," an otherwise permitted use or disclosure is permitted as long as the covered entity has adopted reasonable safeguards as required by the Privacy Rule. For example, a hospital visitor may overhear a provider's confidential conversation with another provider or a patient or may glimpse a patient's information on a sign-in sheet or nurses' station whiteboard.

Public Interest and Benefit Activities The Privacy Rule permits the use and disclosure of PHI without an individual's authorization or permission for 12 national priority purposes, including subpoenas and court orders, certain law enforcement purposes, approved research purposes, public health purposes, organ donations, use by coroners or funeral homes, or compliance with workers' compensation laws.

Limited Data Set Use A **limited data set** is PHI from which certain specified direct identifiers of individuals and their relatives, household members, and employers have been removed. A limited data set may be used and disclosed for research, healthcare operations, and public health purposes, provided the recipient enters into a data use agreement promising specified safeguards for the PHI within the limited data set.

When patient authorization is required or optionally used, specific core elements and required statements must be included in the authorization, including the date the authorization expires and a statement that the authorization is revocable. Covered entities should use a standard patient authorization form drawn up by legal counsel that includes all of the elements required by law.

Privacy Rule and State Laws

State laws that contradict the Privacy Rule are overruled by the Federal requirements, unless an exception applies.

These exceptions include if the state law:

- provides greater privacy protections or rights with respect to individually identifiable health information.

- allows for the reporting of injury, illness, child abuse, birth, death, or for public health surveillance, investigation, or intervention.

- requires health plan reporting, for example, for management or financial audits.

In these examples, a covered entity is not required to comply with a contrary provision of the Privacy Rule.

CHECKP⊕INT 6.1

1. True/False: A healthcare provider may not release patient health information without a specific authorization or consent signed by the patient.

2. True/False: HIPAA regulations only cover health information documented on paper.

3. The HIPAA Privacy and Security Rules apply only to health plans, healthcare clearinghouses, and healthcare providers who transmit health information in electronic format. What term is used for these plans, clearinghouses, and providers?

Minimum Necessary Concept

Covered entities must make reasonable efforts to limit the use, disclosure of, and requests for the minimum amount of PHI necessary to accomplish the intended purpose. This concept is called **minimum necessary** and is required by the Privacy Rule.

An example of a covered entity *not* following the minimum necessary concept is as follows: An insurance company needs to determine whether or not physical therapy services were necessary for a patient residing in a nursing home, so one of its representatives requests a copy of the patient's entire medical record, including physician progress notes, laboratory and radiology results, medical history and physical examination findings, physical therapy progress notes, nutrition progress notes, and case management reports. This is more information than is needed. The insurance company representative should be able to determine whether physical therapy was necessary based on the history and physical, physician's orders, and physical therapy progress notes.

An example of a covered entity that *adheres to* the minimum necessary concept is as follows: A new patient is scheduled for a hemodialysis run tomorrow at an outpatient dialysis clinic. The hospital where he had hemodialysis discharged him yesterday. The outpatient dialysis clinic needs a copy of the last hemodialysis run sheet to plan the patient's hemodialysis run for tomorrow. The dialysis clinic requests only the last dialysis run sheet from the hospital.

Privacy and the Release of Information

Go to the Course Navigator to launch Activity 6.1. As an RHIT, practice releasing a patient's information using the EHR Navigator.

Privacy Rule Enforcement

As with any law, there are consequences when the HIPAA Privacy and Security Rules are not followed. Within the HHS is the **Office for Civil Rights (OCR)**, which is responsible for enforcing the HIPAA Privacy and Security Rules. The enforcement process begins with a complaint and follows through to a resolution with the Department of Justice when violations are criminal, or the OCR when violations are civil, as illustrated in Figure 6.2.

Violations of the Privacy Rule fall into one of two categories, civil or criminal violations. The major difference between civil and criminal violations involves the intent behind the violation.

Figure 6.2　HIPAA Privacy and Security Rule Complaint Process

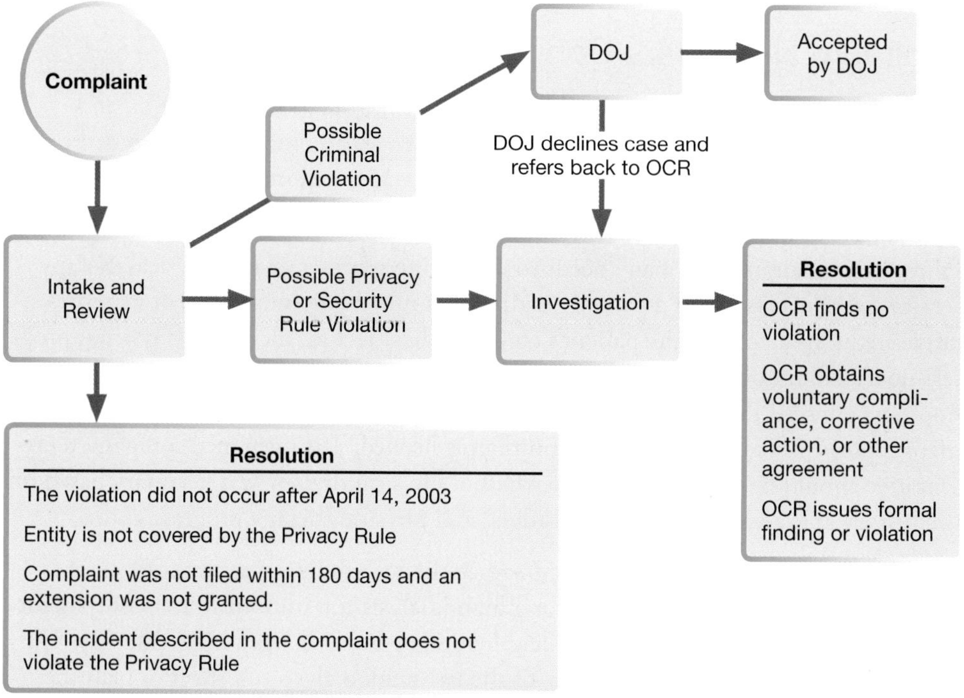

Complaint

Possible Criminal Violation

DOJ

Accepted by DOJ

DOJ declines case and refers back to OCR

Intake and Review

Possible Privacy or Security Rule Violation

Investigation

Resolution

OCR finds no violation

OCR obtains voluntary compliance, corrective action, or other agreement

OCR issues formal finding or violation

Resolution

The violation did not occur after April 14, 2003

Entity is not covered by the Privacy Rule

Complaint was not filed within 180 days and an extension was not granted.

The incident described in the complaint does not violate the Privacy Rule

Civil Violations

If a person *mistakenly* obtained or disclosed individually identifiable health information in violation of HIPAA and the covered entity corrected the violation within 30 days of when it knew or should have known of the violation, then a penalty is not imposed. Since the HITECH ACT, civil monetary penalties of $100 to $50,000 per failure may be imposed on a covered entity failing to comply with a Privacy Rule requirement. The cumulative penalties may not exceed $1.5 million per year.

Criminal Violations

If a person *knowingly* obtains or discloses individually identifiable health information in violation of HIPAA, this is considered a criminal violation and the person can be penalized with a fine of $50,000 and one year of imprisonment. Criminal penalties increase to $100,000 and up to five years of imprisonment if the wrongful conduct involves false pretenses. The penalties increase up to $250,000 and up to ten years of imprisonment if the wrongful conduct involves the intent to sell, transfer, or use PHI for commercial advantage, personal gain, or malicious harm.

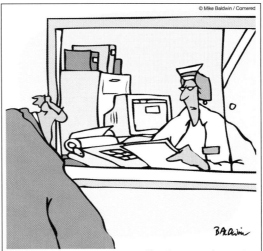

"Somehow your medical records got faxed to a complete stranger. He has no idea what's wrong with you either."

In addition to monetary penalties and imprisonment, the federal government can also require a **Resolution Agreement** with a covered entity, which is a contract signed by the federal government and a covered entity in which the covered entity agrees to perform certain obligations (e.g., staff training regarding privacy and confidentiality, audits of all releases of health information to ensure compliance) and to send reports to the federal government for a certain time period (typically three years). During this period, the federal government monitors the compliance of the covered entity with the obligations it has agreed to perform.

Cases of Privacy Rule Breaches

In recent years, many high-profile cases of enforcement have included significant monetary penalties and resolution agreements.

In March 2008, Massachusetts General Hospital lost documents for 192 patients and was fined $1 million by the U.S. federal government. A Massachusetts General Hospital employee left a patient schedule containing patient names and medical records on the subway. The employee also left billing encounter forms for 66 patients, containing names, birth dates, insurance policy numbers, and patient diagnoses. The violation was inadvertent on the part of the employee; however, because Massachusetts General Hospital did not have policies and procedures in place to ensure that PHI was protected when removed from the hospital, and because employees were not adequately trained, the hospital was fined.

EXPAND YOUR LEARNING
Describe two recent breaches of the Privacy or Security Rules. A list can be found at www.paradigmcollege.net/expoloring ehr/breaches.

On July 16, 2008, the federal government entered into a Resolution Agreement with Seattle-based Providence Health & Services to settle potential violations of HIPAA Privacy and Security Rules. The incidents giving rise to the agreement involved two entities within the Providence Health System, namely Providence Home and Community Services and Providence Hospice and Home Care. On several occasions between September 2005 and March 2006, backup tapes, optical disks, and laptops, all containing unencrypted electronic PHI, were removed from Providence premises and left unattended. The media and laptops were subsequently lost or stolen, compromising the PHI of more than 386,000 patients. The investigation focused on the failure of Providence to implement policies and procedures to safeguard this information. The healthcare facility agreed to pay $100,000 and implement a detailed corrective action plan to ensure that it would appropriately safeguard identifiable electronic patient information against theft or loss. It also agreed to revise its policies and procedures regarding physical and technical safeguards (e.g., encryption) and off-site transport and storage of electronic media containing patient information.

In April 2010, Cignet Health of Prince George's County, MD, violated the rights of 41 patients by denying them access to their medical records when requested. This violation cost Cignet Health $1.3 million. Then, because Cignet refused to cooperate with the investigation, it was fined an additional $3 million by the federal government.

In July 2013, the managed care company, WellPoint Inc., agreed to pay HHS $1.7 million to settle potential violations of the HIPAA Privacy and Security Rules. OCR's investigation indicated that WellPoint did not implement appropriate administrative and technical safeguards as required under the HIPAA Security Rule. The investigation indicated WellPoint did not adequately implement policies and procedures for authorizing access to the online application database; perform an appropriate technical evaluation in response to a software upgrade to its information systems; or have technical safeguards in place to verify the person or entity seeking access to electronic PHI maintained in its application database. As a result, the investigation indicated that WellPoint impermissibly disclosed the PHI of 612,402 individuals via access over the Internet.

A laptop should not contain healthcare information unless it is encrypted.

Although major cases with high-dollar penalties such as those described receive considerable media attention, they are the exception rather than the rule.

From the HIPAA compliance date in April 2003 through September 30, 2012, the federal government received 74,554 HIPAA privacy complaints. Of these complaints, 17,767 (24%) went through the investigative and enforcement phases, whereas the other 56,787 (76%) complaints were either not violations or were determined not to be eligible for the HIPAA enforcement process. Of the 17,767 cases that were investigated, all required changes in privacy practices, other corrective actions by the covered entities, or both. Many different types of entities, including national pharmacy chains, major medical centers, group health plans, hospital chains, and small provider offices, were part of the 17,767 cases investigated.

The most often investigated compliance issues are listed below in order of frequency:

1. Impermissible uses and disclosures of PHI

2. Lack of safeguards of PHI

3. Lack of patient access to his or her PHI

4. Uses or disclosures of more than the minimum necessary PHI

5. Lack of administrative safeguards of electronic PHI

The most common types of covered entities required to take corrective action are listed below in order of frequency:

1. Private practices

2. General hospitals

3. Outpatient facilities

4. Health plans (group health plans and health insurance issuers)

5. Pharmacies

As patients and the public at large have become more familiar with HIPAA privacy rights, there has been a steady increase in the number of complaints made to OCR, as shown in Figure 6.3.

Figure 6.3 Complaints Made to the OCR by Calendar Year (Through 2011)

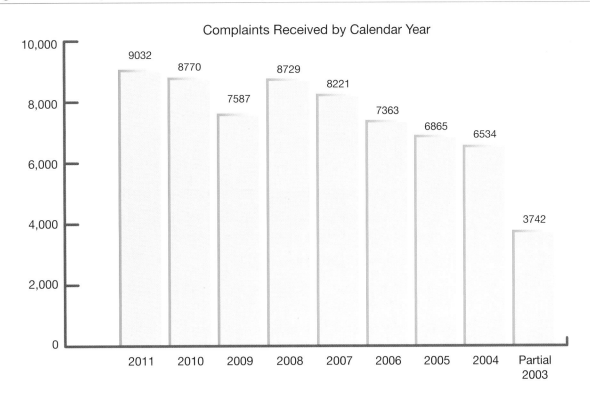

CHECKPOINT 6.2

1. Name three of the top five investigated compliance issues.

   a. _____

   b. _____

   c. _____

2. What is the difference between a civil violation and a criminal violation?

   _____

   _____

   _____

Breach Notification Rule

Implemented in August 2009, breach notification regulations require HIPAA-covered entities and their business associates to provide notification to affected individuals following a breach of unsecured PHI.

Generally speaking, a **breach** is an impermissible use or disclosure under the Privacy Rule that compromises the security or privacy of PHI such that the use or disclosure poses a significant risk of financial, reputational, or other harm to the affected individual.

Breach Notification Requirements

Following a breach of unsecured PHI, covered entities must provide notification of the breach to affected individuals, to the federal government (specifically, the HHS), and, in certain circumstances, to the media. In addition, business associates must notify covered entities that a breach has occurred.

Notice to Individuals

Covered entities must notify affected individuals following the discovery of a breach of unsecured PHI and must provide individual written notifications within 60 days following the discovery of a breach. These notifications must include the following items:

1. A description of the breach

2. A description of the types of information involved in the breach

3. The steps affected individuals should take to protect themselves from potential harm

4. A brief description of what the covered entity is doing to investigate the breach, mitigate the harm, and prevent further breaches

5. Contact information for the covered entity

Notice to the Media

Covered entities experiencing a breach affecting more than 500 residents of a state or jurisdiction are required to notify the affected individuals and provide notice to prominent media outlets serving the state or jurisdiction. Covered entities will likely provide this notification in the form of a press release to appropriate media outlets serving the affected area. Like individual notices, they must provide this media notification within 60 days following the discovery of a breach and must include the same information required for the individual notice.

HIPAA Security Rule

Privacy of health information is one of the main subjects addressed by HIPAA. Another important component of HIPAA is the security of health information. Just as the Privacy Rule was developed to address the privacy provisions of HIPAA, the **Security Standards for the Protection of Electronic Protected Health Information** were developed to address the security provisions of HIPAA and are commonly known as the **Security Rule**. Security Rule provisions pertain exclusively to electronic health information. The Security Rule required all HIPAA-covered entities (the same covered entities discussed earlier in this chapter) to reach compliance no later than April 20, 2005, with the exception of small health plans, which had until April 20, 2006, to comply with the rule.

Prior to HIPAA, no national security standards or general requirements existed to protect health information. With healthcare delivery systems moving away from paper records and toward electronic systems to process claims, manage health information, and document clinical and administrative activities, it became clear that federal guidance was necessary to protect patient information. Covered entities are using Web-based applications and other portals that give physicians, clinical staff, administrative staff, health plan employees, and pharmaceutical companies greater access to electronic health information. In addition to Web-based products, an increasing number of healthcare providers use internal EHR software to varying degrees. As the United States moves toward its goal of a **Nationwide Health Information Network (NwHIN)** and a greater use of EHRs, protecting the confidentiality, integrity, and availability of **electronic protected health information (ePHI)** becomes even more critical. The security standards in HIPAA were developed for two primary purposes: (1) to protect certain electronic healthcare information that may be at risk, and (2) to promote the use of electronic health information in the healthcare industry.

Protecting an individual's health information, while permitting appropriate access and use of that information, ultimately promotes the use of electronic health information in the healthcare industry.

Objectives of the Security Rule

Although HIPAA established the two broad purposes of health information security standards as noted above, the Security Rule was adopted to more specifically define the objectives that covered entities would need to attain to be in compliance with HIPAA. In the General Rules section of the Security Rule, the four major objectives include:

1. Each covered entity must ensure the confidentiality, integrity, and availability of ePHI that it creates, receives, maintains, or transmits.

2. Each covered entity must protect against any reasonably anticipated threats and hazards to the security or integrity of ePHI.

3. Each covered entity must protect against reasonably anticipated uses or disclosures of such information that are not permitted by the Privacy Rule.

4. Each covered entity must ensure compliance by the workforce.

Major Differences Between the Privacy and Security Rules

When HHS developed the Security Rule, it chose to closely align it with the provisions in the Privacy Rule. Because both rules were developed in response to HIPAA, it made sense to ensure that the two rules were in sync with each other. Therefore, it is easier for covered entities to implement the provisions of both rules and achieve the goals of HIPAA. However, although the two rules are closely aligned, there are two areas of distinction:

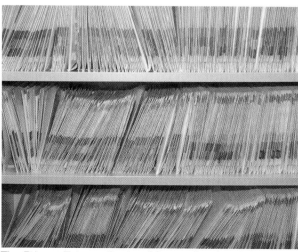

The Privacy Rule applies to all forms of patients' PHI, including paper records. The Security Rule covers PHI that is in electronic form.

1. The Privacy Rule applies to all forms of patient PHI, whether that information is in electronic, written, or oral format. In contrast, the Security Rule only covers PHI in electronic form, including ePHI that is created, received, maintained, or transmitted. For example, ePHI may be transmitted over the Internet or stored on a computer, a CD, a disk, magnetic tape, or other related means. The Security Rule does not cover PHI transmitted or stored on paper or provided in oral form.

2. The Privacy Rule contains minimum security requirements for the protection of PHI, whereas the Security Rule provides comprehensive security requirements.

Sections of the Security Rule

The standards of the Security Rule are divided into six main sections: General Rules, Administrative Safeguards, Physical Safeguards, Technical Safeguards, Organizational Requirements, and Policies and Procedures and Documentation Requirements.

General Rules

The **General Rules** section includes general requirements that all covered entities must meet. This section establishes the flexibility of approach that covered entities have when implementing the standards and identifying the standards required and the standards addressable. Information in this section also addresses the required maintenance of security measures to continue reasonable and appropriate protection of ePHI.

Administrative Safeguards

Generally speaking, the **Administrative Safeguards** section includes the assignment or delegation of security responsibility to an individual and the need for security training for employees and users. Employees must be trained in security and covered entities must have appropriate policies and procedures for security (e.g., a disaster backup plan, incident reporting of security breaches).

Physical Safeguards

The **Physical Safeguards** section includes mechanisms necessary to protect electronic systems and the data they store from threats, environmental hazards, and unauthorized intrusion. These safeguards include restricting access to ePHI and retaining off-site computer backups.

Technical Safeguards

The **Technical Safeguards** section covers primarily the automated processes used to protect data and control access to data. These processes include the use of authentication control to verify that the person signing onto a computer is, in fact, authorized to access that ePHI or encryption and decryption of data as it is being stored, transmitted, or both.

Organization Requirements

The fifth major section of the Security Rule, includes the **Organizational Requirements**, includes standards for business associate contracts and other arrangements and the requirements for group health plans.

Policies and Procedures and Documentation Requirements

The section titled **Policies and Procedures and Documentation Requirements** addresses the implementation of reasonable and appropriate policies and procedures to comply with the Security Rule standards. The covered entity must maintain written documentation and records that include policies, procedures, actions, activities, or assessments required by the Security Rule.

CHECKPOINT 6.3

1. List the six main sections of the Security Rule.

   a. _____

   b. _____

   c. _____

   d. _____

   e. _____

   f. _____

2. Encryption of healthcare data before transmission is an example of which type of security safeguard?

   _____

3. Security training of employees is an example of which type of security safeguard?

   _____

Security Standards Matrix

The Centers for Medicare & Medicaid Services (CMS) created a Security Standards Matrix, which is Appendix A of the Security Rule, to assist covered entities in the assessment of their compliance with the Security Rule. See Figure 6.4.

Note that the first column (left to right) is a description of the Security Standard. The second column lists the section of the Security Rule published within the *Federal Register*. The third and fourth columns list a more specific reference to a portion of the security standards along with a designation of *R* (Required) or *A* (Addressable). The **required standards** indicate the portions of the standards that each covered entity must achieve compliance. The **addressable** portions of the standards indicate that the covered entities must address each standard to determine if it is a reasonable and appropriate safeguard in the entity's environment. These standards should not be considered optional.

Because HIPAA is applicable to a variety of organizations classified as covered entities, HIPAA includes flexibility that allows covered entities to tailor security measures to their own situations while still keeping health information secure. Determining whether an addressable portion of the standard is applicable to a particular covered entity can be challenging. It involves analyzing the standard in reference to the likelihood of protecting the entity's ePHI from reasonably anticipated threats and hazards.

If the covered entity does not implement an addressable standard based on its assessment, the covered entity must document the reason why the implementation of the standard is not appropriate or reasonable. For example, a solo practitioner without any employees would likely not need to implement the Administrative Safeguards of the Security Rule. This specification states that employees should be sent security reminders about potential security threats via email, newsletters, etc. Because there are no employees to be notified, this safeguard is not applicable.

EXPAND YOUR LEARNING

Conduct an Internet search and identify a certification for a healthcare privacy or security specialty. Who offers the certification? What are the qualifications or requirements for the certification?

Figure 6.4   The Security Standards Matrix

1 Security 101 for Covered Entities

Security Standards Matrix (Appendix A of the Security Rule)

ADMINISTRATIVE SAFEGUARDS

Standards	Sections	Implementation Specifications (R)= Required, (A)=Addressable	
Security Management Process	164.308(a)(1)	Risk Analysis	(R)
		Risk Management	(R)
		Sanction Policy	(R)
		Information System Activity Review	(R)
Assigned Security Responsibility	164.308(a)(2)		(R)
Workforce Security	164.308(a)(3)	Authorization and/or Supervision	(A)
		Workforce Clearance Procedure	(A)
		Termination Procedures	(A)
Information Access Management	164.308(a)(4)	Isolating Health Care Clearinghouse Functions	(R)
		Access Authorization	(A)
		Access Establishment and Modification	(A)
Security Awareness and Training	164.308(a)(5)	Security Reminders	(A)
		Protection from Malicious Software	(A)
		Log-in Monitoring	(A)
		Password Management	(A)
Security Incident Procedures	164.308(a)(6)	Response and Reporting	(R)
Contingency Plan	164.308(a)(7)	Data Backup Plan	(R)
		Disaster Recovery Plan	(R)
		Emergency Mode Operation Plan	(R)
		Testing and Revision Procedures	(A)
		Applications and Data Criticality Analysis	(A)
Evaluation	164.308(a)(8)		(R)
Business Associate Contracts and Other Arrangements	164.308(b)(1)	Written Contract or Other Arrangement	(R)

Implementation Specifications (R)= Required, (A)=Addressable	
Contingency Operations	(A)
Facility Security Plan	(A)
Access Control and Validation Procedures	(A)
Maintenance Records	(A)
	(R)
	(R)
Disposal	(R)
Media Re-use	(R)
Accountability	(A)
Data Backup and Storage	(A)

Implementation Specifications (R)= Required, (A)=Addressable	
Unique User Identification	(R)
Emergency Access Procedure	(R)
Automatic Logoff	(A)
Encryption and Decryption	(A)
	(R)
Mechanism to Authenticate Electronic Protected Health Information	(A)
	(R)
Integrity Controls	(A)
Encryption	(A)

Every covered entity is responsible for complying with the required and addressable standards or documenting why it does not need to comply with certain addressable elements. Covered entities should conduct an internal review of their compliance with the security standards.

Activity 6.2 EHRNAVIGATOR

Denied Access

Go to the Course Navigator to launch Activity 6.2. As a lab technician, you will experience what happens when you try and access a restricted area in the EHR Navigator.

Activity 6.3 EHRNAVIGATOR

Resetting a Password

Go to the Course Navigator to launch Activity 6.3. As an office manager, practice resetting a staff member's password using the EHR Navigator.

Because electronic data can be changed at the touch of a keystroke, EHR systems have the ability to track and record user activity. Consequently, once clinical documentation has been entered and authenticated (i.e., the author's signature is applied, confirming the accuracy of the data to the best of the author's knowledge), documented entries cannot be modified. Attempts to change a health record can easily be identified by an administrator by viewing the activity log.

Activity 6.4 EHRNAVIGATOR

Reviewing a User Activity Log

Go to the Course Navigator to launch Activity 6.4. As an IT administrator, practice reviewing a user activity log using the EHR Navigator.

HIPAA Security Rule Enforcement

Enforcement of the Security Rule follows the same process as enforcement of the Privacy Rule. The OCR has the responsibility for the enforcement, and the enforcement process starts with a complaint and follows through to a resolution with the Department of Justice when violations are criminal or the OCR when violations are civil.

From April 2008 through December 2011, more than 700 complaints of violations of the Security Rule were made, about 25% of which were breaches of the Security Rule. Theft and loss of data contributed to 67% of these breaches, with unauthorized access/disclosure at 21%, hacking at 6%, improper disposal at 5%, and other breaches at 1%.

Cases of Security Rule Breaches

Just as there were many high-profile examples of breaches of the Privacy Rule, there have been many large breaches of the Security Rule in recent history.

In June 2010, a laptop containing the health information of 21,000 patients was stolen from Thomas Jefferson University Hospital in Pennsylvania.

In February 2011, at least 667 patient records—which included names, dates of birth, and healthcare data—were stolen from an unencrypted laptop belonging to the Rancho Los Amigos National Rehabilitation Center in California.

On March 15, 2011, Health Net announced that it had lost digital records containing personal data from 1.9 million current and former policyholders. Health Net reported that nine server drives went missing from its data center in Rancho Cordova, CA, and those missing drives contained personal data on its employees, healthcare providers, and policyholders. The insurer noted that the data might have included names, Social Security numbers, addresses, and health and financial information.

One of the largest medical records security breaches in U.S. history occurred in September, 2011, when backup tapes storing PHI for 4.9 million people from a military EHR system were stolen from the car of a Science Applications International Corporation (SAIC) employee. At the time, SAIC was under contract with TRICARE, a U.S. military insurance carrier, to provide off-site data storage and backup data security.

In September, 2013, data thieves hacked into a physician office EHR. The hackers not only gained access to the healthcare information of more than 7,000 patients but also made the data completely inaccessible for the physician practice. The thieves then posted an electronic ransom note demanding that the physicians pay to get access to their data.

Organizations can learn many lessons from these reported breaches, such as:

- the opportunity to reduce risk through network or enterprise data storage as an alternative to local devices. **Enterprise data storage** is a centralized system (online or offline) that businesses use for managing and protecting data.

- the importance of encryption of ePHI on any desktop or portable device.

- the need for clear and well-documented administrative and physical safeguards on the storage devices and media that handle ePHI.

- the need to raise employee awareness of security and to promote good data stewardship. **Data stewardship** can be defined as the authority and responsibility associated with collecting, using, and disclosing health information in its identifiable and aggregate forms. The principles of data stewardship apply to all the personnel, systems, and processes engaging in health information storage and exchange within and across organizations.

EXPAND YOUR LEARNING

For more information about enterprise data storage, see www.paradigmcollege.net/exploringehr/enterprise_storage.

EXPAND YOUR LEARNING

For more information about data stewardship, refer to the article found at www.paradigmcollege.net/exploringehr/data_stewardship.

Consider This

An employee of the State Department of Health and Social Services left a portable electronic storage drive device (USB device) in a car that was later stolen. The USB device contained ePHI, so the State Department of Health and Social Services submitted a report to the OCR, as all covered entities are required to do when a breach of health information security has occurred. When the OCR investigated, it found evidence that the department did not have adequate policies and procedures in place to safeguard ePHI and that the department had not completed a risk analysis, implemented sufficient risk management measures, completed security training for its workforce members, implemented device and media controls, or addressed device and media controls or encryption as required by the HIPAA Security Rule.

Does the State Department of Health and Social Services have to follow the HIPAA Security Rule? Why? Is there a possibility that the department would be fined in this scenario? What do you think the findings of the OCR should be in this scenario?

Chapter Summary

Privacy and security of health information is a major focus of healthcare entities implementing and using electronic health records (EHRs). Healthcare entities must carefully follow all of the Privacy and Security Rules of the Health Insurance Portability and Accountability Act of 1996 (HIPAA) when selecting and installing EHRs and must remain continually vigilant in the monitoring of the use of protected health information (PHI) and electronic PHI (ePHI) in their organizations. Workers must receive initial and ongoing training in the proper use and release of PHI and ePHI, as well as the importance of keeping healthcare data safe and secure. Inappropriate release or loss of PHI, whether purposeful or inadvertent, may result in significant damage and lead to fines and/or imprisonment for the individual and/or organization responsible for the breach.

EHR Review

Check Your Understanding

To check your understanding of this chapter's key concepts, read the following multiple-choice and true/false questions and then record your answers on a separate sheet of paper. Write your answers as modeled in these examples: 1a; 2b; 6T; 7F; etc.

1. What is an example of a *noncovered entity*?

    a. Nursing home

    b. Workers' compensation carrier

    c. Military healthcare program

    d. Healthcare clearinghouse

2. The acronym *TPO* stands for

    a. treatment, protection, organization

    b. transmission, privacy, operations

    c. treatment, payment, healthcare operations

    d. type, patient, officials

3. A breach is

    a. the transmission of health information in an electronic format.

    b. an impressible use or disclosure under the Privacy or Security Rule.

    c. a data set used for healthcare research.

    d. a punishment enforced by the OCR.

4. After a Privacy Rule breach, _____ must be notified.

    a. the individual, the federal government, and the media

    b. the individual, the healthcare organization, and the insurance company

    c. the healthcare organization and the federal and state governments

    d. the federal and state governments and the media

5. De-identified health information:

    a. can never be used in marketing or research.

    b. neither identifies an individual nor provides a reasonable basis to identify an individual.

    c. does not directly identify an individual, but it may provide information that could be used to identify an individual.

    d. cannot be electronically transmitted.

6. True/False: Users of electronic health records are not required to follow the laws and regulations of the Health Insurance Portability and Accountability Act of 1996 (HIPAA).

7. True/False: If an entity does not meet the definition of *covered entity*, then it does not have to comply with the Privacy or Security Rule.

8. True/False: The Office for Civil Rights (OCR) has the responsibility for the enforcement of the HIPAA Privacy and Security Rules.

9. True/False: The major difference between criminal and civil punishments and penalties involves the intent behind the violation.

10. True/False: As patients and the public at large have become more familiar with HIPAA privacy rights, the number of complaints made to the OCR has steadily increased.

Learn the Terms

Go to the Course Navigator to access the flashcards for Chapter 6 of *Exploring Electronic Health Records*.

COURSE
NAVIGATOR

Acronyms

CMS: Centers for Medicare & Medicaid Services

ePHI: electronic protected health information

HHS: United States Department of Health & Human Services

HIPAA: Health Insurance Portability and Accountability Act of 1996

HITECH Act: Health Information Technology for Economic and Clinical Health Act

NwHIN: Nationwide Health Information Network

OCR: Office for Civil Rights

PHI: protected health information

TPO: treatment, payment, healthcare operations

EHR Application

Go on the Record

To build on your understanding of the topics in this chapter, complete the following short answer questions.

1. What is the major purpose of the Privacy Rule?

2. What are the two situations in which disclosure of protected health information is required?

3. Describe a *limited data set* for purposes of research, public health, or healthcare operations.

4. Describe the differences between civil and criminal acts in violation of the Health Insurance Portability and Accountability Act of 1996 (HIPAA).

5. List the top five compliance issues that have been investigated by the federal government since HIPAA went into effect.

Navigate the Field

To gain practice in handling challenging situations in the workplace, consider the following real-world scenarios and then use the guiding questions to help you formulate your responses.

1. Hans Frank, office manager of Mountainview Surgical Clinic, was working on year-end reports at his home over the weekend. He spent several hours on Sunday compiling reports related to the 3,000 surgical patients who received treatment from Mountainview Surgical Clinic during the previous year. Unfortunately, while on his way to work on the subway on Monday, he inadvertently left his work laptop under his seat. In a panic, Mr. Frank tried to locate his laptop but was unsuccessful. Because this is clearly a breach of unsecured protected health information (PHI), what notification processes must Mountainview Surgical Clinic initiate?

2. Green Hills Valley Hospital has hired you to be the Electronic Health Records Security Officer. As you tour the hospital during your first week of employment, you notice that many of the nurses and other staff members are sharing user IDs and passwords to log on to the EHR system. As the Security Officer, what actions should you take to resolve this situation?

EHR Evaluation

Think Critically

Continue to think critically about challenging real-world scenarios and complete the following activities.

1. Interview a privacy or security officer at an acute care hospital to obtain insight regarding the challenges of complying with the Health Insurance Portability and Accountability Act of 1996 (HIPAA) in a hospital that uses an EHR system.

2. Nearly everyone has seen news reports of cyberattacks against nationwide utility infrastructures or the information networks of the U.S. Pentagon. Healthcare providers may believe that if they are small and low profile, they will escape the attention of the criminals running these attacks. Yet, every day, new attacks are specifically aimed at small- to mid-size organizations because they are low profile and less likely to have fully protected themselves. Criminals have been highly successful at penetrating these smaller organizations, carrying out their activities while their victims remain unaware until it is too late. Review the Office of the National Coordinator for Health Information Technology's cybersecurity checklist and discuss five best practices for a small healthcare environment to protect an EHR system. The checklist can be found at the following website: www.paradigmcollege.net/exploringehr/security_checklist.

Make Your Case

Consider the following scenario and create a presentation on the following topic.

Describe the main components of the Privacy Rule.

Explore the Technology

COURSE NAVIGATOR

To expand your mastery of EHRs, explore the following online activities and complete the EHR Navigator assessments.

Ensure you are comfortable with the functionality presented in the EHR Navigator activities, such as releasing information, experiencing the denied access feature, resetting a password, and reviewing a user activity log. Then, complete the EHR Navigator assessments for Chapter 6 located on the Course Navigator.

The people you will encounter in the workforce will likely have different levels of comfort surrounding technology. The technology adoption lifecycle model describes five different groups of people and their attitudes toward new technology. There are the "innovators," who are the first group to use a new product, followed by "early adopters." After that come the "early majority," "late majority," and finally the "laggards," who are the last to become comfortable with new technology.

How will these different kinds of people work together in an environment that implements an EHR system?

What will need to be considered for these populations as health information management (HIM) roles and functions evolve?

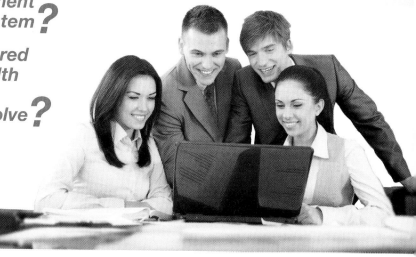

Beyond the Record

In 2013, the top five electronic health record (EHR) vendors by number of users were:

- eClinicalWorks
- Care 360
- Epic
- Allscripts
- McKesson

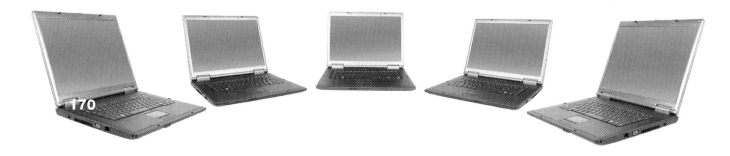

HIM Roles and Functions in the EHR Environment

Master Patient Index Then

Master Patient Index Now

- Depict how health information management (HIM) roles and functions are evolving as a result of implementation of electronic health records (EHRs).

- Demonstrate use of a master patient index.

- Explain the tracking of paper medical records.

- Discuss the advantages and disadvantages of coding from an EHR.

- Explain how transcribed reports interface and become part of the EHR.

- Discuss the benefits and challenges of using speech recognition technology.

- Demonstrate release of information (ROI) functions carried out by HIM staff in the EHR environment.

- Demonstrate how to produce an accounting of disclosures log.

- Demonstrate the monitoring and completion of EHRs.

- Describe the process of scanning paper records, including document identification and preparation, indexing, and quality control.

Implementation of electronic health records (EHRs) affects every healthcare worker who uses patient data and information. Physicians, nurses, dentists, psychologists, and many other clinicians will now use a keyboard instead of a pen. File clerk positions will be eliminated. Even coding, billing, and payment processing will eventually be performed exclusively through technological solutions and enhanced automation. The manual processes of chart analysis, data gathering, and data reporting will be replaced by electronic data capturing and reports.

Perhaps the healthcare workers facing the most changes in procedures due to the implementation of EHRs are health information management (HIM) professionals. Depending on the size of the organization, these staff members might face elimination of some HIM positions, the creation of new HIM positions, and evolving tasks associated with the existing HIM positions. For example, as the need for file clerks decreases, the need for document imaging staff will increase. As the need for assembly and analysis clerks decreases, the need for data quality staff will increase. This chapter examines the roles and functions of HIM professionals in the transition from paper records to EHRs.

The Master Patient Index

As discussed in Chapter 4, healthcare organizations maintain a master patient index (MPI) to have a permanent record of every episode of care for every patient treated at the facility. The MPI is a database of basic patient demographics such as:

- Patient name
- Date of birth
- Sex
- Social Security number
- Medical record number (MRN)

- Patient account number
- Admission date
- Discharge date
- Hospital service

Each patient receives an MRN upon his or her first encounter with the healthcare facility, and he or she retains this same MRN for all subsequent encounters. This procedure ensures that each patient is represented only once in the MPI. See Figure 7.1 for an example of an MPI.

MPIs have been used by larger healthcare organizations for several decades. Prior to the creation of electronic MPIs, the process of maintaining an MPI included cards that were filed alphabetically by patient last name. The admission clerk initiated an index card with a new patient's information upon the patient's first admission or encounter at the facility. The clerk then updated the index card as subsequent admissions and encounters occurred. While most MPIs today are electronic, some traditional, non-electronic MPIs still exist in smaller physicians' offices, nursing homes, and so forth.

Figure 7.1 Master Patient Index

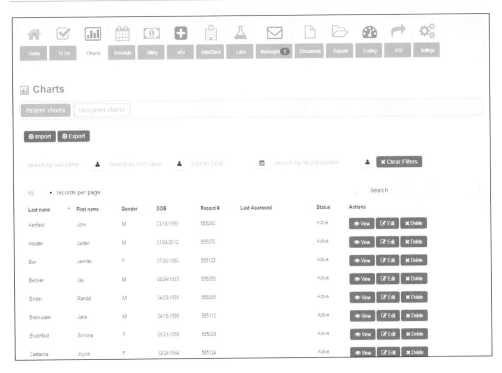

The electronic MPI is the hub of any EHR system because it is the first data entry point for a patient's episode of care. It links subsequent data entries and subsequent episodes of care to the patient's MRN, creating the EHR. A patient should be represented in the MPI only once, with one unique MRN and different patient account numbers for each encounter with the facility.

Large healthcare systems or enterprises comprised of several facilities may use an **enterprise master patient index (EMPI)**, which is the same as an MPI except that it is used for multiple facilities. Using an EMPI allows one enterprise to link all patient information across all of their facilities.

Consider This

Roosevelt Healthcare consists of an acute care hospital, a rehabilitation hospital, a nursing home, an ambulatory surgery center, and a large physician's practice of more than 60 doctors. It experiences more than 700,000 patient encounters per year. Would patient care be better served if Roosevelt Healthcare utilized a separate MPI for each facility (i.e., one MPI for the acute care hospital, one MPI for the rehabilitation hospital, one MPI for the nursing home, and so forth), or would it be better to have one EMPI that includes all the facilities? Why?

Duplicate MPI Records

Certain deficiencies in electronic MPI or EMPI may cause admissions or registration staff to inadvertently ignore a patient's previous encounter within the healthcare organization and create a second MPI entry in error. Duplicating MPI records is a problem because it results in the decentralization of a patient's health records. This creates a patient safety concern because the records attached to the alternate MPI for the same patient can remain unrecognized by providers during episodes of care.

How does this happen and how is it corrected? Duplicate MPI entries typically occur when an admission clerk uses the patient search function as the first step in the admission and registration process but is unable to find the patient in the MPI or fails to select the patient's name in the search results. The admission clerk then creates a new MPI entry for the patient, resulting in a duplicate medical record assignment. This must be corrected so that all of the patient's health records can be linked to one MRN.

Members of the HIM staff are responsible for auditing additions to the MPI on a daily basis and correcting or merging duplicate entries. This is accomplished by using a record-linking computer algorithm to compare patient demographic data—usually name, birthdate, and Social Security number—and look for matches or transpositions of numbers and letters that can indicate duplicated MRNs. Staff can then generate reports from the demographic comparison, review potential duplications, and merge duplicate records by copying a patient's information to the first MRN assigned, thus preventing data entry to the second MRN. The second MRN with the associated patient name is never completely deleted because it serves as a reference that the record has been merged with the initial MRN. A select few employees should be granted access to merge and delete medical record numbers to ensure compliant management of the MPI.

Chart Tracking

Having an EHR system does not necessarily mean that the healthcare facility has gone "paperless"—at least in the beginning stages of EHR implementation. Some hospitals and other healthcare organizations implement portions of EHR software over a period of time, creating hybrid health records. For example, a healthcare facility may implement a medication administration system as the first part of the EHR system, followed by the computerized physician order entry system, then assessments, progress notes, and so on. In addition, HIM staff must scan into the EHR system any paper health records that were created prior to the EHR implementation, or, alternatively, keep them as paper files according to the retention period established by state law and the policies of the healthcare organization.

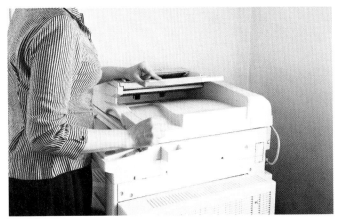

Medical staff scan paper charts into the EHR system.

The capability to track and locate paper health records is essential for every healthcare organization. **Chart tracking software** that is part of, or integrated into, the EHR system can help. Chart tracking software that can track at least 500 paper medical records typically uses **bar coding technology**. This means that the software generates bar code labels with a patient's name, MRN, volume number, and patient account number. The bar code labels are then affixed to chart folders and scanned by medical personnel when the chart moves to a new location. In paper or hybrid environments, consistent use of chart tracking software is necessary to accurately and securely account for the location of paper charts.

If the system contains fewer than 500 charts, bar coding technology is not necessary. Healthcare staff members can track charts by keying MRNs and locations into the chart tracking software. Staff can query the chart tracking database to reveal the location of the chart, the date it was signed out, and the date it is expected to be returned.

As healthcare staff members scan paper records into the EHR system, move them to off-site storage, or shred them (per retention guidelines), they update the chart tracking software to reflect the chart's scanning date, off-site storage location, or date of destruction.

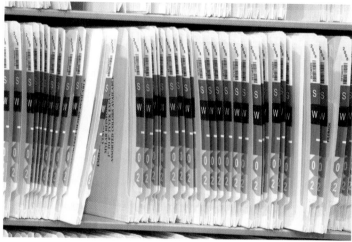

Barcodes on patient chart folders are generated by chart tracking software and scanned as they move through the healthcare facility.

Coding

Coding is the practice of assigning specific codes to written descriptions of diagnoses or procedures. The codes combine letters and numbers and belong to different coding classification systems, such as *International Classification of Diseases, 9th revision, Clinical Modification* (ICD-9-CM); *International Classification of Diseases, 10th revision, Clinical Modification* (ICD-10-CM); *International Classification of Diseases, 10th revision, Procedure Coding System* (ICD-10-PCS); Healthcare Common Procedure Coding System Level II (HCPCS); and Current Procedural Terminology (CPT). Coding will be explored more in Chapter 9.

The same ICD-9-CM, ICD-10-CM, ICD-10-PCS, HCPCS Level II, and CPT guidelines apply to every type of health record, whether paper, hybrid, or electronic. The coders' process is also the same for every type of record, because they must read the entire record, including the discharge summary, history and physical (H&P) examination results, progress notes, physician's orders, radiology and diagnostic tests, laboratory reports, and medication administration records and follow the applicable guidelines in selecting the codes. Whether codes are created from paper health records, hybrid health records, or an EHR, it is important that the documentation from which they are created is accurate and complete. Each clinician caring for each patient is responsible for documenting in a timely, accurate, and thorough fashion.

While EHRs have made coding easier in many ways, they also have created several new challenges of which coders should be aware.

Advantages to Coding from an EHR

There are many benefits to coding from an EHR, including the following:

- EHR documentation is more legible than handwritten paper records, eliminating errors caused by misinterpretation of handwriting.

- documentation may be more timely. Many medical staff members now choose to type the progress notes, history and physical examinations, consultation notes, and procedure notes that they would have previously dictated. This makes the reports immediately available because there is no delay transcription and filing.

- diagnostic reports automatically interface to the EHR, eliminating errors due to incorrect filing and lag time waiting for reports to be filed.

- electronic physician queries can be answered in a timelier manner and are therefore available sooner to the coding staff.

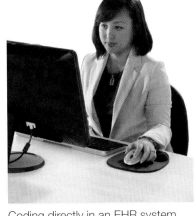

Coding directly in an EHR system instead of from a paper record has many benefits.

- EHRs that use templates for the documentation of progress notes, history and physical examination results, consultation notes, procedure notes, and discharge summaries may elicit more complete information if clinicians are required to fill out all data items in the template.

- physicians may be more likely to document more information in an EHR as opposed to a paper record because the EHR takes less time to fill in than a paper file.

- coders can work within a record at any time because EHRs can be simultaneously accessed by more than one individual.

- coders do not have to wait for a discharged chart to be physically collected from the nursing station before they can begin their work.

- coders do not have to wait for the HIM staff to assemble and analyze the discharged chart before having access to the record for coding.

While there are many benefits to coding from an EHR, support and training of users is crucial for these benefits to be fully realized.

Consider This

Record the time it takes you to read the following progress note in Figure 7.2.

Figure 7.2 Handwritten Progress Note

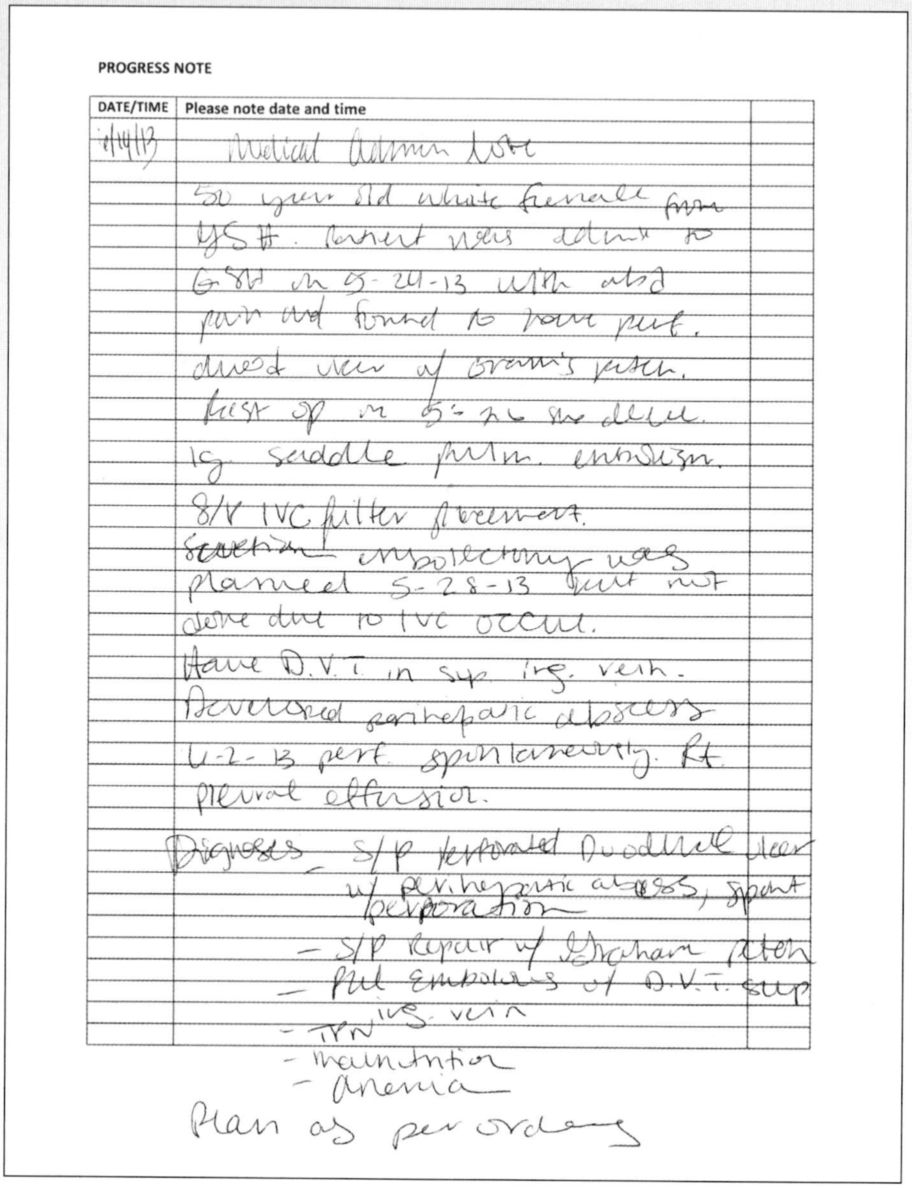

Now, record the time it takes you to read the progress note in Figure 7.3.

Chapter 7 HIM Roles and Functions in the EHR Environment

Figure 7.3 Electronic Progress Note

Progress Note

6-14-13   Medical Adm Note

50-year-old white female transferred from G.S.H. Patient was admitted to G.S.H. on 5-24-13 with abd pain and found to have perforated duodenal ulcer. Had esoph laparoscopy 5-28-13 and repair of perforated duod ulcer with Graham's patch. Post op on 5-26 she developed large saddle pul embolism. S/P I.V.C filter placement. Suction embolectomy was planned 5-28-13 but not done due to I.V.C. occlusion. Have D.V.T. in sup ing vein. Developed perihepatic abscess 6-2-13 perforated spontaneously. Rt. pleural effusion.

Diagnoses: S/P Perforated Duodenal ulcer with perihepatic abscess, spont perforation

S/P Repair with Graham patch

Pul Embolus with D.V.T. sup. ing. vein

T.P.N.

Malnutrition

Anemia

Plan as per orders

How much longer did it take you to read the handwritten progress note? Were you able to decipher every word in it? Did you realize that the two progress notes contain the same information?

The activity you just completed illustrates one of the benefits of coding from an EHR.

Disadvantages to Coding from an EHR

Although the EHR provides a number of significant advantages for the coder, coding from an EHR is not without potential problems. The disadvantages to coding from an EHR include the use of cloned notes and the automatic population of "normal." Issues may also arise when coders are not fully comfortable with the new technology.

Cloned Notes

Cloned notes, also known as copycat charting, are identical notes resulting from copying and pasting information from one encounter or visit to another. Copying and pasting notes that accurately reflect the care and treatment rendered to the patient is an appropriate time-saving technique, but the danger in using cloned notes can arise when a healthcare provider copies and pastes notes among patient encounters without reviewing and updating them to reflect the accurate care and treatment rendered at each visit. This creates problems for coders trying to accurately capture diagnoses and procedures, and it also represents an issue for the reimbursement process. Medicare and other payers have clearly stated that inaccurate cloned documentation may result in loss of reimbursement. In addition, and most importantly, inaccurate or outdated information contained in cloned notes may adversely impact patient care.

Automatic Population of "Normal"

Many EHR systems are programmed to automatically populate all the fields in a template as "Normal" once "Normal" has been selected in one of the template areas. If the healthcare provider filling out the template is not attentive to the automatic population function, then the note may lack documentation of any abnormal findings.

CHECKPOINT 7.1

1. List three advantages of coding from an EHR versus a paper health record.

   a. _____

   b. _____

   c. _____

2. List two disadvantages of coding from an EHR versus a paper health record.

   a. _____

   b. _____

EXPAND YOUR LEARNING

Review the job description of a data integrity analyst found on the AHIMA website at www.paradigm college.net/exploringe hr/data_integrity_ analyst.

Data Integrity

Data integrity is a term used to refer to the accuracy, completeness, and reliability of clinical documentation in the EHR. Appropriate checks and balances are necessary for every organization utilizing an EHR system to ensure data integrity. EHRs that use the automatic population of fields and allow the cloned notes function should have specific policies and procedures in place for reviewing and auditing EHR documentation. Some healthcare organizations may employ a data integrity analyst whose job is to carry out these policies and procedures.

Medical Transcription

The practice of medical transcription has existed for as long as physicians have been documenting the treatment they provide to their patients. In fact, the earliest medical transcription was found on cave walls in the form of pictographs. Today, **medical transcription** is defined as the process of typing medical reports from voice-recorded formats that have been dictated by physicians and other healthcare providers.

EXPAND YOUR LEARNING

What is the future of medical transcription with the move toward EHRs? Visit the following website to view a video on the position of the Association for Documentation Integrity regarding the future of medical transcription: www. paradigmcollege.net/ exploringehr/med_ transcription

Medical Transcription and the EHR

The advent of the EHR has forced the process of medical transcription to advance. In both the paper and EHR environments, the healthcare provider dictates the report and a medical transcriptionist transforms the report into a readable format. Hospitals and healthcare organizations that already had computer systems in place prior to EHRs typically printed transcribed reports to the area where the medical record was located. The reports were then filed by a staff member. The EHR system takes that process a step further: instead of printing a piece of paper that must be physically filed into a record, it automatically "files" the transcribed report directly into the patient's EHR.

Different EHR systems require different types of interfaces. The two most common are Health Level 7 (HL7), discussed in Chapter 1, which directly drives reports into the EHR, and **File Import** or **File Monitor Utility**, which sends documents to the facility's network, where an EHR program imports them into the system.

A hospital or healthcare organization may choose have medical reports transcribed in-house, or they may outsource this work to **medical transcription service organizations (MTSOs)**, which are companies that contract their medical transcription services. These organizations provide a toll-free number to use for dictating and then utilize off-site medical transcriptionists, who may be located across the world, to transcribe the reports. The reports are automatically interfaced to the facility's EHR via a secure Internet link.

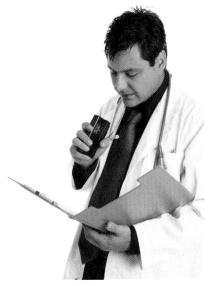

Doctors dictate notes and medical transcriptionists type the reports from the dictation.

You may wonder why medical transcription is necessary in an EHR environment since healthcare providers can type directly into the system. However, just because healthcare providers *can* type directly into an EHR does not necessarily mean that they *will*. Many physicians do not have the time or inclination to make notes directly into the EHR, so they will still require the services of a medical transcriptionist. The Association for Healthcare Documentation Integrity (AHDI) has rebranded the job title of medical transcriptionist to healthcare documentation specialist. This new title reflects that professionals now and in the future may transcribe reports or edit reports produced by speech-recognition software to ensure quality in health record documentation.

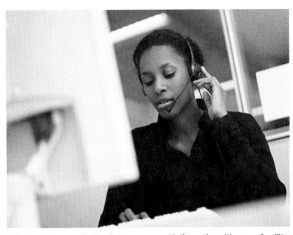

Medical transcriptionists may work for a healthcare facility or for a medical transcription service organization.

Consider This

A physician can choose to use three minutes of his or her time dictating history and physical examination results or 15 minutes typing those same notes into the EHR. Considering that most physicians feel that they never have enough time to spend at the patient's bedside, do you believe most physicians will dictate or type those notes? Explain your response.

Speech Recognition

Speech recognition is a technology widely used in many industries. You have used speech recognition when stating a number or word in response to an automated telephone system. Speech recognition technology works well when the speaker enunciates in the way expected by the speech recognition software; however, problems may arise when the speaker does not speak in the expected way, or speaks at a pace that is either too quick or too slow for the software to recognize. For these reasons, speech recognition technology has made slow inroads into the healthcare industry. In the healthcare environment, speech recognition technology can be implemented through front-end or back-end speech recognition software.

Front-end speech recognition allows the dictator to dictate, edit, and sign the report in the same process because the transcribed words appear directly on the screen as the healthcare provider is dictating. Using front-end speech recognition results in the report being available immediately in the EHR.

Back-end, or **deferred, speech recognition** is the most common type of speech recognition used in healthcare. This process requires the healthcare provider to use a digital dictation system that sends the recording through a speech recognition machine and into a draft document. The document is then routed along with the original voice recording to an editor, also known as a medical language or healthcare documentation specialist, where it is edited, finalized, and saved to the EHR. Medical language and healthcare documentation specialist positions are often filled by medical transcriptionists.

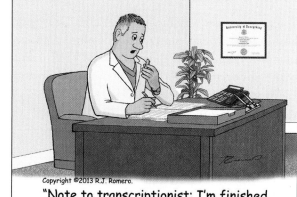

Copyright ©2013 R.J. Romero.

"Note to transcriptionist: I'm finished mumbling and rambling. I expect you to produce a coherent medical report, correct diagnosis and treatment plan."

Successful use of speech recognition technology in healthcare can result in many benefits, including:

- reduced document turnaround times.

- transcription cost savings.

- enhanced patient care through increased document accuracy and access.

- increased healthcare provider and staff satisfaction.

Activity 7.3   EHRNAVIGAT⊕R

Viewing Transcribed Reports

Go to the Course Navigator to launch Activity 7.3. As a nurse, practice reviewing a patient's transcribed reports using the EHR Navigator.

CHECKP⊕INT 7.2

1. True/False: Deferred speech recognition is the most common type of speech recognition used in healthcare.

2. What does MTSO stand for?

3. Define the term *data integrity*.

Protected Health Information

Because EHRs provide increased access to health records, there is an increased need for monitoring and oversight regarding the disclosure and release of protected health information (PHI).

The following sections discuss specific considerations related to PHI.

Release of Information

In Chapter 6, the HIPAA Privacy Rule was discussed in detail, including occasions when it is appropriate to release clinical information. You engaged in activities in which you released health information to a healthcare organization for continuity of patient care and to an insurance company for billing purposes. These are Release of Information (ROI) scenarios that a healthcare provider or a billing clerk at the organization could handle, but the HIM staff handles the majority of ROI activities.

Typically, HIM professionals, in conjunction with compliance and information technology professionals, ensure that all healthcare staff members are educated in the organization's ROI policies and procedures.

Rules and regulations related to the release of PHI are the same whether you are releasing information from a paper record or an EHR. However, the ROI process is significantly more streamlined in an EHR environment for many reasons, including the following:

- physical records do not need to be located, resulting in significant time savings for HIM staff.

EXPAND
YOUR LEARNING

To view a sample letter for request of health information visit www. paradigmcollege.net/ exploringehr/sample_ letter.

- records can be printed to paper, saved to CD, or emailed directly from the EHR rather than being copied or scanned by hand, resulting in significant time savings for HIM staff.

- records can be released in a more timely manner because the process takes less time.

The ROI workflow process follows these steps:

1. A requester submits a written ROI request.

2. For verbal requests, the HIM staff completes a Verbal Request for Information.

3. The HIM staff logs the request into the EHR system.

4. A staff member scans the request, along with other pertinent documents such as patient authorization, into the patient's EHR.

5. A staff member reviews the request to verify the legitimacy for release of information. He or she looks at items such as identification of the patient whose information is being requested, types of documents requested, service dates, etc.

6. The HIM staff produces the records in the format requested (paper or electronic).

7. A staff member generates a correspondence letter to accompany the records.

8. The HIM staff mails or ships the records.

Activity 7.4   **EHR**NAVIGAT✚R

Authorizing the Release of Patient Information

Go to the Course Navigator to launch Activity 7.4. As an RHIT, practice authorizing the release of patient information using the EHR Navigator.

Accounting of Disclosures

As you learned in Chapter 6, the Privacy Rule states that a patient has the right to receive an accounting of disclosures of his or her PHI made by the covered entity. These accountings of disclosure are provided by the covered entity. ROI software that is either part of the EHR system or interfaces with the EHR system makes the release of an accounting of disclosures relatively simple because the ROI software automatically produces these documents.

A sample accounting of disclosures log is found in Figure 7.4.

Figure 7.4 Sample Accounting of Disclosures Log

EMC MEDICAL CENTER

Accounting of Disclosures Log

**EMC
Medical Center**

Patient Name:_____

Medical Record Number: _____

Date Requested	Name of Requestor	Address	Authorization or Written Request (Y/N)	Purpose	PHI Disclosed	Date Disclosed	Disclosed By

---

Activity 7.5 — EHRNAVIGATOR

Producing an Accounting of Disclosures Log

Go to the Course Navigator to launch Activity 7.5. As an RHIT, practice printing an accounting of disclosures log using the EHR Navigator.

Analyzing the EHR for Completeness

Each healthcare organization should establish policies and procedures that define a complete health record. These policies and procedures should incorporate all federal and state regulations and statutes as well as all applicable accreditation standards pertaining to the organization. These procedures are outlined in the Medical Staff Bylaws. The HIM staff must review the EHRs of all patients to ensure compliance with organizational policies and procedures. EHR systems automatically produce reports based on the completion policies and procedures set by the practice, and notify healthcare providers of the need to complete records to avoid negative actions. If a medical staff member does not comply with completion policies and procedures and, thus, has incomplete records, the organization may suspend his or her medical staff privileges or take disciplinary action against him or her.

Parameters of a Complete EHR

Although each organization establishes its own definition of a complete EHR, the most common elements used to determine whether an EHR is complete in a hospital setting are as follows:

- all entries are signed.

- history and physical examinations are complete within 30 days prior to admission or within 24 hours after admission; if a surgery is scheduled, the history and physical examination is dictated and on the patient chart prior to initiation of surgery.

- consultation reports are complete.

- operative and procedure reports are complete.

- entries requiring a co-signature are signed.

- a discharge summary has been completed within 30 days after discharge.

One of the most significant benefits of the EHR related to the completion of health records involves the signing, or authentication, of telephone orders. Accreditation standards require that telephone orders be authenticated within a specific amount of time. The EHR allows physicians, physician assistants, and nurse practitioners to authenticate orders from any computer, which saves time.

Another benefit that the EHR provides for health record completion involves the dating and timing of documentation. Accrediting bodies require that all health record documentation be marked with the date and time. This can be difficult with paper records because it is up to the healthcare provider to remember to note the date and time. However, within an EHR system, the computer automatically dates and times all entries and activities, thus helping healthcare providers to comply with these requirements.

Incorporating Paper-Based Medical Records into the EHR System

With the implementation of an EHR system, a healthcare organization must make decisions regarding how to incorporate its paper-based records. Some organizations may decide to scan all paper-based records into the EHR system at once, while others will choose to scan each patient's record when he or she next experiences contact with the organization. Healthcare facilities may also choose to be selective in what they scan. For example, instead of scanning all records, a physician's office may decide to only enter pertinent historical data, a current problem list, and current treatment data. In the setting of a physician office, scanning may be limited to documents such as immunization records, hospital reports, and diagnostic test results.

Incorporation Procedures

Whatever decisions are made regarding the documents to be scanned, healthcare organizations must establish procedures early on to ensure proper document preparation, indexing, and scanning. For example, **preparation** may involve activities such as putting the paper records in order, straightening the paper, and removing paper clips or staples. **Indexing** is the process of assigning a code to each type of document that is part of the paper medical record and associating the code with the location in the EHR where the document should digitally reside. When the record is scanned, the system matches the code from the indexed paper with the one in the EHR and places the document in the correct digital location (e.g., the image of a scanned history and physical paper record will appear under the history and physical tab in the EHR). Failure to establish these procedures may result in document loss or inaccurate patient document assignment. Most organizations will utilize their HIM staff members to conduct the scanning process; however, depending on the size of the scanning workload, some organizations may choose to outsource the scanning process or hire temporary staff. Another important function is quality control, which should be performed concurrently as paper records are being scanned. Typically, quality control is performed after every 10 images scanned. During this process, the HIM professional reviews the digital images for quality by focusing on the completeness of the scanned pages, clarity and focus of the information on the pages, and correct indexing.

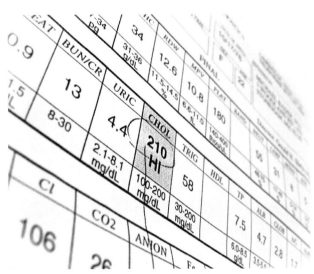

Lab test results are one of the documents that might be scanned into an EHR.

Chapter Summary

Health information management (HIM) professionals play an important role in the successful maintenance of health records. HIM staff are responsible for auditing additions to the Master Patient Index (MPI) and merging duplicate Medical Record Numbers (MRNs). An EHR environment isn't necessarily paperless, and HIM staff play an important role in transitioning from paper records to EHRs. HIM staff will use chart tracking software to help them track paper records during the transition from paper records to EHRs.

The coding process and guidelines are the same whether the record is paper or electronic, but EHRs provide many benefits such as more complete and legible documentation. Coding from an EHR may also present challenges.

As EHRs evolve within healthcare organizations, so does the role of the HIM professional. Although some duties and procedures will be eliminated, others will be created. Some of the new roles filled by HIM professionals include health information analysts (responsible for merging of duplicate medical number records and analyzing data for quality and consistency), auditors (responsible for reviewing and releasing appropriate protected health information and reviewing codes assigned by automated systems to assure accuracy), and overseers in the EHR environment (responsible for ensuring that medical staff complete EHR documentation in a timely manner and monitoring use or misuse of EHRs). The use of new technologies, such as speech recognition software, will require additional procedures to be performed by HIM staff.

The HIM staff is responsible for the majority of Release of Information (ROI) activities and must also analyze EHRs for completeness.

When implementing an EHR, a healthcare facility must make decisions about how to incorporate paper records. Healthcare organizations must establish procedures to ensure proper document preparation, indexing, and scanning.

Check Your Understanding

To check your understanding of this chapter's key concepts, read the following multiple-choice and true/false questions and then record your answers on a separate sheet of paper. Write your answers as modeled in these examples: 1a; 2b; 6T; 7F; etc.

1. Front-end speech recognition

    a. allows the dictator to dictate, edit, and sign the report in the same process.

    b. allows the dictator to dictate and edit in the same process, but he or she must separately sign the report.

    c. does not work as well as back-end speech recognition.

    d. is more common than back-end speech recognition.

2. Which of the following is *not* a common characteristic of a complete hospital record?

    a. All consultation reports are complete.

    b. All data has been reviewed by a physician.

    c. All operative and procedure reports have been complete.

    d. Entries requiring a co-signature have been signed.

3. Data integrity refers to

    a. whether or not a physician has reviewed the data.

    b. the procedures that govern how a paper chart should be scanned into an EHR system.

    c. the accuracy, completeness, and reliability of clinical documentation in the EHR.

    d. whether or not data has been reviewed by the medical facility's legal department.

4. The _____ states that a patient has a right to know whether his or her protected health information has been released (known as the accounting of disclosures).

    a. AHIMA Law

    b. HIPAA Security Rule

    c. CCHIT Doctrine

    d. HIPAA Privacy Rule

5. Which of the following describes a benefit of using an EHR rather than a paper chart for coding?

    a. Documentation is more comprehensive due to the use of templates.

    b. The EHR is more legible.

    c. The EHR can be accessed at any time.

    d. All of the above

6. True/False: Chart tracking software that tracks fewer than 500 paper medical records typically utilizes bar coding technology.

7. True/False: The advent of EHRs is forcing medical transcription services to advance.

8. True/False: Some hospitals and other healthcare organizations implement portions of EHR software over a period of time, creating hybrid health records.

9. True/False: Physicians may be more likely to document more information in an EHR than in a paper record.

10. True/False: One drawback to using cloned notes is that a healthcare provider might copy and paste notes from one patient encounter to another without reviewing and updating them, thus resulting in inaccuracies.

Learn the Terms

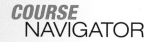

Go to the Course Navigator to access flashcards for Chapter 7 of *Exploring Electronic Health Records*.

Acronyms

AHDI: Association for Healthcare Documentation Integrity

CPT: Current Procedural Terminology

EMPI: Enterprise Master Patient Index

H&P: History and Physical

HCPC: Healthcare Common Procedure Coding System Level II

HIM: Health Information Management

HIPAA: Health Insurance Portability and Accountability Act

HL7: Health Level 7

ICD: International Classification of Diseases

MPI: Master Patient Index

MRN: Medical Record Number

MTSO: Medical Transcription Service Organization

PHI: Protected Health Information

ROI: Release of Information

EHR Application

Go on the Record

To build on your understanding of the topics in this chapter, complete the following short answer questions.

1. List and discuss the benefits of using speech recognition.

2. List five patient demographic data elements that are part of the MPI.

3. How are EHRs impacting the medical transcription job position?

4. Explain why a healthcare facility that uses an EHR system cannot necessarily be considered paperless.

5. Discuss the disadvantages of using an EHR system for coding health records.

Navigate the Field

To gain practice in handling challenging situations in the workplace, consider the following real-world scenarios and then use the guiding questions to help you formulate your responses.

1. As a part of the implementation of EHRs, Remington Medical Center loaded the data from its old MPI into its new EHR system. Upon doing so, it found 250,000 duplicate records. Are there steps that Remington Medical Center should have taken before merging the old MPI data into the new system? What steps would you suggest the Remington Medical Center HIM staff take to "clean up" the 250,000 duplicate MPI records?

2. It is estimated that only about one-half of physician offices in the United States have implemented an EHR system. One of the main reasons this statistic is so low may be physician reluctance to embrace EHRs. Physicians are concerned about the amount of time they will have to spend with the data entry of progress notes, consultation notes, and history and physical examination notes. You are the HIM manager at a large physician practice. You have heard physicians' complaints about the amount of time they spend on data entry, and you have identified speech recognition software as a possible solution. Prepare a report to the office manager outlining the details of your proposed solution.

EHR Evaluation

Think Critically

Continue to think critically about challenging real-world scenarios and complete the following activities.

1. Interview an HIM manager in a facility that uses speech recognition technology. Identify the pros and cons of the technology based on your conversation.

2. Review the document titled "Medical Transcription: Proven Accelerator of EHR Adoption," which was collaboratively written by the Association for Healthcare Documentation Integrity and the Medical Transcription Industry Association. Discuss how the medical transcription/clinical documentation sector can contribute to successful EHR implementation.

   www.paradigmcollege.net/exploringehr/med_transcription_EHR_Adoption

Make Your Case

Consider the following scenario and create a presentation on the following topic.

Create a presentation for the HIM staff at an acute care hospital that explains the changes in departmental procedures that will occur after an EHR system is implemented at the hospital.

Explore the Technology

To expand your mastery of EHRs, explore the following online activities and complete the EHR Navigator assessments.

COURSE
NAVIGATOR

Ensure you are comfortable with the functionality presented in the EHR Navigator activities, such as merging duplicate medical record numbers, tracking a patient's chart, viewing transcribed reports, authorizing the release of patient information, and producing an accounting of disclosures log. Then, complete the EHR Navigator assessments for Chapter 7 located on the Course Navigator.

Are You Ready?

A successful job search in the allied health field requires diligence and preparation. One area in which preparation is particularly critical is the job interview. The interview allows you to make a good first impression, emphasize your personal strengths and skills, and explain why you are the best candidate for the available position. With that in mind, do your homework before your interview by completing the following tasks:

- research the company so that you are knowledgeable about the organization's history, structure, philosophy, and mission.

- take time to practice your answers to typical interview questions regarding your personal characteristics, strengths and weaknesses, valuable work experiences, and professional goals.

- prepare samples of your work and have them available to share with the interviewer.

- plan your attire for the interview and ensure your clothing is appropriate for the position you are seeking.

The more prepared that you are, the easier the interview may be. For more interviewing tips, visit Jist Publishing's website at www.jist.emcp.com.

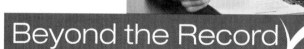

Beyond the Record

- Nurses using electronic health record (EHR) systems have seen reductions in documentation time by up to 45%.

- EHR systems allow nurses to spend 15% to 26% more time monitoring patients.

- A survey conducted by the Centers for Disease Control and Prevention found that 75% of physicians said their organizations' EHR systems enhanced patient care.

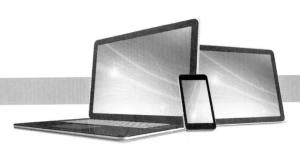

8

Clinical Inputs and Outputs

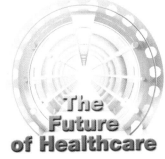

The Future of Healthcare

According to the U.S. federal government's official website for health information technology, future technologies may offer many different ways for patients and their doctors to monitor and manage healthcare. These new practices could include:

- use of global positioning system technology and real-time reminders and alerts to prevent and treat health conditions.

- the ability to send health data to clinics from personal devices such as tablets and smartphones.

- more virtual doctor's visits and health coaching tailored to issues based on clinical data in a patient's electronic health record (EHR).

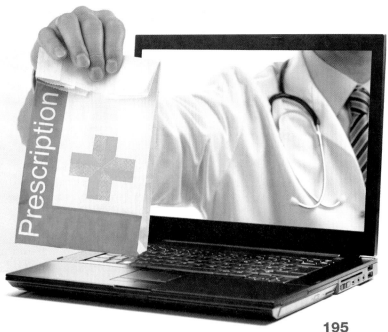

- Define and discuss *structured* and *unstructured* data.
- Define *data mining* and its relationship to structured and unstructured data.
- Explain manual and automated methods of data collection.
- Identify the elements of a history and physical examination.
- Understand how to enter progress notes into an EHR, as well the role of assessments, orders, test results, and other clinical documentation in the EHR system.
- Define *cloned notes* and their related concerns.
- Define *e-prescribing* and its benefits and challenges.
- Modify an e-prescription and override a drug allergy notification.
- Understand clinical results reporting and discuss manual and automatic methods of results entry into the EHR.
- Understand how EHR systems support public health initiatives.
- Create a Meaningful Use Report via the EHR Navigator.
- Report an immunization.

The movement to replace traditional paper health records with EHRs is building momentum. This textbook has explored many of the scheduling, administrative, and health information management data activities in an EHR system. This chapter will focus on clinical inputs and outputs.

Clinical inputs are data related to the patient's clinical status that is entered into the patient's EHR or paper record. Data entered into an EHR can be classified as either structured or unstructured. **Structured data** is stored in a fixed field in a database. Examples of structured data include date of birth, sex, race, lab results, International Classification of Diseases (ICD) codes, etc. Unstructured data is the opposite of structured data and is information that is not contained in a traditional fixed field database. Examples of **unstructured data** include primarily the narrative portions of the EHR such as progress notes, test interpretations, operative reports, and the like.

The implementation of the EHR has streamlined data entry and allowed interoperability of data access. Depending on the compatibility of the clinical system interface with other systems such as radiology, laboratory, pharmacy, and transcription services, healthcare staff members enter patient and clinical data either automatically or manually to create the EHR. Examples of clinical data include the history and physical examination (H&P), progress notes by all clinicians, immunizations information, laboratory test results, and medications. The clinical input of medication information via the e-prescribing feature of EHR systems has improved the safety and efficiency of drug administration. You will learn more about e-prescribing later in the chapter.

Clinical outputs are data that can be extracted from a patient record and compiled in a meaningful way. For example, HIM staff might run a cumulative report of the laboratory results of a patient to easily determine if trends in laboratory values need to be addressed by the patient's physician. The transcribed reports of an H&P as well as consultations and radiology reports are additional examples of clinical output. All clinicians involved in the patient's care can then use this data.

Data mining is the process of searching for and examining data to organize it into useful patterns and trends. Data mining and reporting of structured data can be accomplished quickly and easily using an EHR system because the fixed nature of structured data makes it easy to search for, query, and quantify. Data mining of unstructured data is a more challenging process that researchers and developers are working hard to conquer. A wealth of information is buried in the narrative provider notes of the EHR, waiting to be manipulated and studied.

Data Collection

Data collection for the EHR occurs through a combination of manual and automated methods. **Manual data collection** of demographic and insurance information is often initiated by a staff member upon initial patient contact with a healthcare facility. The data is typically obtained from a preprinted form the patient has completed or during an in-person interview; however, at times, the information is collected over the telephone. A staff member subsequently enters this information into the EHR system. Some healthcare organizations ask patients to enter their own demographic data through a secure, personal Internet link that a staff member sends to the patient to begin developing the EHR.

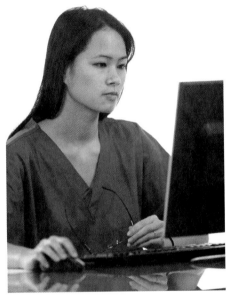

Healthcare workers manually enter demographic and insurance information into the EHR. On subsequent visits this information is automatically copied over to the next patient encounter

Automated data collection occurs when the data from the initial patient encounter is automatically copied over to each new patient encounter using an automated data capture. Automated data collection is the preferred method of data capture because it requires less personnel time, avoids repetitive requests of information from patients, and may allow for more consistent data entry. The era of patients entering EHR data highlights the importance of front-line review for errors and duplications of data. The success of patient-initiated entry of demographic data relies on a healthcare facility's structured auditing and correction procedures to reconcile data errors and/or duplications. As EHR technology evolves, more data collection will be automated and healthcare professionals may have to enter less information manually.

EXPAND YOUR LEARNING

The Standards and Interoperability Framework within the Office of the National Coordinator for Health Information Technology was formed to gather input from both public and private sectors regarding the creation of standardized health information technology specifications for use throughout the United States. In January 2013, the Standards and Interoperability Framework launched the Structured Data Capture initiative. Read about this initiative at the following website. Why is this initiative important to the interoperability of EHRs?

www.paradigmcollege.net/exploringehr/data_capture

History and Physical Examination

A **history and physical examination (H&P)** is a part of most patient encounters with healthcare providers and is a valuable tool for the healthcare providers in identifying and treating patient diagnoses. The H&P consists of two main elements: a **subjective element** and an **objective element**.

History

The **history** is the subjective element of the H&P because it is obtained from the patient or a family member as well as a review of previous medical records. **Subjective** information is based on personal reporting and opinions. The history is made up of the following components:

- History of present illness
- Past medical history
- Allergies
- Medications currently prescribed to the patient
- Family and social histories

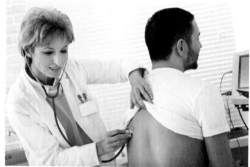
The physical examination is the objective portion of the history and physical.

Physical Examination

The **physical examination** is the objective element of the H&P. **Objective** information is based on facts and not subject to interpretation like subjective information. This procedure is conducted by the nursing or medical staff and consists of an investigation of the patient's body systems, an assessment of his or her condition, and a treatment plan. The examination of each body system is called the **review of systems (ROS)**. The ROS consists of the following system assessments:

1. General (documents the general appearance of the patient, e.g., "A 66-year-old Caucasian woman in no acute distress. Patient is alert and able to discuss medical history.")

2. Vital signs (includes the patient's blood pressure, pulse, respiratory rate, pulse oximetry, and body temperature)

3. Head, ears, eyes, nose, and throat (HEENT)

4. Respiratory

5. Cardiovascular

6. Abdominal

7. Gastrointestinal

8. Genitourinary

9. Musculoskeletal

10. Neurologic

Depending on the reason for the patient's visit, the physician may conduct a complete ROS or a selective ROS that focuses on the body systems involved with the patient's chief complaint(s). The **chief complaint** is articulated by the patient as his or her reason for seeking health services. For example, a high school student whose chief complaint is that he or she wishes to participate in sports will likely need a complete ROS to ensure his or her health status is appropriate for participation in the sport. However, a 10-year-old whose chief complaint is throat pain will likely only receive a general examination along with a check of vital signs and a review of the HEENT system.

Once the healthcare provider has reviewed the history of the patient, physically examined the patient, and evaluated all recent laboratory and diagnostic test results, he or she makes an assessment of the patient's diagnoses and decides on a **treatment plan** to alleviate the patient's condition.

Depending on the preference of the healthcare provider, he or she may type the H&P directly into the EHR or dictate a report and have a transcriptionist type and upload the report into the patient's EHR. **Uploading** is the process of transmitting a file from one computer to another computer or portal.

Activity 8.1 — EHRNAVIGATOR

Viewing a History and Physical Report

Go to the Course Navigator to launch Activity 8.1. As an occupational therapist, practice reviewing a patient's history and physical report using the EHR Navigator.

EHR Templates and Data Collection

Many of the clinical inputs in an EHR system are accomplished using a **template**, which is a preformatted file that provides prompts to obtain specific, consistent information. For healthcare providers, the use of a template:

- indicates required fields that must be completed during the documentation process.

- ensures consistent data-gathering techniques among users.

- allows for efficient data entry through the use of structured input options such as drop-down menus and check boxes.

- provides immediate data population of the EHR system.

- avoids the added expense of hiring a transcriptionist to document patient information.

- facilitates easy access to data due to its consistent format, thus avoiding time-consuming searches.

- enables faster and more precise reporting and analysis of data due to its format and consistent elements.

Clearly, EHR templates offer several advantages. However, their use should never hinder thorough documentation by a healthcare provider. For any selections not available in drop-down menus, a provider will need to input patient information to ensure accuracy and completeness of the patient record.

CHECKPOINT 8.1

1. Provide two reasons why automated data collection is the preferred method of data capture.

_____

_____

2. Define history and physical and identify the two main elements of an H&P.

_____

_____

Specialized Templates

Certain patient diagnoses or conditions may dictate the creation of specialized templates that offer information fields tailored to specific documentation needs. Specialized healthcare providers may also need specialized templates. For example, a detailed eye examination template like the one shown in Figure 8.1 would be a useful tool for an ophthalmologist. Depending on the policies of a healthcare organization, staff members may conduct special assessments to determine these special needs.

Figure 8.1 Specialized Template

Choose an item. Visual Acuity OD
Choose an item. Pinhole OD
Yes ☐No ☐Afferent Pupillary Defect OD
Yes ☐No ☐Dilated OD
☐ IOP OD
☐ CVF OD
Yes ☐No ☐Lid OD WNL
Choose an item. Lid OD
Yes ☐No ☐Conjunctiva/Sclera OD WNL?
Choose an item. Conjunctiva/Sclera OD

Choose an item. Visual Acuity OS
Choose an item. Pinhole OS
Yes ☐No ☐Afferent Pupillary Defect OS
Yes ☐No ☐Dilated OS
☐ IOP OS
☐ CVF OS
Yes ☐No ☐Lid OS WNL
Choose an item. Lid OS
Yes ☐No ☐Conjunctiva/Sclera OS WNL?
Choose an item. Conjunctiva/Sclera OS

Progress Notes

Progress notes are the portion of the health record in which healthcare providers of all disciplines document the patient's progress, or lack thereof, in relation to the established goals of the care plan. Healthcare providers may choose to write or transcribe progress notes in any format. For healthcare organizations that have adopted an EHR system, this task can be easily completed through the use of customized templates.

Progress Note Templates

These templates provide information fields that cater to certain disciplines and specialties. For example, a template for a physical therapy progress note may include checkboxes to indicate whether the patient can bear weight on the right side and on the left side and drop-down menus with options for indicating the patient's range of motion and pain level. A progress note template for a cardiologist may allow healthcare providers to select different causes of syncope (i.e., cardiac, metabolic, neurologic). Use of a progress note template lessens data entry time and ensures the inclusion of all pertinent data elements.

Activity 8.2	EHRNAVIGAT✛R

Entering a Progress Note

Go to the Course Navigator to launch Activity 8.2. As a nurse, practice entering a progress note into a patient's chart using the EHR Navigator.

Cloned Progress Notes

As you learned in Chapter 7, one area of concern related to EHR progress notes has been the increased use of cloned progress notes. A **cloned progress note** is a note that has been partially or totally copied from an existing progress note. The copied note is then updated by the healthcare provider to include any new information. This shortcut may save time, but it can also result in inaccurate or outdated documentation regarding a patient's health status and progress if the healthcare provider forgets to make the necessary updates to the existing note. Consequently, other healthcare providers may make inappropriate medical decisions based on incorrect patient information, which could have dire consequences for the patient.

Cloned progress notes may also impact the process of coding diagnoses and procedures for reimbursement purposes. Coding classification systems such as International Classification of Diseases (ICD) and Current Procedural Terminology (CPT) require detailed documentation for accurate coding. Cloned progress notes that do not accurately reflect patient diagnoses and treatment may result in inaccurate code assignment, which, in turn, could lead to reduced reimbursement and increased focus and monitoring from payer sources.

The U.S. federal government's Office of the Inspector General (OIG) is responsible for combating healthcare fraud, waste, and abuse, as well as for working to improve healthcare efficiency. To that end, the OIG routinely audits the billing and coding practices of healthcare organizations. Health record documentation must support code assignment and bills submitted for Medicare and Medicaid reimbursement. The OIG establishes an annual **Workplan** of areas of healthcare documentation and billing practices to be addressed and audited during the year. The topic of cloned documentation was a focus of the OIG's 2012 and 2013 Workplans and will likely be included in the 2014 Workplan as more EHR systems are implemented. The goals of the OIG are to ensure that healthcare organizations maintain accurate coding and billing records and that documentation is consistent throughout the records.

e-Prescribing

Another documentation feature available to users of EHR systems is electronic prescribing, commonly known as **e-prescribing**. This feature allows a physician, nurse practitioner, or physician assistant to electronically transmit a new prescription or renewal authorization to a pharmacy. The healthcare provider enters the medication order along with the location of the patient's pharmacy into the patient's EHR, and the e-prescription is automatically transmitted to the pharmacy, where it is filled for patient pickup. All EHR systems must have the e-prescribing feature because meaningful use requires that more than 40% of all permissible prescriptions written by an eligible healthcare provider are electronically transmitted using certified EHR technology.

Benefits of e-Prescribing

For healthcare providers, the benefits of e-prescribing include improved prescribing accuracy and efficiency, a decreased potential for medication errors and prescription forgeries, and more accurate and timely billing. Using e-prescriptions lessens the risk for potential medication errors due to unclear handwriting, illegible faxes, or misinterpreted prescription abbreviations. EHR systems also have the ability to alert a healthcare provider if he or she prescribes a drug to which the patient is allergic, resulting in improved medication safety. In fact, many studies indicate that the use of the e-prescribing feature of EHR systems has reduced medication errors by 12% to 15%. E-prescriptions also benefit patients in terms of improved accuracy in medication administration, more effective and efficient communication between patients and prescribers, and timely notifications for refills. Overall, e-prescription functionality improves patient care quality and reduces healthcare costs. Figure 8.2 on the following page illustrates an e-prescription.

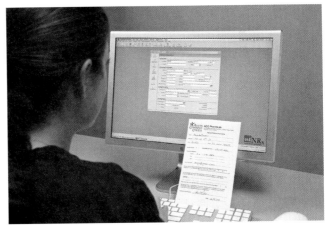

Practitioners enter orders for medications along with the patient's pharmacy location into the patient's EHR and the prescription is automatically transmitted to the pharmacy.

e-Prescribing Alerts

The e-prescribing component of an EHR includes an alert function that notifies the prescribing healthcare provider of drug-to-drug interactions, drug-to-food interactions, and patient's allergies to medications. These alerts are grouped into a hierarchy of potential risk and seriousness of the interactions or allergies, and healthcare prescribers may override less serious interactions or allergies and continue to prescribe the medication. For example, if there is only one medication that will be effective in treating a life-threatening illness and the potential drug-to-drug interaction may result in a minor drop in blood pressure, the physician may determine that the need for the medication is worth the minor drop in blood pressure.

Figure 8.2 E-Prescription

```
----------------------------------------------------------------
!!! -- START SECURED ELECTRONIC PRESCRIPTION TRANSMISSION -- !!!
----------------------------------------------------------------
FROM THE OFFICES OF PHIL JACKSON, MD; ETHEL JACOBSON, MD;
                   PETER JARKOWSKI, PA; EUGENE JOHNSON, DO

OFFICE ADDRESS:          67 EAST ELM
                         CEDAR RAPIDS, IA 52411
OFFICE TELEPHONE:        (319) 555-1212  TRANSMIT DATE: FEB 20, 2015
OFFICE FAX:              (319) 555-1313  WRITTEN DATE:  FEB 20, 2015
----------------------------------------------------------------
TRANSMITTED TO           THE CORNER DRUG STORE
PHARMACY ADDRESS:        875 PARADIGM WAY
                         CEDAR RAPIDS, IA 52410
PHARMACY TELEPHONE:      (319) 555-1414
----------------------------------------------------------------
PATIENT NAME:            JEFFREY KLEIN     D.O.B.: OCT 18, 1979
PATIENT ADDRESS:         1157 NORTH PLAZA AVE
                         CEDAR RAPIDS, IA 52411
----------------------------------------------------------------
PRESCRIBED MEDICATION:   FLUOXETINE 20 MG
SIGNA:                   i PO QD
DISPENSE QUANTITY:       30
REFILL(S):               PRN
----------------------------------------------------------------
PHYSICIAN SIGNATURE:     [[ ELECTRONIC SIGNATURE ON FILE ]]
                         [[ FOR DR. ETHEL JACOBSON ]]
----------------------------------------------------------------
!!! -- END SECURED ELECTRONIC PRESCRIPTION TRANSMISSION -- !!!
----------------------------------------------------------------
```

Challenges of e-Prescribing

Although e-prescribing affords many benefits to both patients and healthcare providers, there are also some challenges associated with the use of this technology. The biggest obstacle for prescribers involves the laws governing the dispensing of controlled substances. A **controlled substance** is a drug (primarily a narcotic) declared by U.S. federal or state law to be illegal for sale or use by the general public but legal if dispensed per a healthcare provider's prescription. The basis for determining whether a drug is a controlled substance is the drug's potential for addiction, abuse, or harm.

Although U.S. federal and state laws governing the distribution of controlled substances were in place prior to 1970, in that year the drug counterculture of the 1960s led the U.S. government to enact stronger legislation regarding the manufacture and distribution of narcotics, stimulants, depressants, hallucinogens, anabolic steroids, and chemicals used in the illicit production of controlled substances. This legislation, known as the **Controlled Substances Act of 1970**, placed tight controls on the pharmaceutical and healthcare industries and outlined five schedules of controlled substances based on potential for harm. This legislation established additional procedures for healthcare providers writing prescriptions for controlled substances. These procedures dictate that prescribers must use hard-copy or printed prescriptions when ordering Schedule II controlled substances. Consequently, the use of e-prescriptions for these substances must be approved by individual U.S. state boards of pharmacy before this technology can be implemented.

Another challenge associated with e-prescribing is the lack of interoperability between healthcare facility EHR software and some pharmacy software. An e-prescription is not useful to a patient if he or she is unable to fill it at the pharmacy. If a pharmacy's software does not communicate with the healthcare facility's EHR, a traditional, handwritten prescription must be used.

Activity 8.3   **EHR**NAVIGAT✚R

Modifying a Patient's e-Prescription

Go to the Course Navigator to launch Activity 8.3. As a physician, practice modifying a patient's e-prescription using the EHR Navigator.

Activity 8.4   **EHR**NAVIGAT✚R

Overriding a Drug Allergy Notification

Go to the Course Navigator to launch Activity 8.4. As a physician assistant, practice adding an e-prescription and overriding a drug allergy notification using the EHR Navigator.

Consider This

Prescriptions that have been handwritten by physicians or other prescribers pose a number of potentially serious problems. The combination of handwriting style and the use of abbreviations can lead to difficulty in reading and filling the prescription accurately. This difficulty can result in mistaken drug names, dosage, and strength. Another issue with handwritten prescriptions is that they can be easily altered by drug seekers. In light of these issues, how does the use of e-prescribing decrease the potential for medication errors and prescription forgeries?

CHECKP✚INT 8.2

1. List three benefits of e-prescribing.

2. Discuss two challenges facing the complete implementation of e-prescribing.

Clinical Results Reporting

Clinical results reporting is an EHR system function that allows healthcare providers to view laboratory and diagnostic test results immediately, provided there is an interface between the clinical results system and the EHR. This feature satisfies one of the National Patient Safety Goals (NPSGs) of The Joint Commission, an organization that surveys and accredits hospitals and other types of healthcare facilities. Hospitals accredited by The Joint Commission are required to comply with the NPSGs, which were established to help hospitals address specific areas of concern in regard to patient safety. The first set of NPSGs became effective on January 1, 2003, and the goals are annually updated by The Joint Commission based on the recommendations of the Patient Safety Advisory Group, a panel of widely recognized patient safety experts that includes nurses, physicians, pharmacists, risk managers, clinical engineers, and other professionals with hands-on experience in addressing patient safety issues. Reporting the critical results of tests and diagnostic procedures in a timely manner has been included in the NPSGs for several years and will continue into 2014. Such reporting is likely to remain on the list of NPSGs for many years.

According to surveyors from The Joint Commission, "There is an increased awareness that poor communication is at the heart of medical errors and lawsuits, which is why The Joint Commission is emphasizing the role of communication in critical value reporting." This goal is meant to ensure that laboratories report important clinical results to healthcare personnel in a timely manner, thereby allowing them to expediently treat patients. Hospitals must have policies and procedures in place that specify the timeframe during which healthcare providers must be advised of test results that are considered critical. Each healthcare organization is responsible for specifying the values and circumstances that define a critical test result. These specifications should be clearly defined in facility policy and medical staff bylaws. For example, the hematocrit laboratory value might be considered critical if it was below 18% or greater than 55% for an adult. A chest X-ray with a suspicious shadow may also be considered critical.

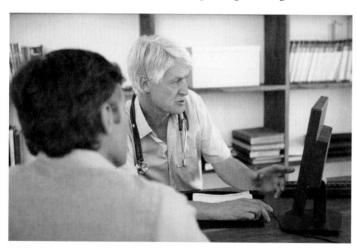

With clinical results reporting, clinicians are able to view and discuss lab results with patients immediately upon completion.

Automated Clinical Results Reporting

The clinical results reporting feature of EHR systems addresses a longstanding problem associated with phone and fax communications of test results, which is the inability for healthcare providers to receive these communications during times they are not in their offices (such as weekends, holidays, and night-time hours). When EHR systems are able to interface with laboratory computers and other computers that output test results, healthcare providers can use personal computers or mobile devices to access test results and order medications, treatments, or further tests to address the reported results. This is an example of the **automatic method** of results entry. In addition, many EHR systems are able to generate email or text alerts to notify providers of critical test results or other important information.

Manual Method of Clinical Results Reporting

In an environment that does not have an EHR system interfaced with laboratory computers, the laboratory sends a printed report via fax to the prescriber's office, and then a staff member scans the report into the EHR. This is an example of the **manual method** of results entry. However, the preferred method for retrieving lab and test reports would be via automatic transmission or an interface between the laboratory systems and the EHR.

Eventually, most laboratory and other diagnostic company computers will be interfaced with all EHR systems, but this process will take many years to accomplish. In the meantime, telecommunications continues to be the best way to obtain test results for facilities whose laboratory computers cannot interface or transfer clinical results. Until total interface and interoperability is achieved, scanning of results is a manageable process and the best option available for some EHR users.

Activity 8.5   **EHRNAVIGATOR**

Viewing Clinical Results in the EHR

Go to the Course Navigator to launch Activity 8.5. As a medical assistant, practice viewing a patient's lab results using the EHR Navigator.

Activity 8.6   **EHRNAVIGATOR**

Signing a Scanned Diagnostic Report

Go to the Course Navigator to launch Activity 8.6. As a physician, practice signing a scanned diagnostic report using the EHR Navigator.

Meaningful Use

As you have learned throughout this text, there are core measures of meaningful use that must be achieved by healthcare organizations if they plan to receive incentive payments for EHR adoption. Stage 1 and 2 requirements of meaningful use have been implemented or are in the process of being implemented by healthcare organizations. EHR systems are able to demonstrate compliance with these requirements by collecting data and running reports that indicate core measure compliance as well as those core measures still requiring achievement.

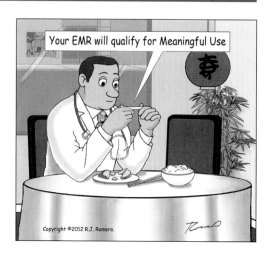

EHRs and Public Health Objectives

Stage 1 of meaningful use has three public health objectives that require the capability of the EHR system to submit electronic data to public health agencies for:

- Immunization registries

- Reportable laboratory results

- Syndromic surveillance (**syndromic** describes a group of symptoms that, when grouped together, are characteristic of a specific disorder or disease)

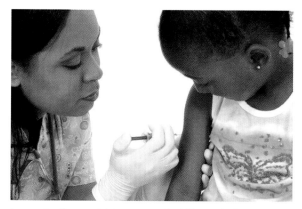

Immunization registries are part of Stage 1 of meaningful use.

EXPAND YOUR LEARNING

To read about engaged physicians whose time commitments to the EHR implementation at their practice have resulted in positive outcomes, visit www .paradigmcollege.net /exploringehr/physic ian_commitment.

The U.S. federal government included these meaningful use requirements for EHRs to improve collaboration between clinical and public healthcare organizations at both the local and state levels. Consequently, these public healthcare agencies (PHAs) may utilize the electronic data to improve the quality of healthcare, reduce healthcare disparities among various groups, and improve public health. An EHR system allows this data exchange to automatically occur with minimal interaction from healthcare personnel.

Immunization Registries

Healthcare clinics can report confidential, anonymous vaccination data about their patients to public health agencies. Immunization registries are important tools to help remind patients when vaccines are past due and consolidate immunization records for patients who may have multiple healthcare providers.

EHRNAVIGAT✛R

Reporting an Immunization

Go to the Course Navigator to launch Activity 8.7. As a medical assistant, practice reporting an immunization using the EHR Navigator.

Reportable Laboratory Results

Reportable laboratory results reporting for meaningful use is the electronic transfer of data from laboratories to public health agencies (PHAs). Reporting on conditions of concern to public health is a cornerstone of public health surveillance and includes the reporting of laboratory results that may be indicative of a notifiable condition. The Council of State and Territorial Epidemiologists determines the list of reportable conditions that are nationally notifiable on a voluntary basis to the Centers for Disease Control and Prevention (CDC) by state PHAs. Some examples of conditions that are reportable include anthrax, measles, rubella, polio, smallpox, and botulism.

Using the EHR system for laboratory results reporting has many benefits, including improved timeliness of reportable conditions, reduction of manual data entry errors, and more complete information provided to PHAs.

Syndromic Surveillance

Syndromic surveillance is the process of using health and health-related data in near "real-time" to make information available on the health of a community. This information includes statistics on disease trends and community health behaviors. Syndromic surveillance is particularly useful to local, state, and federal PHAs for the awareness of public health trends, identifying when emergency response is needed, and identifying an outbreak or potential outbreak of disease. Patient-encounter data from healthcare settings are a critical input for syndromic surveillance, which is greatly enhanced with the transfer of patient data occurring via EHRs. Clinical data are provided by hospitals and urgent care centers to PHAs for all patient encounters. The PHAs then use the Public Health Information Network, which is a national system for the electronic exchange of data operated by the CDC, to electronically exchange data and information across organizations and jurisdictions (e.g., clinical care to public health, public health to public health, and public health to other federal agencies).

EXPAND YOUR LEARNING

For more information on reportable conditions visit www.paradigmcollege.net/exploringehr/cdc and www.paradigmcollege.net/exploringehr/reportable_conditions.

Chapter Summary

Clinical data inputs and outputs are at the core of the EHR system, making this system an interactive repository of timely, valuable, and, in some cases, even lifesaving data.

Data collection for the EHR occurs through a combination of manual and automated methods, with automated data collection being the preferred method of data capture, as it requires less personnel time, avoids repetitive requests of information from patients, and allows for more consistent data. Patient demographic data is usually entered manually at the patient's first encounter with the healthcare organization and is automated at subsequent visits. History and physical examination results, progress notes, assessments, consultations, and operative reports are examples of documents that may be manually or electronically added to the EHR. An area of concern related to EHR progress notes has been the increased use of cloned progress notes. Healthcare providers must ensure that their documentation is accurate at all times.

Diagnostic tests such as laboratory results are ideally interfaced from the laboratory computer to the EHR. E-prescribing has greatly benefited patients and providers, with improved accuracy in medication administration and efficiencies related to communications and refills.

Without the capability for exchange of clinical data inputs and outputs, the EHR system would function merely as a static, electronic file folder. From filling e-prescriptions to the emergency review of laboratory results, the electronic exchange of clinical information has proven to be invaluable to patients and their caregivers.

Healthcare organizations must achieve core measures of meaningful use if they plan to receive incentive payments for EHR adoption. Stage 1 requires EHRs to have the ability to submit electronic data to public agencies for immunization registries, reportable laboratory results, and syndromic surveillance.

EHR Review

Check Your Understanding

To check your understanding of this chapter's key concepts, read the following multiple-choice and true/false questions and then record your answers on a separate sheet of paper. Write your answers as modeled in these examples: 1a; 2b; 6T; 7F; *etc.*

1. *Uploading* is
   a. the transmission and filling of prescriptions.
   b. the process of transmitting a file from one computer to another.
   c. the auditing of computer files.
   d. the transmission of computer viruses.

2. Which document contains the results of the examination of a patient's body systems?
   a. Operative report
   b. Radiology report
   c. Laboratory report
   d. History and physical examination (H&P)

3. Which of the following statements concerning e-prescribing is true?
   a. E-prescribing is the electronic generation and transmission of prescriptions.
   b. E-prescribing increases the efficiency of healthcare practices.
   c. E-prescribing assists prescribers by telling them which medication they should order for each diagnosis.
   d. both *a* and *b*

4. The abbreviation ROS means a
   a. review of systems on the history and physical examination.
   b. record of steroid use in e-prescribing.
   c. report of substance abuse.
   d. review of syndromic surveillance.

5. Which of the following is *NOT* one of the meaningful use stage 1 public health objectives?
   a. immunization registries
   b. reportable laboratory results
   c. prescription fraud prevention
   d. syndromic surveillance

6. True/False: The e-prescribing feature of an EHR system is an optional meaningful use function.

7. True/False: A template is a preformatted file that provides prompts to obtain specific, consistent information.

8. True/False: If a physician's office does not have an interface with a laboratory's computer, there is no way to incorporate laboratory results into the EHR system.

9. True/False: A physician who copies and pastes documentation from one progress note to another is creating cloned notes.

10. True/False: Per U.S. law, Schedule II controlled substances cannot be ordered via e-prescribing.

Learn the Terms

COURSE NAVIGATOR

Go to the Course Navigator to access flashcards for Chapter 8 of *Exploring Electronic Health Records*.

Acronyms

CDC: Centers for Disease Control and Prevention

CPT: Current Procedural Terminology

H&P: History and physical examination

HEENT: Head, ears, eyes, nose, and throat

ICD: International Classification of Diseases

NPSG: National Patient Safety Goals

PHA: Public health agency

OIG: Office of the Inspector General

ROS: Review of systems

EHR Application

Go on the Record

To build on your understanding of the topics in this chapter, complete the following short answer questions.

1. Explain why a healthcare provider might use cloned progress notes.

2. Describe the benefits of e-prescribing.

3. List three body systems examined during an H&P.

4. Describe the two elements of an H&P.

5. Explain how Northstar Medical Center can prove that its EHR system meets the core requirements of meaningful use.

Navigate the Field

To gain practice in handling challenging situations in the workplace, consider the following real-world scenarios and then use the guiding questions to help you formulate your responses.

1. You are the health information manager at a local hospital. A physician on the medical staff does not understand how to add H&P notes to a patient's EHR. He explains that he "always used to handwrite the H&P." You explain to the physician that he can no longer handwrite his H&P notes and you give him two options of how he can add his H&P notes to the EHR. Describe these two options.

2. You are a laboratory manager at a local hospital. Your laboratory systems can interface with the hospital's EHR system to automatically provide test results. However, there are times when this process does not function properly and results have to be entered manually. As the laboratory manager, you want to develop a procedure for doing this. What steps might you include in this procedure? Write a one-page procedure for manually entering laboratory results into the hospital's EHR system when the laboratory computer cannot automatically interface the laboratory results to the hospital's EHR system.

Think Critically

Continue to think critically about challenging real-world scenarios and complete the following activities.

1. As the quality manager at a local hospital, you are conducting an audit of physician progress notes to ensure that the progress notes accurately reflect the condition of the patient and are not simply cloned notes depicting inaccuracies.

   Patient Scenario #1: Progress Note of 10/4/15, 07:45: Infectious disease note: No fevers/chills. Tolerating antibiotics without difficulty. Lungs clear. Abdomen soft with positive bowel sounds. PICC without phlebitis. Vanc trough value of 10/2/15 is 14.0.

   Which of the following progress notes is accurately written according to the patient scenario #1 if the patient's status is completely the same as it was on 10/4/15?

   _____ a. Progress note of 10/5/15, 10:00: Infectious disease note: No changes from progress note of 10/4/15, 07:45.

   _____ b. Progress note of 10/5/15, 16:00: Infectious disease note: No fevers/chills. Tolerating antibiotics without difficulty. Lungs clear. Abdomen soft with positive bowel sounds. PICC without phlebitis. Vanc trough value of 10/2/15 is 14.0.

   _____ c. Progress note of 10/5/15, 14:00: Infectious disease note: Temp of 101.8°F today. Tolerating antibiotics without difficulty. Lungs clear. Abdomen soft with positive bowel sounds. PICC without phlebitis. Vanc trough value of 10/2/15 is 14.0.

Patient Scenario #2: Progress Note of 04/12/16, 8:10: Pulmonary note: Patient doing well on trach collar. Afebrile. Chest clear. No edema. Chronic respiratory failure. Change trach to #6 and start capping speech to evaluate for swallowing.

Which of the following progress notes is accurately written according to Patient Scenario #1 if the patient's status is completely the same as it was on 4/12/16, except the patient now has a fever of 101.4°F?

_____ a. Progress Note of 04/13/16, 14:15: Pulmonary note: Patient doing well on trach collar. Fever of 101.4°F. Chest rales heard. No edema. Chronic respiratory failure. Change trach to #6 and start capping speech to evaluate for swallowing.

_____ b. Progress Note of 04/13/16, 14:10: Pulmonary note: Patient doing well on trach collar. Afebrile. Chest clear. No edema. Chronic respiratory failure. Change trach to #6 and start capping speech to evaluate for swallowing.

_____ c. Progress Note of 04/13/16, 11:10: Pulmonary note: Patient doing well on trach collar. Temp of 101.4°F. Chest clear. No edema. Chronic respiratory failure. Change trach to #6 and start capping speech to evaluate for swallowing.

2. Perform an Internet search to determine the laboratory results that must be reported to your state public health agency. Select another state and perform an Internet search to determine the laboratory results that must be reported to that state's public health agency. How do the required test results compare? What tests are in common? Which are different? Why do you think some required test results vary from state to state? Why are some tests similar?

EHR Evaluation

Make Your Case

Consider the following scenario and create a presentation on the following topic.

You are a nurse at a medical office committed to community outreach and education. Your office uses e-prescribing software and wants to conduct a meeting for patients and guests to explain this technology. Develop a presentation for the meeting that explains the functions and benefits of using e-prescribing.

Explore the Technology

To expand your mastery of EHRs, explore the following online activities and complete the EHR Navigator assessments.

COURSE NAVIGATOR

Ensure you are comfortable with the functionality presented in the EHR Navigator activities, such as viewing H&Ps, entering a progress note, modifying a patient's e-prescription, overriding a drug allergy notification, viewing clinical results, signing a scanned diagnostic report, and reporting an immunization. Then, complete the EHR Navigator assessments for Chapter 8 located on the Course Navigator.

Beyond the Record

- The International Classification of Diseases, Ninth Revision (ICD-9) classification system has 13,000 diagnosis codes, whereas the Tenth Revision (ICD-10) has almost 68,000 diagnosis codes.

The ICD-10 codes are updated to reflect the latest medical conditions. Because there are so many new codes, they may need to invent one for healthcare professionals spending a lot of time typing on a computer!

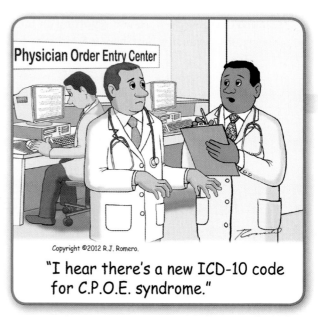

Copyright ©2012 R.J. Romero.

"I hear there's a new ICD-10 code for C.P.O.E. syndrome."

ICD Timeline

- **1837**–William Farr became the first medical statistician at the General Register Office of England and Wales. The office worked to secure better classifications of diseases and causes of death and pushed for international uniformity in these classifications.

- **1893**–French physician and statistician Jacques Bertillon presented the *Bertillon Classification of Causes of Death* at the International Statistical Institute of Chicago.

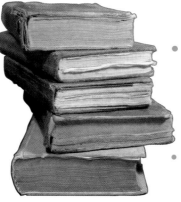

- **1900**–The first international conference convened to revise the International List of Causes of Death. Delegates from 29 countries reviewed the document and made revisions to the 179 causes of death.

- **1948**–The World Health Organization endorsed the sixth revision of the classification and assumed responsibility for updating it every 10 years. The name was changed to *Manual of the International Statistical Classification of Diseases, Injuries, and Causes of Death*.

- **1955**–The seventh revision occurred in 1955 and resulted in the revised name *International Classification of Diseases* (ICD) that we continue to use today.

- **1965**-The eighth revision occurred in 1965. This edition was more radical than the seventh but it did not change the structure of ICD.

- **1975**–The ninth revision (ICD-9) was published and contained a great deal of changes, including four-digit subcategories and five-digit subdivisions. The revision also included an optional alternative method of classifying diagnosing statements.

- **1979**–Clinical Modification codes (ICD-9-CM) are required for Medicare and Medicaid claims in the United States.

Chapter 9

Coding, Billing, and Reimbursement

ICD-10 goes into much greater detail as to the types of injuries patients sustain, including some rather uncommon injuries, such as:

- Struck by a sea lion, initial encounter

- Pedestrian on foot injured in collision with roller skater, subsequent encounter

- Stabbed while crocheting

- Struck by a turtle, subsequent encounter

- Hurt at the opera

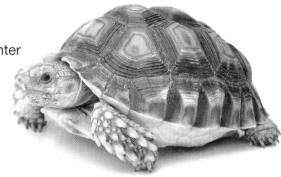

- **1990**—The tenth revision (ICD-10) was endorsed by the Forty-Third World Health Assembly.

- **2012**—The U.S. Department of Health and Human Services proposed to delay the United States' adoption of ICD-10-CM and ICD-10-PCS from October 1, 2013, to October 1, 2014.

- **2014**—ICD-10-CM and ICD-10-PCS implemented in the United States in October 2014.

Field Notes

As a billing specialist, electronic health records (EHRs) has made it much easier to verify what we can bill for after a visit. Instead of having to hunt around for a paper chart in the shelves, I don't even have to leave my desk to find the documentation I need.

– Diana Fischer, Billing Specialist

The transition to EHRs in my clinic has been incredibly valuable for streamlining the patient experience of scheduling appointments, billing insurance, requesting records, and tracking patient visits. EHRs create a deeper sense of accountability of accuracy in documentation and also eliminates the constant search for runaway paper charts.

Kyle Meerkins, Volunteer Coordinator

- Define *nomenclature* and identify the role of nomenclature in the electronic health record (EHR).

- Define *classification systems* and identify specific classification systems used for coding for each healthcare delivery system.

- Discuss the purposes of diagnostic and procedural coding.

- Discuss the classification systems used to code diagnoses and procedures, including the *International Classification of Diseases*, Current Procedural Terminology, Healthcare Common Procedure Coding System, the *Diagnostic and Statistical Manual of Mental Disorders, Fifth Edition*, and Current Dental Terminology.

- Discuss how EHRs affect coding and billing processes.

- Define and describe *computer-assisted coding*.

- Define and discuss important coding and billing terms such as *discharged not final billed* and *present on admission*.

- Demonstrate coding and billing processes utilizing EHR software.

Whether in an inpatient healthcare setting such as a hospital, nursing home, or long-term acute care hospital, or an outpatient setting such as an ambulatory surgical center or behavioral health clinic, there are individuals tasked with assigning or validating diagnostic and procedural codes to represent the patient's diseases or conditions and the treatment rendered. These individuals are known as **clinical coders**, medical coders, or coders and are responsible for assigning accurate codes based on health record documentation and coding guidelines. These codes are then used for reimbursement, research, decision-making, public health reporting, quality improvement, resource utilization, and healthcare policy and payment.

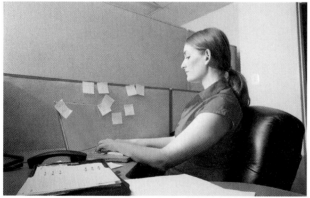

Clinical coders (or medical coders) are responsible for assigning accurate codes based on health record documentation.

The practice of accurately coding diagnoses and procedures is a complicated process but can be facilitated by the use of electronic health records (EHRs). The adoption of an EHR system allows coders in every healthcare setting to easily access patient health data as well as billing and reimbursement systems. This improved access, along with the increased legibility of documentation, results in a more streamlined approach to coding and billing. However, EHRs will only be of assistance in the reimbursement process if clinical and support staff members are properly trained in complete and accurate documentation.

Nomenclature Systems

Nomenclatures and classification systems are two terms frequently—but incorrectly—used interchangeably. **Nomenclature** refers to a common system of naming things. When used in a discussion of EHRs, nomenclature refers to a system of common clinical and medical terms, with codes to represent diseases, procedures, symptoms, and medications. Systemized Nomenclature of Medicine, Clinical Terms (SNOMED-CT) became a federally sanctioned standard in 2003. Another common nomenclature system is MEDCIN. Nomenclatures are developed by private companies and are adopted or approved for use by government agencies or professional organizations depending on the intended use.

SNOMED-CT

SNOMED-CT is a standardized vocabulary of clinical terminology used by healthcare providers for clinical documentation and reporting, and it is considered the most comprehensive healthcare terminology in the world.

Federal and private developers of EHR systems can purchase a license to incorporate SNOMED-CT in their systems. SNOMED-CT was recommended and adopted as a federal Consolidated Health Informatics standard. However, even with the federal adoption of SNOMED-CT as a standard, EHR systems have not consistently implemented SNOMED-CT. For example, some facilities use the nomenclature system MEDCIN in their EHR systems.

EXPAND
YOUR LEARNING
To learn more about the SNOMED-CT, and its applications with EHR systems, go to www.paradigmcollege.net/exploringehr/SNOMED to view an informational video.

MEDCIN

MEDCIN, which is a naming system primarily used in physicians' offices, was developed by MediComp Systems, Inc. and is derived from the U.S. Centers for Medicare & Medicaid Services (CMS) guidelines for evaluation and management coding/charges. Because MEDCIN's vocabulary has been mapped to the evaluation and management Current Procedural Terminology (CPT) codes that physicians use for billing their services, EHR systems using MEDCIN assist with the coding and billing processes. Physicians use nearly 300,000 clinical elements in MEDCIN at the point of patient care. In addition to a standard vocabulary, MEDCIN has a developed medical terminology interface that facilitates interoperability in regard to patient information exchange.

Classification Systems

A **classification system**, as used in healthcare, is a standardized coding method that organizes diagnoses and procedures into related groups to facilitate reimbursement, reporting, and clinical research. The two most widely used classification systems are the *International Classification of Diseases* (ICD) and **Current Procedural Terminology (CPT)**. Hospitals, medical offices, long-term care facilities, ambulatory care centers, and many other healthcare institutions use ICD and CPT. Other classification systems include the *Diagnostic and Statistical Manual of Mental Disorders, Fifth Edition* (DSM-5), used to classify psychiatric disorders, the **Healthcare Common**

Procedure Coding System (HCPCS), used to code ancillary services and procedures, and **Current Dental Terminology (CDT)**, used to code dental procedures.

Under the Health Insurance Portability and Accountability Act of 1996 (HIPAA), the U.S. federal government adopted specific code sets for diagnoses and procedures required of healthcare facilities for all billing transactions. These specific code sets include ICD for diagnosis coding in all settings and hospital inpatient procedure coding, CPT for physician services procedures, CDT for dental claims, HCPCS for ancillary services and procedures, and National Drug Codes for drugs.

Purposes of Diagnostic and Procedural Coding

The use of standardized classification systems such as ICD and CPT has a direct impact on healthcare, because the data is used for:

- Reimbursement—enabling healthcare facilities and providers to bill for services and treatment rendered.

- Research—helping researchers with studies and clinical trials.

- Decision making—supporting healthcare systems with operational and strategic planning.

- Public health—assisting the Centers for Disease Control and Prevention (CDC) and other public health programs to monitor contagious diseases and other health risks.

- Quality improvement—aiding healthcare providers with clinical, safety, financial, and operational quality improvement activities.

- Resource utilization—supporting administrative and financial healthcare executives with tracking and monitoring utilization of resources.

- Healthcare policy and payment—assisting government and private agencies with establishing and updating healthcare policies and payment systems.

ICD Coding

The history of ICD can be traced back to the eighteenth century during which a classification system was developed in England and implemented for the statistical study of infant mortality rates. Although the classification system was rudimentary, it served its purpose at the time and accurately estimated an appalling trend: England's 36% child mortality rate before the age of 6 years. William Farr (1807–1883), one of the first medical statisticians, worked with the General Register Office in England and became interested in disease and mortality statistics. Farr used the classification system to categorize diseases by anatomic site and to monitor mortality rates.

Bertillon and the *International List of Causes of Death*

In 1891, the International Statistical Institute of Chicago commissioned Chief of Statistical Services of the City of Paris Jacques Bertillon to create a classification system based on Farr's work. This new classification system, presented to the Institute in 1893, became known as the *Bertillon Classification of Causes of Death* and was referenced as such until its first revision in 1900 when it was renamed the *International List of Causes of Death*. Twenty-six countries, including the United States, began to use and revise the *International List of Causes of Death*.

Emergence of ICD

The *International List of Causes of Death* continued to evolve through several revisions until 1948, when the First World Health Assembly of the World Health Organization (WHO) endorsed the sixth revision of the classification system and renamed it the *Manual of the International Statistical Classification of Diseases, Injuries, and Causes of Death*. This sixth revision marked the beginning of a new era in international vital and health statistics. Governments began to establish national committees on vital and health statistics, correlate statistical activities within their countries, and coordinate statistical activities with other countries and the WHO.

The seventh revision occurred in 1955 and resulted in the revised name *International Classification of Diseases* (ICD), a title in continued use today. The eighth revision (ICD-8) occurred in 1965 and the ninth revision (ICD-9) was published in 1975.

ICD-9

By 1977, the U.S. National Center for Health Statistics convened a steering committee to provide expertise and advice in the development of a clinical modification of ICD-9 to be solely used by the United States. This clinical modification would make it more applicable to the diseases experienced by U.S. patients and would include the level of detail requested by the country's researchers and statisticians. The U.S. version was titled ICD-9, Clinical Modification (ICD-9-CM).

There have been annual updates to the 1977 version of ICD-9-CM to include new codes, delete codes, and modify existing codes. The Coordination and Maintenance Committee of the ICD-9-CM is responsible for maintaining the classification system and is composed of four cooperating parties (American Hospital Association [AHA], CMS, the American Health Information Management Association [AHIMA], and the National Center for Health Statistics). In addition to developing new and revised ICD-9-CM codes, the committee also provides coding guidance for ICD-9-CM and publishes clarifications of coding issues in *Coding Clinic*, published by the AHA. The clarifications of coding questions and issues that are published in *Coding Clinic* are considered official interpretations and guidance of coding issues and must be followed for accurate coding.

ICD-10

None of the revisions to ICD-9 and ICD-9-CM were extensive until the tenth revision (ICD-10) was adopted by the World Health Assembly in 1990. ICD-10 is vastly different from ICD-9. There are approximately 68,000 codes in ICD-10 as compared with approximately 13,000 codes in ICD-9 to allow for more specific coding and reporting of diagnoses and procedures. The format of the ICD-10 codes is also much different than the ICD-9 format. The codes in ICD-9 are primarily numeric (000.1–999.99), with combination alphanumeric codes being limited to three sections, namely the Morphology of Neoplasms (M codes), External Causes of Injury and Poisoning

(E codes), and Factors Influencing Health Status and Contact with Health Services (V codes). All of the ICD-10 codes are alphanumeric codes (A00-T98, V01-Y98, and Z00-Z99). In the United States, ICD-10-Clinical Modification/Procedure Coding System (ICD-10-CM/PCS) must be implemented by all healthcare organizations on October 1, 2014. The ICD-10-CM/PCS classification system was originally scheduled for implementation in the United States on October 1, 2013. Both the AHA and the American Medical Association (AMA) requested a delay to allow healthcare providers and organizations time to fully prepare and test systems to ensure a smooth transition from ICD-9 to ICD-10.

ICD-11

EXPAND YOUR LEARNING

The WHO was created by the United Nations in 1948 and is responsible for providing leadership on global health matters, shaping the health research agenda, setting norms and standards, articulating evidence-based policy options, providing technical support to countries, and monitoring and assessing global health trends. The WHO also provides training tools for projects such as ICD-10. To identify these tools, conduct a search of the organization's website at www.paradigmcollege.net/exploringehr/WHO_ICD.

ICD-11 is in development and will likely be implemented in the United States sometime around 2020. Experts have realized that waiting 38 years to update from ICD-9 to ICD-10 was not in the best interest of the healthcare industry or the population as a whole, and are now committed to more frequently updating the ICD classification system. Such updates are vital to keep up with the progress of medicine and healthcare information technology, as well as to improve the foundation for international comparisons. Emerging diseases and scientific developments, combined with advances in service delivery, medical technologies, and health information systems, require a revision of this global classification system. One major need is to improve the relevance of the ICD system in primary care settings, such as clinics and physician offices, which are the sites where most people are treated. The alpha draft process of ICD-11 began in 2009, with the beta draft process following shortly in 2011. The ICD-11 final draft will be submitted to the WHO by 2014, with an expected worldwide implementation date of October 2015. However, the United States will be an exception to the global adoption of ICD-11, because the country is not expected to implement ICD-11 until sometime after the year 2020. The reason for this delay is the projected time frame (five years or longer) to clinically modify the WHO version of ICD-11.

CPT Coding

CPT is the classification system that describes medical, surgical, and diagnostic services and is used to report the procedures and services rendered to patients, including all surgical, radiologic, and anesthetic procedures, as well as other diagnostic screenings such as laboratory and pathology studies. The sites of these services include hospitals, nursing homes, medical offices, and other patient care facilities. CPT codes are used to report procedures and services when billing both private and public insurance companies.

CPT is published by the AMA and is in its fourth edition. The AMA is also responsible for the creation and maintenance of the CPT codes. A CPT editorial panel meets three times per year to discuss issues associated with new and emerging technologies as well as difficulties encountered with procedures and services and their relation to CPT codes. The panel is composed of 17 members. Eleven are nominated by the AMA and the remaining six individuals are nominated by entities such as private insurance companies or professional healthcare organizations.

The CPT Coding Manual is updated every January; therefore, individuals who use CPT codes must stay current and always use the most current manual to bill for services. There are approximately 7,800 CPT codes ranging from 00100 through 99499.

In addition, two-digit modifiers may be added to certain CPT codes to clarify or modify the description of the procedure.

HCPCS

CPT codes are part of the Healthcare Common Procedure Coding System (HCPCS). HCPCS—pronounced "hick picks"—is divided into Levels I and II. Level I of HCPCS is composed of CPT codes and is used to bill physician services and procedures. Level II of HCPCS is commonly referred to as National Codes and is primarily used to bill for products, supplies, and services not included in the CPT codes, such as ambulance services, durable medical equipment, prosthetics, orthotics, and supplies. HCPCS codes are published annually by the CMS.

CDT Coding

The Code on Dental Procedures and Nomenclatures that is used in the United States is Current Dental Terminology (CDT). CDT is maintained and published by the American Dental Association (ADA). CDT is a set of dental procedural codes used to report all dental services, with the exception of some oral surgery procedures. Dentists use ICD codes to report diagnoses and CDT to report the dental procedures and services. The ADA updates the CDT annually.

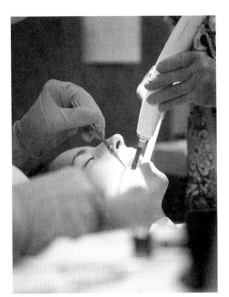

Current Dental Terminology (CDT) is used to code dental services.

DSM-5 Coding

DSM-5 refers to the *Diagnostic and Statistical Manual of Mental Disorders, 5th Edition*. DSM-5, published by the American Psychiatric Association (APA), is a manual that contains codes for every known behavioral health condition. The manual is designed to coincide with ICD, but the two coding systems are not exactly identical. ICD diagnoses codes are used for billing purposes, but they are not detailed enough for researchers, clinicians, policy makers, health insurance companies, pharmaceutical companies, and psychiatric drug regulatory agencies. DSM codes are not included as an approved code in the HIPAA transaction and code set standards for electronic data interchange for billing purposes. Mental health providers rely on DSM as a supportive diagnostic tool; to submit claims for reimbursement purposes, DSM codes are cross-walked to ICD codes. **Crosswalking** is the act of translating a code in one code set to a code in another code set.

CHECKP⊕INT 9.1

1. List three purposes of diagnostic and procedural coding.

   a. _____

   b. _____

   c. _____

2. What is the implementation date of ICD-10 in the United States? _____

3. In what year is ICD-11 expected to be implemented in the United States? _____

WHO USES WHAT

ICD-9-CM/PCS and **ICD-10-CM/PCS** are used in the United States to code for diagnosis coding in all settings and hospital inpatient procedure coding.

CPT is used in the United States to code outpatient procedures for facility coding, as well as all physician services rendered (regardless of the setting).

DSM-5 codes are used by the psychiatric community to more specifically code disorders such as major mental, learning, substance abuse, and personality disorders; intellectual disabilities; acute medical conditions; physical disorders; and psychosocial and environmental factors that contribute to the mental disorders for nonbilling purposes.

CDT is used to code dental procedures. The CDT codes are used in conjunction with ICD codes for billing purposes.

Code Assignment

Traditionally, coders have used hard- or soft-cover coding manuals to assign ICD, CPT, and DSM-5 diagnostic and procedure codes. Depending on the classification system, coders have used as many as three books at a time, such as when coding with ICD-9-CM. For those healthcare organizations with a low volume of health records to code, the use of coding manuals may be effective. However, with high volumes of health records to code, using several cumbersome manuals slows down the coding process. To remedy the situation, clinical encoders/groupers were adopted by these high-volume facilities in the 1990s. However, it is important to note that many coding certification exams require the test taker to code from coding books. Therefore, classroom instruction often focuses on coding from manuals to ensure that students understand how the coding classification systems work and how to apply that knowledge when they take their certification exams.

Clinical Encoders and Diagnostic-Related Groups

A **clinical encoder** is a software program that helps coding professionals navigate coding pathways with the end result of assigning codes and **diagnostic-related groups (DRGs)**. A DRG is a patient classification system that groups hospital patients of similar age, sex, diagnoses, and treatments. Each DRG is associated with a specific dollar amount that the hospital expects to be reimbursed for in relation to the treatment provided. The first DRG system—Medicare **Inpatient Prospective Payment System (IPPS)**—was implemented in 1983 to reimburse acute care hospitals for the treatment of Medicare patients. Since then, many other payers, such as Medicaid and commercial payers, have adopted the Medicare DRG system for the reimbursement of inpatient care of their insured members. The purpose of a DRG system is to relatively equalize payments to hospitals for providing the

Medicare and Medicaid patients may be grouped together using a Diagnostic Related Group classification system for coding purposes.

same care to patients with the same clinical characteristics. Prior to the implementation of the Medicare DRG system, acute care hospitals were reimbursed for whatever they charged Medicare or other payers. Take a look at a simplified example of pre-DRG and post-DRG payments for two patient scenarios in the "Consider This" box below.

Consider This

Patient A
Final principal diagnosis:
acute respiratory failure
Principal procedure: mechanical ventilation, more than 96 hours

Patient B
Final principal diagnosis:
acute myocardial infarction
Principal procedure: coronary artery bypass

Hospital Name	Patient A Reimbursement Prior to Medicare DRG ($)	Patient A Reimbursement After Medicare DRG ($)	Patient B Reimbursement Prior to Medicare DRG ($)	Patient B Reimbursement After Medicare DRG ($)
City Hospital	63,588	47,184	24,160	33,238
Tender Care Hospital	52,140	47,184	44,321	33,238
Bayview Hospital	38,690	47,184	45,870	33,238
Grace Hospital	47,545	47,184	63,923	33,238

DRG = diagnostic-related group.

Analyze the table above. Why do reimbursement rates for Patients A and B vary among hospitals in the time prior to the Medicare DRG implementation? Why are the reimbursement rates the same for Patients A and B among the hospitals, under the Medicare DRG system? Under the Medicare DRG system, why is the reimbursement for Patient A not the same as Patient B?

Consider This

Through the Medicare Inpatient Prospective Payment System (IPPS), the U.S. federal government spends $90 billion to $100 billion every year in payments to acute care hospitals for inpatient care. Because the IPPS depends on diagnostic and procedural coding to calculate the payments to the acute care hospitals, what would happen if coding staff incorrectly coded charts 10% of the time?

EXPAND
YOUR LEARNING

Learn more about the IPPS by visiting to following link:

www.paradigmcollege.net/exploringehr/medicare_IPPS

Coding and the EHR

The use of an EHR system has a positive impact on the coding of health records. It provides efficient concurrent and final coding processes, greater accuracy in code assignments, and improved access to health records.

Efficient Concurrent and Final Coding

For coders, an EHR system can perform **concurrent coding**, which is the task of coding while a patient is still receiving treatment in a hospital. This concurrent coding process accelerates the final coding process that is completed upon discharge of the patient, by allowing coders to query healthcare providers for necessary documentation regarding diagnoses and procedures over the course of a particular patient's stay. Consequently, the coder has all the documentation needed upon patient discharge to allow for final coding.

The financial managers of healthcare organizations promote concurrent coding because the process speeds up final billing procedures, thereby reducing the number of unbilled accounts. Health information management (HIM) departments and coding staff, in particular, are held accountable for the inability of an organization to produce final bills to payers due to a lack of final coding.

"Discharged Not Final Billed" Accounts

Final bills are typically held in a suspended status for three days after patient discharge to allow for final charge entry, documentation, insurance verification, and final coding. Patient accounts not able to be final billed to the insurance company or responsible party due to a lack of final coding, insurance verification, or other data errors are considered **Discharged Not Final Billed (DNFB)**. These accounts of discharged patients that have not been final billed are flagged as DNFB and are included on a data report produced by the EHR system. This report is monitored daily by health information managers, coders, and other staff members in healthcare organizations. For coders, this report highlights the oldest outstanding accounts and the accounts with the highest unbilled account balances. The EHR system further assists the coder by providing coding **work-list** reports. These reports present the patient accounts for coding in a priority order, beginning with the oldest accounts with the highest balances. For those coders who use physical paper records rather than an EHR system, the main contributor to a DNFB list is the delay in locating the paper record.

Accuracy in Code Assignments

As you have already learned in Chapters 1 and 2, EHRs eliminate the problems of illegible handwriting that exist in most paper health records. Illegible handwriting can result in inaccurate coding when coders miss or miscode diagnoses because they cannot read the healthcare provider's handwriting. The EHR also improves coding through more accurate documentation. Physicians may be prompted to enter more information based on their entries in the EHR system. EHRs can therefore reduce the number of errors due to incomplete or vague diagnostic or procedural information.

Clinical encoder software windows are open and functional as the coder navigates through the EHR. As a result, the clinical coder can read and enter the patient's diagnoses and procedures rendered to a patient into the encoder resulting in the applicable codes. The coder may automatically generate physician queries and highlight or make notations to the EHR that do not change or affect the legality of the health record. A **physician query** is a request, typically from a coder or a case manager, to add documentation to the health record that clarifies a diagnosis or procedure performed. Physician queries may be issued to providers concurrently or retrospectively. AHIMA has published best practice guidance on the query process in its *Guidelines for Achieving a Compliant Query Practice*. In an EHR, all physician queries are automatically routed to the appropriate physician's message inbox and displayed when the physician logs in to the system.

The use of clinical encoders and physician queries assists coders in establishing the most accurate code assignments. Accurate code assignments, in turn, result in appropriate reimbursement for healthcare organizations. Although organizations must ensure that health record documentation is complete and accurate, its staff members cannot educate or encourage physicians to document simply for the purpose of claiming a higher paying DRG and, therefore, increased reimbursement. This maneuver is referred to as **upcoding** and is illegal. Unintentional upcoding is considered **abuse**, whereas intentional upcoding is considered **fraud**. Those convicted of fraud or abuse may receive monetary fines or jail time.

Computer-Assisted Coding Programs

Some EHR systems incorporate **computer-assisted coding (CAC)** programs that automatically assign diagnosis and procedure codes based on electronic documentation, which can increase the productivity of a coder by up to 20%. However, the use of a CAC program does not mean that the coding process is completely automated. When CAC programs are used, the coder assumes the role of a reviewer or an auditor. The coder must validate the codes, ensure that coding guidelines have been followed, and validate whether or not the coded diagnoses were **present on admission (POA)**, meaning the patient had the diagnoses when he or she was admitted to the facility. All primary and secondary diagnoses require POA indicators to be reported on the Medicare claims of IPPS general acute care hospitals. POA indicator assignment is determined by the coder based on clinical documentation entered into the health record by the provider.

Coders must exercise care in assigning POA indicators. Medicare patients who experience diagnoses and conditions that are **hospital acquired**, meaning that they developed when the patient was an inpatient in the hospital, must not be reported as POA. The care and treatment of these hospital-acquired diagnoses and conditions (e.g., hospital-acquired pressure ulcer, urinary tract infection, pneumonia) are typically not reimbursed by Medicare.

EXPAND
YOUR LEARNING

To learn more about present on admission indicators and reduced Medicare reimbursement for hospital-acquired conditions, review the following websites:

www.paradigmcollege
.net/exploringehr/
medicare_POA

www.paradigmcollege
.net/exploringehr/
medicare_HAC

Improved Access to Health Records

For coders, an EHR system affords easy access to health records from any work site. Consequently, coding can be performed by **remote coders** who value the autonomy and flexibility of working from home. This work setup also benefits healthcare organizations by allowing hiring personnel to recruit top-notch coders from across the country.

Although implementation of an EHR system can be challenging for both healthcare organizations and personnel, the use of this type of technology can streamline coding as well as other record-keeping processes.

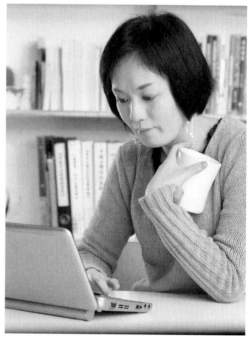

Remote coders are able to code from home using an EHR system.

CHECKP⊕INT 9.2

1. List three ways in which the EHR benefits the coding process.

   a. _____

   b. _____

   c. _____

2. True or False: A successful healthcare organization uses upcoding to ensure that the best DRG is selected for billing. Discuss why you chose true or false.

   _____

   _____

Activity 9.1 | **EHR**NAVIGAT⊕R

Coding a Patient's Record

Go to the Course Navigator to launch Activity 9.1. As an RHIT, practice coding a patient's record using the EHR Navigator.

Billing and Reimbursement

The billing process in healthcare is part of the **revenue cycle management**. The Healthcare Financial Management Association (HFMA) defines the revenue cycle as "all administrative and clinical functions that contribute to the capture, management, and collection of patient service revenue." The revenue cycle begins with the registration or admission of a patient and ends with collection and posting of payments. Figure 9.1 shows the revenue cycle management process. A healthcare organization that has a well-managed revenue cycle will experience a timelier, increased cash flow which in turn translates into higher revenues. To understand revenue cycle management or the billing process for medical claims, healthcare personnel should be familiar with the reimbursement process. Healthcare reimbursement is a complex subject in a state of constant flux. Patients have witnessed this changing landscape as they struggle to keep abreast of the varying health insurance rules. Employers have also had to navigate changes in healthcare insurance coverage and escalating costs. Consequently, they have had to frequently shop around to find the best insurance plans for their employees while keeping costs in mind. Healthcare delivery systems must also take into account Medicare and Medicaid laws, insurance contracts, workers' compensation

Figure 9.1 Revenue Cycle Management

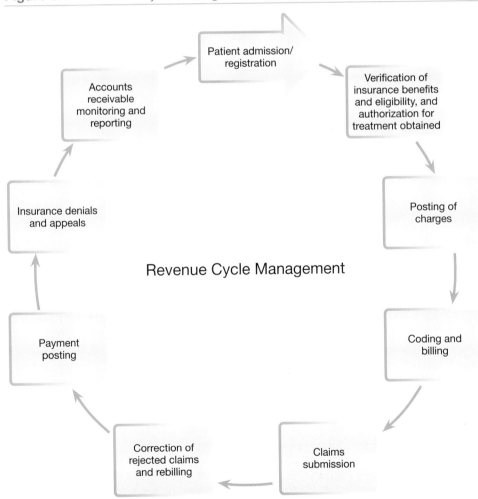

laws, Veterans Administration regulations, and other payer rules. Billers and reimbursement staff must stay well informed of all billing rules and contracts to effectively perform their jobs. Staying current in the changing healthcare environment can be a daunting task. To meet this challenge, billers and reimbursement specialists must participate in formal and informal education and training to achieve compliance.

The main sources of reimbursement for the provision of healthcare services include government-sponsored insurance plans (Medicare, Medicaid, TRICARE, Civilian Health and Medical Program of the Veterans Administration), commercial insurance plans, and self-pay plans.

Patients who participate in some type of healthcare insurance plan are called **insured patients**. Patients who do not have any type of insurance coverage must pay for healthcare services themselves and are called **self-pay patients**.

Types of Insurance Plans

The insurance plans of insured patients are classified as either managed care plans or indemnity plans. A **managed care plan** is a type of insurance plan offered by a carrier who has negotiated and contracted with healthcare providers to provide healthcare services for their subscribers. The insured patient (called the subscriber) is responsible for following the rules of the managed care plan, including receiving services from the contracted healthcare providers. The trade-off for this lack of flexibility in selecting providers is cost-effective insurance coverage. An **indemnity plan** is commonly thought of as a traditional insurance plan. Insured patients have the freedom to obtain healthcare from the providers of their choice in exchange for higher premiums, deductibles, and out-of-pocket expenses. Understanding the scope of these types of insurance plans is critical to billers and reimbursement specialists as they perform their daily tasks and procedures.

Billing and Reimbursement Process

As you learned in Chapter 4, **admission/registration clerks** (sometimes also called patient access specialists) are generally responsible for entering insurance information into the EHR system at the time the patient is admitted to an inpatient hospital or scheduled for treatment at an outpatient facility or physician's office. Following insurance data entry, the admission/registration clerk or **insurance verifier** must confirm with the insurance company the patient's insurance coverage. The purpose of this insurance verification process is twofold: (1) to ensure that the patient has active coverage, and (2) to determine important billing aspects of the insurance plan such as the guarantor, guarantor information, covered dependents, co-payments, deductibles, and any other limitations or payment rules.

The **guarantor** is the individual responsible for payment. An example might be a man who obtains health insurance coverage through his employer for himself as well as his spouse and children. In such an example, the man is the guarantor or subscriber, and the spouse and children are **covered dependents**.

A **co-payment** is the amount that an insured individual must pay for healthcare services received, typically office visits, urgent care visits, or emergency department encounters. These services might be provided by staff members in a healthcare facility or by personnel in a pharmacy. A co-payment must be paid by the insured patient upon each visit to one of these facilities.

A **deductible** is the amount an insured individual must pay out of pocket before the insurance will pay. This payment must be met before insurance coverage can be applied to healthcare services. For example, a family insurance plan may have a $25 co-payment every time a parent takes his or her sick child to the pediatrician. That same family may have a deductible of $800 a year for healthcare services such as laboratory tests, X-rays, and hospitalizations before their insurance provider pays the remaining balance of any services rendered. Once the bill has been submitted to the insurance company, the deductible is calculated. The insurance company sends payment to the healthcare facility and sends the guarantor a copy of the Explanation of Benefits (EOB). The EOB describes the detail of how the insurance company paid the healthcare bill. The healthcare facility subsequently bills the guarantor for the remaining balance of the bill that the insurance company did not pay.

A sample EOB is found in Figure 9.2.

Figure 9.2 Explanation of Benefits

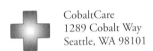

EXPLANATION OF BENEFITS

CobaltCare
1289 Cobalt Way
Seattle, WA 98101

Alana Feltner, MD
Northstar Medical Center
Cincinnati, OH 45202

Date:	02/01/2017
Tax ID #:	01010101
Check #:	10101010
Check amount:	

Patient Name: Minako Saito
Patient Account Number: 129789327
Patient ID#: 1856390
Member ID: 58205

Treatment Date	Product or Service	Submitted Charges	Allowed Amount	Your Responsibility
06/26/2017	Physical Therapy	$135.00	$60.00	$75.00
06/26/2017	X-ray	$200.00	$150.00	$50.00

Posting payments, insurance appeals, and collections is the last step in the billing or revenue cycle. At this point in the revenue cycle, the focus is on making sure the healthcare organization receives the correct amount of reimbursement for the treatment and services rendered. When insurance companies do not pay correctly, healthcare organizations will go through an appeals process to request additional payment from the insurance companies. When individuals owe the healthcare organization monies and do not pay in a timely manner, the healthcare organizations will initiate a formal collections process.

EHR and Billing Operations

Most EHR systems have a billing software component that may or may not be used by the healthcare organization. The decision to use the EHR's billing component depends on the sophistication of the organization's current billing software. Smaller healthcare organizations and physician practices are more likely to utilize the billing software component that comes with the EHR system that they implement. Hospitals and large physician practices are likely to already have a well-functioning billing system and may choose to interface it with the EHR system instead. An **interface** provides communication flow between two or more computer systems. If a healthcare organization chooses to interface the EHR system with the current billing/financial system, the patient record is easily accessible, which is an advantage to the billing staff. Regardless of which approach a healthcare organization chooses, an EHR system can have a positive impact on billing operations, including improved accuracy and efficiency of procedures.

Improved Accuracy

The implementation of an EHR system allows for better accuracy in healthcare claims. The software can check for billing errors as well as speed up the billing process. Faster billing typically improves cash flow for the healthcare facility. Using the EHR system for billing purposes may also eliminate having to chase down papers at the end of the business day. The system allows for daily charges to be reconciled and for staff to more easily determine what services and treatments were provided.

Improved Efficiency

In addition to improved accuracy, the use of an EHR system increases the efficiency of the billing process. No longer are patients and insurance companies provided with paper bills sent via the mail. EHR software provides electronic billing and insurance forms, accesses the Internet to securely send electronic bills or reminders to patients, submits claims to insurance companies and tracks their progress, checks for billing errors, provides data analysis tools related to medical office billing and finance, and more. All of these features allow for increased efficiency of the billing cycle, resulting in fewer rejected claims and a more robust monetary flow for the healthcare practice.

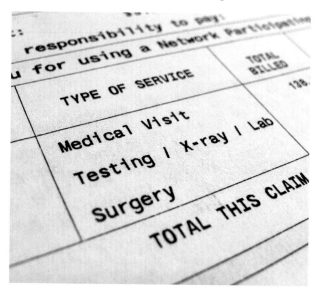

EHRs can eliminate the need for paper bills, improving efficiency of the billing process.

Superbills

A **superbill** (also known as an encounter form) is a staple of every physician office because it is a document that records the diagnosis and treatment for each patient at each visit. The content of superbills varies by healthcare organization and contains the common diagnoses and procedures experienced by the healthcare organization. The superbill contains checkboxes next to the diagnoses, procedures and associated ICD and CPT codes that are marked by the healthcare provider, such as the physician, nurse, or other healthcare provider. Traditionally, a superbill has been a paper document that the patient carries from the check-in desk to the examination room and to areas of testing such as the laboratory and radiology department. The electronic version of the superbill found in many EHR systems for use in the physician office and outpatient setting looks very similar to the paper superbill that physicians and staff are used to. Figure 9.3 illustrates an electronic superbill.

Figure 9.3 Electronic Superbill

Name:	Donaldson, Vance	Insurance:	CobaltCare	DOS:	03/5/2017
Age:	42	Visit Reason:	B-12 injection		

Qty	I/P	Code	Description	Mod	ICD Pointers
			New Patient		
		99201	New PT Level 1		
		99202	New PT Level 2		
		99203	New PT Level 3		
		99204	New PT Level 4		
		99205	New PT Level 5	12	
		99206	Case Code 1		
			Procedures		
		20551	Inj. Tendon		
		20552	TPI 1-2 muscle grps		
		20553	TPI 3 or more muscle grps		
		20600	Inj. Small Joint		
		20605	Inj. Med. Joint		
		20610	Inj. Major Joint		
		27093	Hip Arthrocentosis W. Flouro		
		27098	S1 Joint Injection		

When used correctly the superbill is a useful tool in coding compliance activities. With the selection of the ICD and CPT codes placed in the hands of the individual providing the healthcare service or treatment, coding should be accurate and consistent. When superbills are used, there must still be a review of the healthcare provider's documentation to ensure that the documentation supports the diagnoses and procedures selected on the superbill. The coder that performs this review is verifying that the healthcare provider's superbill diagnoses and procedures selections are appropriate based on the healthcare provider's documentation in the health record. There must be frequent communication between the coder and the provider to ensure that the provider's superbill documentation and health record documentation are in synch.

Bills marked for final billing will automatically be transmitted to the appropriate payer. Prior to transmission to the insurance companies, the bills are checked for errors by a software program called a **claim scrubber**, which checks thousands of edits and billing rules. If the claim scrubber finds an error, it generates an error report for the billing supervisor or staff to review and correct prior to transmission of the final bill to the payer.

Following transmission of the final bill to the payer, the EHR system automatically updates to reflect the name of the payer, the date, and amount billed. The billing supervisor of the physician practice will receive a report automatically delivered to an email address that lists the accounts billed.

Payments from payers may come in the form of electronic funds transfer or a check. The billing supervisor will receive a **Remittance Advice (RA)** that lists the patient's information and amount paid by Medicare or other payer to the physician practice.

Chapter Summary

Electronic health record (EHR) systems are revolutionizing the reimbursement, clinical coding, and billing processes. Some of the benefits of EHR implementation include easy access to clinical records by the coding and billing staff, more efficient methods of coding of health records, a streamlined physician query process, improved documentation by providers and improved fiscal management of healthcare organizations.

Classification systems are used for reimbursement, research, decision making, public health, quality improvement, resource utilization, and healthcare policy and payment. The types of classification systems used depends on the types of services one is coding. Common coding classification systems include International Classification of Diseases (ICD), Current Procedural Terminology (CPT), Diagnostic Statistical Manual of Mental Disorders, Fifth Edition (DSM-5), and Current Dental Terminology (CDT).

To assist with the coding process, a coder may use a clinical encoder software program and classify patients by their diagnostic-related group (DRG).

The billing process in healthcare is part of the revenue cycle management. The revenue cycle begins with registration or admission and ends with collection and posting of payments.

Checks and balances must be put in place in an EHR environment just as they should in a paper environment as coders must still follow official coding guidelines, physicians and healthcare providers must thoroughly and accurately document procedures and diagnoses, and billing staff must generate accurate bills and post proper payments.

EHR Review

Check Your Understanding

To check your understanding of this chapter's key concepts, read the following multiple-choice and true/false questions and then record your answers on a separate sheet of paper. Write your answers as modeled in these examples: 1a; 2b; 6T; 7F; etc.

1. The following are all examples of classification systems *except*:

    a. MEDCIN

    b. *International Classification of Diseases* (ICD)

    c. Current Procedural Terminology (CPT)

    d. *Diagnostic and Statistical Manual of Mental Disorders, Fifth Edition* (DSM-5)

2. Which of the following classification systems is used to code outpatient procedures and inpatient and outpatient provider services?

    a. Current Dental Terminology

    b. ICD-10-CM

    c. DSM-5

    d. CPT

3. How does the implementation of an electronic health record (EHR) system affect the process of coding health records?

    a. It allows for more efficient coding.

    b. It increases the accuracy of code assignments.

    c. It eliminates the physician query process.

    d. It allows for more efficient coding and increases the accuracy of code assignments.

4. How does the use of an EHR system benefit the billing processes?

    a. It improves claims accuracy.

    b. It accelerates the billing process.

    c. It improves efficiency.

    d. All of the above.

5. What software program reviews bills for possible errors prior to their transmission to the insurance companies?

    a. Claim scrubber

    b. Billing checker

    c. Superbill scourer

    d. Remittance reviewer

6. True/False: The term *nomenclature* refers to a standardized method of assigning codes to diagnoses and procedures.

7. True/False: Concurrent coding is an easy process to perform with paper records but is made more difficult with the use of an EHR system.

8. True/False: The insurance plans of insured patients are classified either as managed care or indemnity plans.

9. True/False: The Explanation of Benefits is a report received by a billing supervisor that lists the patient's information and amount paid by Medicare or other payer to the physician practice or healthcare facility.

10. True/False: The use of standardized classification systems has a direct impact on healthcare.

Learn the Terms

Go to the Course Navigator to access flashcards for Chapter 9 of *Exploring Electronic Health Records.*

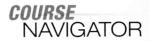
COURSE NAVIGATOR

Acronyms

ADA: American Dental Association

AHA: American Hospital Association

AHIMA: American Health Information Management Association

AMA: American Medical Association

CAC: Computer-Assisted Coding

CDC: Centers for Disease Control and Prevention

CDT: Current Dental Terminology

CMS: Centers for Medicare & Medicaid Services

CPT: Current Procedural Terminology

DNFB: "Discharged Not Final Billed"

DRG: Diagnostic-Related Group

DSM-5: Diagnostic and Statistical Manual of Mental Disorders, Fifth Edition

EOB: Explanation of Benefits

HCPCS: Healthcare Common Procedure Coding System

HFMA: Healthcare Financial Management Association

HIM: Health Information Management

ICD: International Classification of Diseases

IPPS: Inpatient Prospective Payment System

POA: Present on Admission

RA: Remittance Advice

SNOMED-CT: Systemized Nomenclature of Medicine, Clinical Terms

WHO: World Health Organization

EHR Application

Go on the Record

To build on your understanding of the topics in this chapter, complete the following short answer questions.

1. List and describe three purposes of diagnostic and procedural coding.

2. Discuss the differences between *nomenclature* and a *classification system.*

3. Define *clinical encoder* and discuss how this software program assists coding professionals.

4. List three ways in which the electronic health record (EHR) system improves work processes for a coder.

5. Define *physician query* and describe how the process is automated with the EHR system.

Navigate the Field

To gain practice in handling challenging situations in the workplace, consider the following real-world scenarios and then use the guiding questions to help you formulate your responses.

1. You are a coder for Northstar Medical Center. While coding diagnoses for a discharged patient's encounter, you notice that the attending physician has documented that the patient has type 1 diabetes mellitus and a consulting physician has documented that the patient has type II diabetes mellitus. How would you handle this discrepancy?

2. You are the front desk clerk for Northstar Physicians and are in the process of registering a new patient who is a minor. During the registration process, the mother accompanying the patient is confused by the insurance terms *subscriber* and *guarantor*. Consequently, she is unsure how to respond to your requests for information. How should you proceed?

EHR Evaluation

Think Critically

Continue to think critically about challenging real-world scenarios and complete the following activities.

1. As the office manager of a large physician practice, you must ensure that the bills are accurate and reflect the treatment rendered to each patient. In light of recent news events of inaccurate billing by physicians for services not performed, you want to exercise diligence in your billing process. What steps should you take to make sure that the bills generated from your practice are accurate?

2. Conduct an Internet search to identify two clinical encoders that can be interfaced with electronic health record systems. After examining the components of each system, write a proposal to the coding manager of Northstar Physicians that identifies the program you would select and discusses the reasoning behind your choice.

Make Your Case

Consider the following scenario and create a presentation on the following topic.

As the revenue cycle manager for a hospital, you have been asked by the vice president of finance to prepare a short presentation for hospital administrators that addresses how the hospital's electronic health record (EHR) system has benefited the coding and billing processes. For your presentation, include a minimum of five advantages of using an EHR in these processes.

Explore the Technology

To expand your mastery of EHRs, explore the following online and EHR Navigator activities.

COURSE
NAVIGATOR

Ensure you are comfortable with the functionality presented in the EHR Navigator activities, such as coding a patient's record, performing billing activities, and posting a payment from a remittance advice. Then, complete the EHR Navigator assessments for Chapter 9 located on the Course Navigator.

Are You Ready?

Joining a professional organization can help you in every aspect of your career. When you first start out, your connections at a professional organization may alert you to job openings. Professional organizations can help you maintain continuing education requirements associated with professional credentials. As you progress in your career, you may find reaching out to a mentor through a professional organization to be very valuable. You can learn a lot about your field by attending conferences hosted by professional organizations.

What professional organizations serve the health information technology/health information management industry?

What organizations exist for allied health professions in general?

Identify organizations you are interested in and research their membership requirements.

Beyond the Record

- Some common clinical decision support systems (CDSS) include:
  - ESAGIL
  - CADUCEUS
  - DiagnosisPro
  - Dxplain
  - MYCIN
  - RODIA

- A 2005 review of 100 studies showed that CDSSs improved practitioner performance in 65% of the studies.

- CDSSs improved patient outcomes in 13% of the studies.

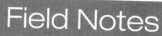

Field Notes

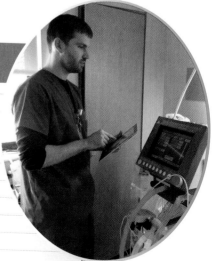

EHR has drastically improved communication and continuity for our pulmonary patients. This integrative technology has allowed clinicians to thoroughly review ventilator weaning tolerance from previous facilities and implement achievable goals in improving patient outcomes.

— Tom Frye, RRT
Manager, Respiratory Therapy

Chapter 10

Clinical Decision Support Systems and Quality Improvement

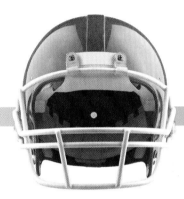

EHRs in the News

The National Football League (NFL) plans to implement an electronic health record (EHR) system for each of its 32 teams by the start of the 2014 season. Because NFL players often move to different teams, an NFL-wide EHR system would allow their records to be accessed no matter what team they are playing on. The system will include features unique to the NFL, such as video footage of injuries occurring and a sideline concussion assessment tool. These features will assist healthcare providers of the NFL in creating treatment plans for players off the field.

- Define *clinical decision support system (CDSS)*.

- Define the two types of CDSSs.

- Discuss the knowledge-based CDSS.

- Discuss the advantages and disadvantages of using a CDSS.

- List the most common uses of clinical decision support in healthcare.

- Explain the requirements of the Centers for Medicare & Medicaid Services (CMS) for the clinical decision support rule as part of meaningful use core measures.

- Demonstrate clinical decision support activities in electronic health record (EHR) software, and discuss the role of EHRs in clinical decision support.

- Discuss the role of the EHR in quality improvement.

As you have learned throughout this text, electronic health records (EHRs) improve the quality of patient care in many different ways. One of the most significant ways is through the incorporation of clinical decision support systems. A **clinical decision support system (CDSS)** assists healthcare providers with decision-making tasks such as determining diagnoses, choosing the best medications to order for a patient, and selecting proper diagnostic tests. The CDSS filters EHR data available for a specific patient, producing information based on current healthcare knowledge and interactions among physicians and other healthcare providers to assist them in making decisions that will result in the highest quality of care. This chapter will discuss CDSSs in detail and explore the federal mandates that require healthcare providers to use EHR systems with CDSSs.

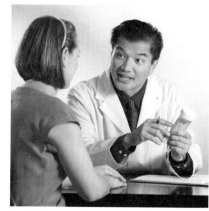

A CDSS can help physicians choose the right medications for a patient.

In addition to CDSSs, the role of EHRs in healthcare quality improvement activities will be discussed. Healthcare providers and organizations constantly strive to improve processes, policies, and procedures that result in higher quality outcomes. Through data gathering and analysis, EHRs play a significant role in assisting healthcare organizations in these quality improvement activities.

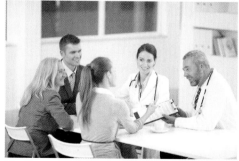

Healthcare organizations work together to improve policies and procedures.

Clinical Decision Support

There are a number of definitions of clinical decision support. The Centers for Medicare & Medicaid Services (CMS) define clinical decision support in relation to the meaningful use standards as, "health information technology that builds upon the foundation of an EHR to provide persons involved in care decisions with general and person-specific information, intelligently filtered and organized, at point of care, to enhance health and healthcare."

The simplest rendition of a CDSS is any tool that helps healthcare providers make a better clinical decision. Examples of CDSS tools include computerized alerts and reminders, clinical guidelines, standardized order sets, patient data results and reports, documentation templates, diagnostic support, and clinical workflow tools.

There are two basic types of CDSSs, knowledge-based and non–knowledge-based. Most CDSSs are **knowledge-based** and utilize inference software and databases containing the most current medical, scientific, and research information. Non–knowledge-based CDSSs utilize artificial intelligence software to study and learn from data and patterns of medical practice.

CDSSs may also be stand-alone systems or an integrated component of an EHR. For purposes of this discussion, this chapter will focus on the knowledge-based CDSS as an integrated component of an EHR.

A knowledge-based CDSS integrated with an EHR is a good example of semantic interoperability. The data may be shared, exchanged, and interpreted. See Figure 10.1 for an example of a knowledge-based CDSS integrated with an EHR. This figure illustrates how the three components of EHR data, scientific evidence and research, and physician experience, work together to make up the CDSS.

Figure 10.1   Knowledge-based CDSS Integrated with EHR

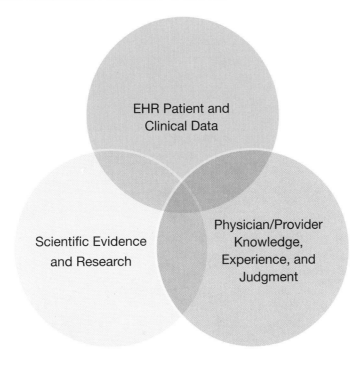

A knowledge-based CDSS integrated with an EHR is effective because it utilizes these three components:

1. Subjective and objective clinical patient data from the EHR

2. State-of-the-art scientific evidence and research

3. Physician knowledge, experience, and judgment

Benefits and Disadvantages of Using a CDSS

Using a CDSS has numerous benefits, the most significant of which improve quality of care and healthcare delivery through:

- reduced risk of medication errors.

- reduced risk of misdiagnosis.

- increased direct patient care time for healthcare providers.

- access to state-of-the-art data, research, clinical pathways, and guidelines.

- reduction of unnecessary diagnostic tests.

- faster diagnoses, resulting in faster treatments.

- prescriptions for lower cost medications.

However, using a CDSS also has potential disadvantages, including the following:

- high costs of maintaining the CDSS with up-to-date medical research, clinical pathways, guidelines, medication costs, and so forth.

- potential over-reliance on computer technology.

- perception by healthcare providers as a threat to clinical knowledge and skills.

- harmful outcomes if software is not thoroughly and continuously updated.

CHECKPOINT 10.1

1. Define a clinical decision support system.

_____

_____

_____

2. List two types of clinical decision support systems.

a. _____

b. _____

3. List three advantages and three potential disadvantages of using a clinical decision support system.

a. _____

b. _____

c. _____

d. _____

e. _____

f. _____

Most Common Uses of a CDSS

The most common uses of a CDSS in healthcare involve clinical needs such as alerting providers to possible drug interactions, assisting with establishment of correct diagnoses, screening for preventable diseases, and accessing state-of-the-art treatment options. In addition to clinical needs, the CDSS also addresses administrative and financial needs of the healthcare organization by assisting with cost reductions and improving patient satisfaction and provider efficiency. This is accomplished by using CDSS tools to minimize length of hospital stay, alert staff of duplicate testing orders, and increase patient–provider communication. Table 10.1 identifies common uses of a CDSS.

Table 10.1 Common Uses of a Clinical Decision Support System

Use	Examples
Alerts	Drug–drug alerts
	Drug–food interactions
	Duplicate testing alerts
	Abnormal laboratory results
Diagnoses	Suggestions for possible diagnoses that match patient signs and symptoms
Treatment Options	Treatment options and guidelines for specific diagnoses
	Medication recommendations
Preventive Care	Immunization due-date alerts
	Diagnostic screening
	Disease management/prevention
Hospital/Provider Efficiency	Care plans and treatment to minimize length of stay
	Standardized order sets
	Suggestions for lower cost medications and testing
Cost Reductions and Improved Patient Satisfaction	Duplicate testing alerts
	Drug formulary guidelines
	Faster diagnoses and treatment

Alerts

CDSS components of the EHR Navigator alert the healthcare provider in the following activity to an attempt to place a duplicate order for computed tomography. Although the healthcare provider has an opportunity to place a duplicate order, alerting him or her to the duplication may avoid unnecessary costs.

Activity 10.1	**EHR**NAVIGAT**+**R

Adding an Order

Go to the Course Navigator to launch Activity 10.1. As a physician, practice adding an order using the EHR Navigator.

A common use of a CDSS is to prevent adverse drug interactions. Interoperability of EHR systems can save time, money, and patient lives. For example, a primary care clinic may enter a patient's common prescriptions into the EHR. However, if the patient goes to the hospital and the emergency department does not have access to that list of medications, then the risk for adverse drug interactions increases. The emergency department staff may prescribe a medication that interacts with the patient's regular prescriptions if the staff is unaware of possible interactions. A CDSS component of an EHR compares the list of the patient's prescriptions with the new prescription, alerting the prescriber if there is a potential interaction.

Consider This

A patient enters an emergency department with shoulder pain and is diagnosed with minor inflammation of his shoulder. The healthcare provider prescribes an anti-inflammatory medication to resolve the inflammation, which eliminates his symptoms of pain.

Two months later, the patient returns to the emergency department with stomach bleeding and pain. He is diagnosed with a bleeding ulcer caused by an interaction between the anti-inflammatory medication he took for his shoulder and his regular hypertension medicine. Did the emergency department use an EHR with access to a list of the patient's medications? How would a CDSS help to prevent this scenario?

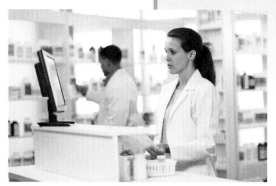

A CDSS alerts prescribers of possible drug interactions.

Alert Fatigue Are more alerts always better? A phenomenon commonly known as alert fatigue has become a significant issue for healthcare organizations following CDSS implementation. Healthcare providers may experience **alert fatigue** after encountering excessive numbers of alerts, such as drug–drug, telemetry, and out-of-normal range laboratory results, within the EHR system. The provider may ignore such alerts without studying each one due to the large amount they encounter in daily practice. The consequences of alert fatigue may be life-threatening if a provider inadvertently ignores a serious alert. Therefore, to reduce the chances of alert fatigue, the thresholds of when an alert is triggered in a CDSS must be set at an appropriate level, which can be accomplished by defining policies regarding the types of results (normal, abnormal, and critical) that trigger an alert. Medical staff should be instrumental in determining thresholds to ensure continued buy-in regarding alert delivery from the CDSS. Constant monitoring of these thresholds is imperative to ensure that healthcare providers are alerted when significant or potentially significant care concerns arise. Provider feedback regarding the types of valuable alerts is also important.

Drug–Drug Interaction

Go to the Course Navigator to launch Activity 10.2. As a physician, experience what happens when a drug–drug alert occurs in the EHR Navigator.

Diagnoses

A CDSS can assist physicians in diagnosing patient conditions based on a variety of factors. For example, a college student may present at the emergency department with a high fever, stomach pains, stomach bleeding, appetite loss, headache, and weakness. Routine laboratory results only reveal an elevated white blood cell count. The patient is then admitted for further testing and diagnosis. The attending physician uses the CDSS integrated with the hospital's EHR system, which searches the patient's EHR, filters the information, and suggests a diagnosis of typhoid fever based on the patient's symptoms and a documented recent trip to Kenya. Based on the suggestion from the CDSS, the attending physician agrees with this possibility and orders a special laboratory study for *Salmonella typhi*. The test result is positive for the bacteria and the physician begins treatment.

Treatment Options

CDSSs can also monitor treatment options and assist physicians in keeping up with the latest advancements in medicine. For example, an oncologist using the CDSS component of his or her practice's EHR system can review the latest research trials for all types of carcinoma treatments and offer his or her patients choices if traditional treatment options are unsuccessful.

Preventive Care

Good preventive care has a host of benefits. Patients stay healthier when they go to their physicians for routine, preventive care, which in turn can help healthcare facilities save money by catching health issues earlier.

For example, a physician's practice may have a patient population with a high percentage of patients with diabetes. Because of the significant health risks associated with undiagnosed diabetes, a physician's practice may routinely use the preventive screening aspect of the CDSS to identify patients at risk for diabetes. According to the American Diabetes Association, anyone with a body mass index above 25 who has additional risk factors such as high blood pressure and high cholesterol

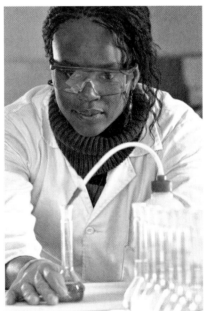

A CDSS allows practitioners to track the latest scientific research.

levels is at risk for diabetes. Therefore, a physician's practice may routinely run reports to identify at-risk patients, sending alerts via their preferred method of contact to ask these patients to make an appointment for diabetes screening.

Identifying patients who meet the pattern of certain diseases would be far more complicated without the assistance of a CDSS.

Activity 10.3   EHRNAVIGAT⊕R

Preventive Care Report

Go to the Course Navigator to launch Activity 10.3. As an office manager, practice running a preventive care report using the EHR Navigator.

Provider Efficiency

CDSSs can contribute to greater efficiencies for the providers. The hospital can incorporate the care plans for certain types of diseases in the system, thus making it easier for physicians and other clinicians to follow them and increase compliance with Medicare or accreditation requirements. For example, for patients presenting with a possible diagnosis of pneumonia, the protocol of care includes a chest X-ray and a blood culture within 24 hours of admission to confirm the diagnosis of pneumonia. Such protocols can be programmed in the CDSS, thus contributing to greater compliance with requirements, quicker diagnosis, quicker treatment, and possible decreased length of stay.

Cost Reduction

Another common role a CDSS plays in healthcare support is reducing costs. Patients are becoming increasingly savvier consumers of healthcare, and often they are invested in keeping costs down. Although many ways exist to help patients and physicians work together to reduce costs, a CDSS plays a key role in achieving cost-effective healthcare. For example, a family physician who understands how important the cost of medications is to her aging patient population may use the CDSS component of the practice's EHR system to select the best, most cost-effective medications covered by her patients' insurance plans.

Meaningful Use Requirement

As you learned in Chapter 1, the Health Information Technology for Economic and Clinical Health (HITECH) Act specifies criteria for meaningful use of EHRs. Clinical decision support is a requirement of an EHR system that meets specified meaningful use criteria. Specifically, Measure 11 of the 14 meaningful use core measures for eligible providers requires that the healthcare facilities' EHR system "implement one clinical decision support rule" and notifications based on the rule(s) to meet this core measure. To meet this specific clinical decision support requirement, the EHR clinical support rule(s) implemented by the healthcare facility must include clinical decision support features that go beyond drug–drug and drug–allergy contraindication checking and must be based on certain data elements, including those in the problem or medication list, demographic information, and laboratory test results. In addition, automated notifications and suggestions for care must be generated based on the clinical decision support rules. Meaningful use core measures for eligible hospitals include even more requirements. For example, it is required that the hospital implements at least one clinical decision support rule for a high priority hospital condition along with the ability to track performance and compliance with that rule.

EXPAND
YOUR LEARNING
Learn more about the Clinical Decision Support Rule Meaningful Use Requirement by accessing the resources found on the HealthIT.gov website, www.paradigmcollege.net/exploringehr/CDS_Meaningful_Use.

Role of EHRs in Quality Improvement Activities

EHRs can play a major role in a healthcare organization's quality improvement activities, but the question remains as to whether the healthcare organization is fully utilizing the data made available through the use of EHRs. Reporting capabilities in EHR systems provide healthcare organizations with important statistics and can help identify opportunities to improve patient care. A routine review of clinical and outcome data and statistics can assist healthcare providers and administrators to identify potential quality issues.

Typical subject areas of statistical review and monitoring in an inpatient facility include infection rates, ventilation wean success rates, lengths of stay, fall rates, morbidity and mortality rates, types and frequency of diagnostic tests per diagnosis-related group (DRG), and medication errors. A CDSS integrated with an EHR can provide

A CDSS integrated with an EHR system can help improve patient care.

statistics on many typical functions of an inpatient facility, so physicians, hospital managers, and other stakeholders can take necessary steps to improve areas in which the inpatient facility falls short.

Typical subject areas of statistical review and monitoring in an outpatient facility or physician practice include mammography, diabetes and colorectal screenings, and routine physical examinations. A CDSS integrated with an outpatient EHR system can provide information on that practice's patient population, allowing healthcare staff to send reminders or schedule follow-up procedures.

1. Discuss the role of EHRs in the quality improvement activities of a healthcare organization.

_____

_____

_____

2. List two examples of subject areas of statistical review and monitoring for an inpatient healthcare organization and two examples of subject areas of statistical review and monitoring for an outpatient facility or physician practice.

_____

_____

_____

_____

Garbage In, Garbage Out

EXPAND YOUR LEARNING

Learn more about improving healthcare through the use of data by reviewing the following article:

www.paradigmcollege
.net/exploringehr
/improving_data

The term "garbage in, garbage out" is commonly used in the field of computer science, and it refers to computers that produce faulty output when input data is inaccurate. If the data entered into an EHR system is inaccurate, then the output data is also non-reliable, non-usable, or as stated in the above expression, "garbage."

Members of the healthcare staff must continually review and monitor EHR documentation processes and systems for pertinence and accuracy. Inaccurate and unreliable data residing in a healthcare organization's EHR system is potentially life threatening because healthcare policies, procedures, treatments, and medication decisions are made based on this data. Strict procedures must be in place to ensure accurate EHR data and the correction of any incorrect data in a timely fashion.

Healthcare facilities should create strict documentation policies and guidelines to comply with governmental, regulatory, and industry standards. Facilities should use a standardized format for healthcare documentation, such as SNOMED-CT to record diagnoses, and create consistent templates in their EHR system for documentation.

In addition to consistent documentation, any corrections to EHR data should also be handled in a consistent manner. Healthcare facilities should establish policies that outline who may amend records and what guidelines should be followed. For example, as a staff member of the healthcare information team, you may be able to change demographic data, but clinical data can only be corrected by clinical staff.

Accurate data is important to patient safety, and plays an important role in a successful CDSS. A CDSS of an EHR system will not properly function if entered data is not accurate. If a patient's medications are not entered into the EHR system, then the CDSS will not detect drug–drug interactions. If the patient's weight and height are not accurate, then the CDSS cannot accurately assess his or her risk for diabetes. It is crucial for healthcare facilities to ensure consistent and accurate documentation if they want a CDSS to provide its many benefits.

Chapter Summary

Clinical decision support systems (CDSSs) play an important role in electronic health record (EHR) systems, elevating the medical record from a stagnant paper chart to an electronic interactive system that assists healthcare organizations with diagnostic decision-making and improves quality of care and healthcare delivery. The benefits of a CDSS include reduced risk of medication errors, reduced risk of misdiagnosis, increased direct patient care time, access to state-of-the-art data, research, clinical pathways, and guidelines, reduction of unnecessary diagnostic tests, faster diagnoses, faster treatments, and prescriptions for lower cost medications.

However, using a CDSS also has potential disadvantages, including high costs of maintaining the CDSS, potential over-reliance on computer technology, perception by healthcare providers as a threat to clinical knowledge, and harmful outcomes if software is not thoroughly and continuously updated. A CDSS component of an EHR is required as a part of meaningful use.

Some of the most common uses of a CDSS are alerts, diagnoses, treatment options, preventive care, hospital/provider efficiency, cost reductions, and improved patient satisfaction.

It is imperative that a CDSS is kept up to date with current trends in medical diagnosis and treatment; otherwise, the CDSS may become more of a liability than an asset. EHRs play an important role in a healthcare organization's quality improvement activities, assisting with the assessment and monitoring of healthcare processes and outcomes. It is also crucial that EHR data is accurate for reliable study and analysis.

EHR Review

Check Your Understanding

To check your understanding of this chapter's key concepts, read the following true/false and multiple-choice questions and then record your answers on a separate sheet of paper. Write your answers as modeled in these examples: 1a; 2b; 6T; 7F; *etc.*

1. All of the following are examples of clinical decision support system (CDSS) tools *except*:

   a. computerized alerts and reminders

   b. clinical guidelines

   c. standardized order sets

   d. email tools

2. Which of the following is a benefit of using a CDSS?

    a. It helps eliminate the need for medical research.

    b. It may promote an over-reliance on computer technology.

    c. It helps reduce the risk of medication errors.

    d. It may produce alert fatigue.

3. The two basic types of CDSS are

    a. knowledge-driven and documentation driven.

    b. knowledge-based and documentation based.

    c. knowledge-driven and non–knowledge driven.

    d. knowledge-based and non–knowledge-based.

4. All of the following are disadvantages of CDSS *except*:

    a. cost of maintenance of the CDSS

    b. over-reliance on computer technology

    c. perceived threat by healthcare providers to their knowledge and skills

    d. software does not need updating

5. Typical subject areas of statistical review and monitoring in an inpatient facility include all of these, *except*:

    a. lengths of stay

    b. ventilation wean rates

    c. number of cardiologists on staff

    d. infection rates

6. True/False: A 2005 review of 100 studies showed that CDSSs improved practitioner performance in 95% of the studies.

7. True/False: A facility's drug–drug interaction software component meets the requirement for a CDSS as required for meaningful use.

8. True/False: The electronic health record (EHR) can play a major role in a healthcare organization's quality improvement activities.

9. True/False: Corrections to EHR documentation are never allowed.

10. True/False: Clinical decision support does not play a role in cost-effective healthcare.

Learn the Terms

Go to the Course Navigator to access the flashcards for Chapter 10 of *Exploring Electronic Health Records*

COURSE NAVIGATOR

Acronyms

CDSS: Clinical Decision Support Systems

CMS: Centers for Medicare & Medicaid Services

DRG: Diagnostic-related Group

HITECH: Health Information Technology for Economic and Clinical Health Act

EHR Application

Go on the Record

To build on your understanding of the topics in this chapter, complete the following short answer questions.

1. Why is the CDSS a necessary component of an EHR system?

2. Describe the two different types of CDSS.

3. Describe three benefits of CDSS.

4. List three common uses of CDSS with examples.

5. Describe Measure 11 of the 14 meaningful use core measures.

Navigate the Field

To gain practice in handling challenging situations in the workplace, consider the following real-world scenarios and then use the guiding questions to help you formulate your responses.

1. As the information technology manager for Northstar Medical Center, you receive a report that physicians have substantially increased their disregard for the clinical decision support system laboratory result alerts. You take this information to the president of the medical staff of the facility. Do you agree that this was the appropriate action to take? If so, what should the president of the medical staff do? If not, what should the IT manager have done?

2. You are the manager of a hospital that has recently incorporated a CDSS. One of your staff members does not want to use the new system, as he feels it makes him overly reliant on technology and not using his knowledge and experience as a physician. How would you explain the advantages of a CDSS and persuade him to use it in practice?

EHR Evaluation

Think Critically

Continue to think critically about challenging real-world scenarios and complete the following activities.

1. Identify *Yes* or *No* if the following are examples of clinical decision support:

   _____ a. Dr. Smith is alerted to a drug–drug interaction.

   _____ b. The dietician for Northstar Physicians mails out diabetic information to patients diagnosed with diabetes mellitus.

   _____ c. Dr. Jones is an orthopedic surgeon who takes a "time out" for "right patient, right procedure, right site."

   _____ d. A pharmacist receives an alert regarding a lower-cost medication to be substituted for a patient's current medication.

   _____ e. A pharmacist looks up a national drug code number to order a medication.

2. Conduct an Internet search to identify the top three clinical decision support systems. Briefly discuss the components of each of these systems and identify the interoperability of each system.

Make Your Case

Consider the following scenario and create a presentation on the following topic.

You are the Office Manager for BayView Physician Group and have been asked to prepare a presentation for the staff regarding the CDSS component of the EHR system that its group uses. The physicians would like you to explain to the staff the following items:

- definition of a CDSS.

- why a CDSS is important.

- whether or not a CDSS is a requirement.

- three examples of how the staff of BayView Physician Group will use the CDSS.

Prepare the presentation for the BayView Physician Group staff.

Explore the Technology

To expand your mastery of EHRs, explore the following online activities and complete the EHR Navigator assessments.

Ensure you are comfortable with the functionality presented in the EHR Navigator activities, such as exploring adding an order, experiencing the drug-drug interaction feature, and running a preventive care report. Then, complete the EHR Navigator assessments for Chapter 10 located on the Course Navigator.

COURSE NAVIGATOR

Are You Ready?

Networking can be one of the best ways to get a job, regardless of the field, but it is especially important in the health information industry. Studies show that approximately 70% to 80% of jobs are obtained through networking. How can you start developing a network in health information or allied health? Consider asking your professors or mentors. Online networking sites such as LinkedIn can be valuable resources. Professional associations also provide networking opportunities.

Beyond the Record

- Approximately 35% of U.S. adults say that they have conducted an online search to determine what medical condition they or someone they know might have.

- A 2013 survey of health-related iPad apps showed that diabetes topped the list at 143 apps. Depression had 60 apps.

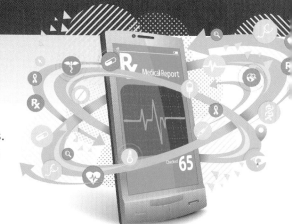

Personal Health Record Time Line

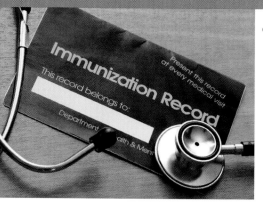

- **1950s**–Patients were encouraged to keep written personal health logs to help track their health information.

- **1978**–The term *personal health record* was first used in an article.

- **2000s**–The idea of storing an electronic personal health record grows in popularity.

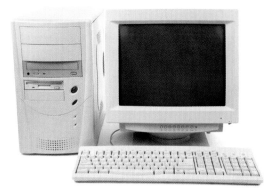

The Personal Health Record and the Patient Portal

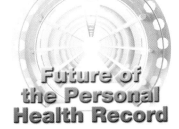

Future of the Personal Health Record

As people do more and more tasks on their smartphones—such as communicating with friends, banking, and shopping—managing health information on a mobile device will likely increase in popularity. The image to the right shows a screen shot of a personal health record on a mobile device.

- **2012**—Stage 2 Meaningful Use encourages patients' participation in their health.

- **2016**—Stage 3 Meaningful Use gives patient access to self-management tools.

Field Notes

Electronic prescribing has had a positive effect on the practice of pharmacy and the quality of care of patients. It allows healthcare providers to send prescriptions to the pharmacy more quickly, meaning medications are ready for the patients when they arrive at the pharmacy, reducing their wait time. Electronic prescribing also reduces medication errors, since handwriting is not a factor. Overall, electronic prescribing is improving patients' quality of care as well as their safety.

– Michelle Waters, Pharm D, Pharmacist

Learning Objectives

- Examine a personal health record (PHR).

- Identify the characteristics (or content) of the PHR.

- Compare the differences in the types of PHRs.

- Discuss the multiple purposes of a PHR.

- Explain the various ways PHRs are stored.

- Explain the ownership of the PHR.

- Discuss the advantages of the PHR.

- Identify the challenges to implementing a PHR.

- Explain the connection between the PHR and the electronic health record (EHR).

- Identify the components of a patient portal.

- Demonstrate use of the Northstar Patient Portal.

Consumers today are faced with many decisions regarding their healthcare. For that reason, they have become better educated about healthcare costs, treatment options, and preventive care measures. In addition to becoming more informed, many individuals have taken control of their healthcare by creating a personal health record or participating in a patient portal. These health information management (HIM) tools have two goals: (1) to have health information available at the point of care and (2) to help foster enhanced communication between the patient and the healthcare provider. This chapter examines these HIM tools and their evolving roles in patient care.

EXPAND
YOUR LEARNING

What does Facebook have to do with your health information? Doctors saved a woman's life by reading some of her health information on her Facebook account. Read the article at www.paradigmcollege.net/exploringehr/facebook to learn how social media helped save a life. What impact can social media tools such as Facebook have on your health?

Personal Health Record

A **personal health record (PHR)** is a tool that enables an individual to plan and manage his or her health information, thus improving overall quality of care. To use this tool, the patient gathers his or her demographic information and health data and enters this information into a formatted document or an online template. The result is a record that contains a complete overview of the individual's health history and current health status. Aside from forming a complete summary of an individual's health, a PHR also allows the patient to:

- Track and update healthcare information from any location via a computer, tablet, or smartphone

- Coordinate care among selected healthcare providers and facilities

- Locate information about diseases and conditions

- Avoid duplication of tests and procedures

- Monitor prescriptions, allergies, wellness, and research

- Share health information with selected providers and healthcare facilities

Rise of the PHR

As you can see by the time line on pages 256–257, PHRs emerged at the turn of this century. Since 2000, there has been a steady rise in both interest and use of PHRs by individuals who want to take control of their healthcare needs. Because of the relatively recent popularity of PHRs and changes in healthcare, national organizations have struggled to come up with a common definition of a PHR (see Table 11. 1).

Table 11.1 National Organizations and Their Definitions of PHRs.

Name of Organization	PHR Definition
National Committee on Vital and Health Statistics (NCVHS)	"The collection of information about an individual's health and health care, stored in electronic format."
American Health Information Management Association (AHIMA)	"…an electronic, universally available, lifelong resource of health information needed by individuals to make health decisions. Individuals own and manage the information in the PHR, which comes from healthcare providers and the individual. The PHR is maintained in a secure and private environment, with the individual determining rights of access. The PHR is separate from and does not replace the legal record of any provider."
U.S. Department of Health & Human Services (HHS)	"An electronic file or record of a [patient's] health information and services, such as …allergies, medications, and doctor or hospital visits that can be stored in one place, and then shared with others, as [the patient] see[s] fit."
Healthcare Information and Management Systems Society (HIMSS)	"…a universally accessible, layperson comprehensible, lifelong tool for managing health information, promoting health maintenance and assisting with chronic disease management via an interactive, common data set of electronic health information and e-health tools. An ePHR [PHR] should be owned, managed, and shared by the individual or legal proxy and must be secure to protect the privacy and confidentiality of the health information it contains. It is not a legal record unless so defined and, therefore, is subject to various legal limitations."

However, what these national organizations can agree on are the attributes that a successful PHR should have. PHRs should give patients ownership of their information and be easily accessible, secure, private, and comprehensive.

To that end, in 2002, the Markle Foundation, an organization that promotes the use of technology to improve people's lives, created Connecting for Health, a public–private collaboration focused on improving health through the use of information technology. Representatives from more than 100 organizations formed this collaboration and were tasked to develop policies that would be shared among patients and healthcare providers. The outcomes of this working group were as follows:

- accelerate the development of the PHR.

- increase the patient's relationship with a healthcare provider and involvement in his or her care and safety.

- develop a common data set.

- develop a variety of approaches to creating a PHR.

To fulfill these goals, Connecting for Health developed seven best practices for a PHR:

1. Each individual would have his or her own PHR.

2. PHRs are to provide a complete medical history for an individual from birth to death.

3. PHRs are to contain information from healthcare providers.

4. PHRs are to be accessible from any place at any time.

5. PHRs are to be private and secure.

6. PHRs are to be transparent. An individual can see who entered data, when the data was entered, and where data was imported or transferred from as well as who is viewing the data in the PHR.

7. PHRs will permit the seamless exchange of information across healthcare systems.

Contents of a PHR

As mentioned earlier, a PHR contains demographic information and health data, such as the individual's current medications, allergies, past hospitalizations, diagnoses, and more. Table 11.2 lists recommended information for inclusion in a PHR.

Table 11.2 Recommended Information for the PHR

Demographic	Name
	Address
	Telephone
	Email
	Date of birth
Emergency Contact	Name
	Address
	Telephone
	Email
Insurance Information	Company name
	Address
	Telephone
	Group number

Table 11.2 Recommended Information for the PHR *(continued)*

Religious Preferences	Name of spiritual leader
	Address
	Telephone
	Email
Advanced Directives	Scanned copies of Do Not Resuscitate Directive,
	Living Will, and Health Care Proxy
Providers	Name
	Address
	Telephone
	Email
	Specialty
Health Issues	List health issues providers are addressing
Dentists	Name
	Address
	Telephone
	Email
Dental Issues	List dental issues providers are addressing
Pharmacy	Name
	Address
	Telephone
	Email
Optometrist	Name
	Address
	Telephone
	Email
Allergies	List of all allergies
Blood Type	List blood type
Current Medications	Every drug or supplement, including vitamins
Past Medications	Every drug or supplement, including vitamins taken in the past
Immunizations, Vaccinations	Flu shots and other vaccinations, including dates
Illnesses, Conditions, Treatments	Diagnoses/treatments/dates of occurrence/failed treatments
Hospitalizations	Inpatient and outpatient services
Pregnancy	All maternity encounters (live, stillbirth, etc.)
Surgeries	All inpatient and outpatient surgeries
Additional Medical Tests	All medical tests
Permission Forms	Release of information and medical procedures
Imaging	X-rays
	Magnetic resonance imaging
	Computed tomography scans
Alternative Therapies	Alternative therapies or treatments
Correspondence	Correspondence among healthcare providers and facilities

The PHR should be organized so it is easily accessible to the necessary parties and covers all pertinent health information. Depending on the type of PHR selection (paper or electronic), the information would either be keyed or scanned to the PHR. Many health information organizations have created templates for individuals to use. For example, the American Health Information Management Association (AHIMA) created the MyPHR website (www.myphr.com) to inform consumers about PHRs, suggest information for them to gather, and provide them with links to PHR templates. Many insurance companies also provide PHRs, as will be discussed below (see Figure 11.1).

Figure 11.1 Sign on Screen of a Typical PHR

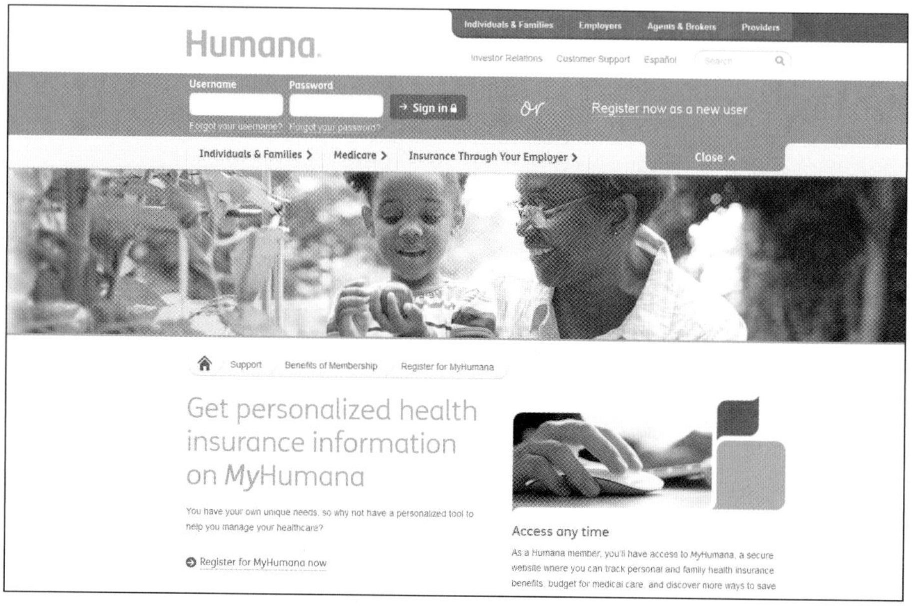

Ownership of a PHR

A patient has complete ownership of a PHR, including the setup and maintenance of the record. In light of this fact, a patient also establishes the parameters for the parties who can view the record and for the data they can access. A patient can limit the type of medical information provided to family, healthcare providers, or healthcare facilities. For example, a patient may choose to have only information about medications and allergies available to family members but may grant his or her healthcare provider or facility access to the entire health record. Patients should be aware, however, that a PHR is not a substitute for a legal medical record that healthcare providers and facilities maintain.

General Types of PHRs

There are three general types of PHRs: paper, computer-based, and web-based. Each type of PHR has certain advantages and disadvantages that individuals need to consider.

Paper PHRs

The traditional paper PHR, a collection of medical documents and personal journals of an individual's health history, rose to prominence in the 1950s as families were encouraged to document medical treatments (including drug therapy), procedures, and vaccinations, and take a vested interest in monitoring and improving their overall health status. This type is losing its appeal as electronic record keeping becomes the norm.

Advantages

A paper PHR has the advantage of being a low-cost method of record keeping. Individuals who continue to use a paper health record also like the privacy and security of keeping the record safe at home rather than out in cyberspace. Although this type of record is portable and can be carried by a patient to healthcare visits, the patient does not always remember to do so.

Disadvantages

There are many disadvantages associated with a paper PHR. For a patient, a paper health record may be difficult to assemble, organize, and update. Without an established format, a paper PHR may also lack the necessary details to provide a complete picture of the patient's health status. Lastly, in an emergency, a paper record is either unavailable for use or difficult to decipher by an attending healthcare provider or emergency facility. Privacy and security of paper PHRs are also drawbacks to this type of record. Unless placed in a secure location, a paper PHR is accessible to others who may invade the privacy of the record's owner.

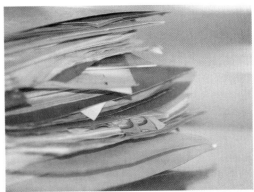

Paper PHR files are difficult to store and organize.

Computer-Based PHRs

Computer- or software-based PHRs are similar to paper PHRs, but they are in an electronic format. Patients can purchase or download PHR software and install it on their chosen electronic device. This type of PHR system is known as a stand-alone or untethered PHR, and it is not designed to send or receive information electronically with other PHR or EHR systems. The patient or his or her designee is responsible for entering the data into the program as well as attaching any documents or images to accompany the data. Therefore, the patient is in control of an untethered PHR. When the patient visits a healthcare provider or facility, he or she can print the health information or transfer the information to a portable storage device, such as a flash drive, memory card, or CD, so that the data can be transferred to the legal health record.

Advantages

In addition to the portability feature mentioned above, computer- or software-based PHRs are often password-protected and are not connected to the Internet, making these health records more secure than paper PHRs. Computer-based PHRs also allow patients to back up their health information, thus helping to prevent a loss of valuable data.

Disadvantages

Of course the data contained in computer-based PHRs is only as accurate as the accuracy of the typist. Patients must exercise caution when inputting information into the health record. Another disadvantage of these records is the lack of Internet connectivity. Although this feature aids security of data, it also makes patients bear the sole responsibility of updating their health records and maintaining their accuracy. Lastly, not all healthcare providers have computer system compatibility that allows them to accept an external media transfer of information into the EHR. If the system is not compatible, then the healthcare provider or facility cannot read or upload the information.

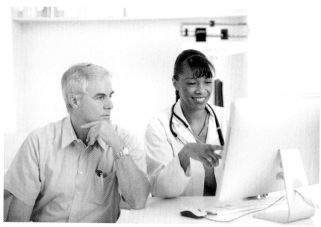
Patients can take their PHR to their healthcare provider to view.

Web-Based PHRs

To use web-based PHRs, patients must have access to a computer or digital device and have an Internet connection. Web-based PHRs are either tethered or untethered. A **web-based tethered PHR** is health information that is attached to a specific organization's health information system. A **web-based untethered PHR** is not attached to a specific organization's health information system.

Tethered PHRs

This web-based PHR may be provided through a patient's health insurance, employer, healthcare facility, or healthcare provider and is stored on a server owned by a third-party organization. To gain access to health data on a tethered PHR, a patient must use a portal. Once access is granted, a patient may only make limited changes to the record, such a change in insurance coverage. Because the PHR is attached to a covered entity, the patient's health information is protected by the Health Insurance Portability and Accountability Act (HIPAA). However, patients should be aware that this type of PHR does not meet the best practices criteria of the Markle Foundation.

Tethered PHRs may be provided by health insurers, healthcare facilities, and employers as discussed below.

Health-Insurer–Provided PHRs Many health insurers offer subscribers the opportunity to participate in their healthcare with tethered PHRs known as **health-insurer–provided PHRs**. A health insurer often populates information about a subscriber, such as insurance claim information, a list of providers, prescriptions, and benefits coverage. However, a subscriber can also enter his or her own data. Subscribers may also access additional resources, such as wellness information on exercise, nutrition, weight loss, pregnancy, smoking cessation, and other topics that will encourage them to make healthy choices to improve their quality of life as well as reduce costs to the health insurer. Because health insurer–provided PHRs are owned by companies rather than patients, these records are not considered to be "true" PHRs. One advantage of a health-insurer–provided PHR is that the health insurer updates the PHR as information becomes available. That way, the patient is not solely responsible for entering the health information updates. Information may be extracted, printed, or saved, as well as provided to various healthcare providers or facilities.

Facility-Provided PHRs Another type of tethered PHR comes from a physician or healthcare facility. This type of PHR, known as a **facility-provided PHR**, links the EHR and the PHR and allows the patient to access the PHR portion online using a username and access code. This type of technology is relatively new and is increasing in popularity. Many of these types of PHRs are static, meaning that the patient may only view the information. There are several features that a tethered PHR from a physician or healthcare facility may include, such as a messaging feature that provides the patient with the opportunity to email a provider, request an appointment, view test results, request a prescription refill, and view reminders. The section titled "Patient Portal" on page 276 walks you through the features of a facility-provided PHR. See Figures 11.2 and 11.3 to view screenshots from this type of portal.

Figure 11.2 Log In Screen of a Facility-Provided PHR/Patient Portal

Figure 11.3 Facility-Provided PHR/Patient Portal

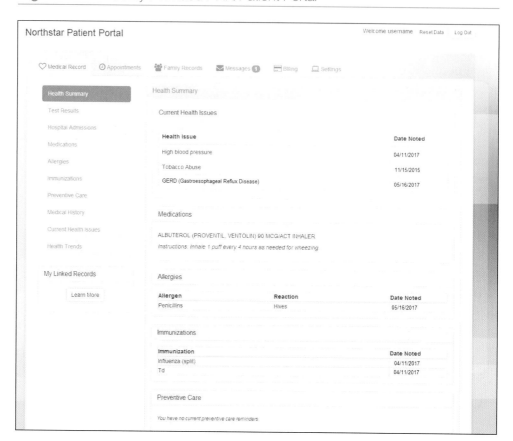

Employer-Provided PHRs Employers are also getting involved in the area of PHRs. In 2006, several companies, such as Intel, BP America, Pitney Bowes, Walmart, and others, formed an organization called Dossia. In 2008, Dossia offered PHRs to employees of the companies that formed Dossia. This type of PHR, known as an **employer-provided PHR**, contains data from hospitals, doctors' offices, health plans, laboratories, and pharmacies as well as information entered by the employee. The goal of employer-provided PHRs is to enable employees to make better health decisions. Achieving this goal is a win–win situation for both employees and employers: Employees improve their health and well-being, and employers reap the benefit of decreased insurance costs and employee absenteeism.

There are several advantages to using an employer-provided PHR. One of the biggest advantages is that this type of PHR is not limited to one healthcare provider or facility. Employees may enter health information from all of their providers and can determine what information can be shared. Another advantage is that, because the PHR is Web-based, patients can access the content anytime and anywhere. So, for example, patients can access their PHRs from providers' offices or healthcare facilities by entering a username and password. Lastly, an employer-provided PHR is available to the employee for life, even if he or she is no longer employed by one of the organizations.

Employer-provided PHRs also have a few disadvantages for employees. One of the disadvantages is that employees are responsible for entering the information and keeping it current. Another potential disadvantage for an employer-provided PHR is that many employees are not comfortable sharing sensitive health information with their employers, or have misgivings regarding how their data will be used.

Untethered PHRs

This type of PHR allows the patient to control the information in the record by customizing access rights for family and providers. The patient can create a username and password to ensure the security of his or her health information. Because the PHR is web-based, the patient can access the record at any time. Web-based untethered PHRs are available for free or by paying a fee.

Networked PHRs

A web-based, networked PHR is the type Connecting for Health imagined. A web-based networked PHR can transfer information to and from various healthcare providers and facilities (for example, doctors, pharmacies, laboratories, insurance companies) and the patient, thus allowing for continuous updates. This interoperability saves the patient time and ensures that the information in the patient's PHR is accurate and current. For example, when a patient visits a dermatologist, the office staff updates the patient's diagnoses and procedures. Then when that patient goes to the pharmacy to retrieve the prescription the dermatologist just prescribed, the pharmacy staff updates the insurance claim information to the networked PHR.

A networked PHR has several advantages:

- this type of PHR is accessible anytime from anywhere as long as the patient has an Internet connection.

- information is shared among multiple providers and facilities, unlike the other types of PHRs previously discussed.

- individuals can select the information that is shared with family, healthcare providers, and facilities.

- the PHR is kept more accurate, up-to-date, and complete because of the input of healthcare staff.

Although the networked PHR offers several advantages, one disadvantage of this type is the issue of privacy and security. The exchange of information over the Internet and among multiple healthcare providers and facilities opens the PHR for potential compromise of health information.

Because of the fluidity of Web-based PHR developers, patients must consider the ramifications of a developer who, for whatever reason, cancels the site. For example, in 2011, Google Health —a free, opt-in web-based PHR that contained voluntary information by the user—was shut down after three years of operation. To find out more about this incident, refer to the Consider This feature box.

Consider This

You are likely familiar with the search engine Google. If you do not know something, you are likely to "Google" it. There are many apps available with Google; however, one app, Google Health, did not catch on as the company thought it would. Read the following blog on why Google's PHR is no longer available:www.paradigmcollege.net/exploringehr/google.

What happened to a user's health information after it was added to Google Health?

CHECKPOINT 11.1

1. What are the advantages and disadvantages of a paper PHR?

   _____

   _____

2. What are the advantages and disadvantages of a computer-based PHR?

   _____

   _____

3. List three types of web-based PHRs.

   a. _____

   b. _____

   c. _____

Evaluation of PHRs

Some clear benefits have emerged as PHRs are being increasingly used by consumers. Indeed, many national healthcare organizations have been outspoken advocates of PHRs and have not only encouraged consumers to use these health records but have also created website templates for their use.

There are several issues that a patient should consider when determining the type of PHR to select, including:

- is remote access available?

- is online storage available?

- if the PHR is web-based, how trustworthy is the site?

- how is your information kept private?

- is your information secure?

Overall Benefits of PHRs

The primary benefit of a PHR is that a patient and his or her healthcare providers can view a complete chronological health history of the patient. Patients can access information about their healthcare providers, treatments, vaccinations, medications, allergies, and other types of health data. Knowing this information allows patients to make informed decisions about their own health and wellness. Healthcare providers can also access the information in a PHR, making all practitioners aware of the patient's past and current health status, test results, medication interactions, overdue preventive tests, and so on. This data access allows providers to work in tandem with each other to provide patients with optimal, safe care. For emergency healthcare providers, in particular, a PHR provides them with the necessary information to act quickly and decisively when treating their patients during a critical time.

The cost of healthcare also benefits from the use of PHRs. For patients, PHRs prevent duplicate tests and treatments and allow them to select lower-cost treatments and medications. For healthcare providers, PHRs allow them to start the correct treatment sooner, which leads to shorter hospital stays or emergency visits.

PHRs that are offered by covered entities, such as healthcare providers and health plans, have the added advantage of being covered under HIPAA. The HIPAA Privacy Rule protects the privacy of the information contained in the PHRs.

NCVHS and the Benefits of PHRs

In 2006, the NCVHS developed a list of key potential benefits for a variety of users of PHRs. This list was presented in the NCVHS's Personal Health Records and Personal Health Record Systems report and recommendations. Table 11.3 lists the key potential benefits of PHRs and PHR systems for patients, providers, payers, employers, and society as a whole.

Advocates of PHRs

As mentioned earlier, many healthcare organizations have voiced their support for the benefits of PHRs. In 2003, the **Veterans Administration** rolled out the MyHealth*e*Vet website, which is a web-based PHR that veterans can use to maintain and update their health information (see Figure 11.4).

A PHR, like MyHealth*e*Vet, improves the continuity of care for veterans who move often and/or visit a variety of healthcare specialists. Figure 11.5 illustrates some of the menu options on the MyHealth*e*Vet website.

Another outspoken advocate for the use of PHRs is the Centers for Medicare & Medicaid Services (CMS). The CMS encourages the use of PHRs to decrease medical errors and reduce healthcare costs. In 2006, the CMS began several pilot programs to encourage Medicare recipients to use PHRs.

Table 11.3 Key Potential Benefits of PHRs and PHR Systems

Roles	Benefits
Consumers Patients Caregivers	• Support wellness activities • Improve understanding of health issues • Increase sense of control over health • Increase control over access to personal health information • Support timely, appropriate preventive services • Strengthen communication with providers • Verify accuracy of information in provider records • Support home monitoring for chronic disease • Support understanding and appropriate use of medications • Support continuity of care across time and providers • Manage insurance benefits and claims • Avoid duplicate tests • Reduce adverse drug interactions and allergic reactions • Reduce hassle through online appointment scheduling and prescription refills • Increase access to providers via e-visits, which are interactions with the healthcare provider via email, phone, or video
Healthcare Providers	• Improve access to data from other providers and the patients themselves • Increase knowledge of potential drug interactions and allergies • Avoid duplicate tests • Improve medication compliance • Provide information to patients for both healthcare and patient services purposes • Provide patients with convenient access to specific information or services (e.g., laboratory results, prescription refills, e-visits) • Improve documentation of communication with patients
Payers	• Improve customer service (transactions and information) • Promote portability of patient information across plan • Support wellness and preventive care • Provide information and education to beneficiaries
Employers	• Support wellness and preventive care • Provide convenient service • Improve workforce productivity • Promote empowered healthcare consumers • Use aggregate data to manage employee health
Societal/Population Health Benefits	• Strengthen health promotion and disease prevention • Improve the health of populations • Expand health education opportunities

Figure 11.4 MyHealtheVet Website

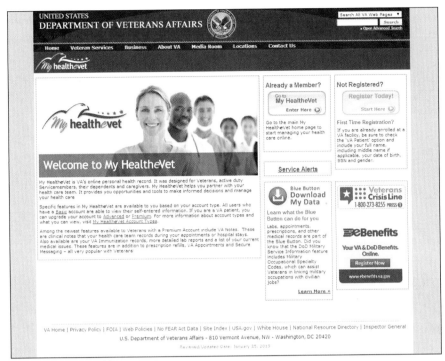

Source: www.myhealth.va.gov

EXPAND
YOUR LEARNING
Visit www.paradig
mcollege.net/exploring
ehr/va to explore the
resources available to
veterans, active service
members, and depen-
dents. How do you
think the MyHealtheVet
will help them manage
their health informa-
tion?

Figure 11.5 MyHealtheVet Menu Options

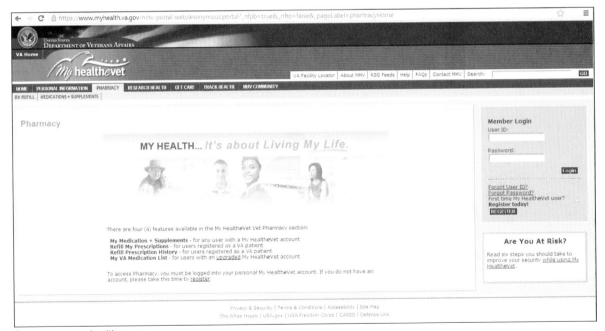

Source: www.myhealth.va.gov

Overall Challenges of PHRs

Similar to the lack of EHR interoperability, PHRs are faced with the same communication challenges. Some networked PHRs can communicate with healthcare provider systems, but most PHRs are not interoperable.

Privacy and security concerns also impact the adoption of PHRs. Those PHRs not offered by HIPAA-covered entities fall under the privacy policies of the PHR vendor, as well as any other applicable laws that govern how information in the PHR is protected. In addition, no federal law exists yet that covers the storage or transmission of PHR content. These privacy and security issues are troubling and must be addressed.

Lastly, depending on the type of PHR, the information in the record may not be accurate, up-to-date, or both. For PHRs to be effective, patients must assume the responsibility of maintaining the record—a task that can be time-consuming.

Consider This

The Centers for Medicare & Medicaid Services (CMS) prepared an article to help consumers select a PHR to meet their needs. To access this article, go to www.paradigmcollege.net/exploringehr/cms_PHR. Read the article and review the questions to ask when choosing a PHR. Consider how you would answer the questions. How would your answers apply to the type of PHR that would fit your situation?

The EHR–PHR Connection

As you have already learned, an EHR system stores information about a patient's health. Depending on the type of PHR a patient establishes, their information may be shared and/or integrated. Although an EHR and a PHR have different characteristics, these records share a common goal: to provide a complete picture of a patient's past and current health status (see Table 11.4). To meet this goal, a connection needs to exist between the two entities, allowing the exchange of information.

Healthcare organizations agree that the key to the effective use of PHRs is the linkage to an EHR system. The Office of the National Coordinator for Health Information Technology (ONC) has determined that a PHR plays an important role in the implementation of the EHR and the Nationwide Health Information Network (NwHIN).

The Institute of Medicine (IOM) also agrees that a PHR can help providers using an EHR system. In its research, the IOM discovered that patients see many different healthcare providers in a variety of healthcare facilities, and often these providers do not have a complete view of the patient's health history because each provider and facility keeps individual records on patients. A networked PHR, discussed earlier, is the tool that allows complete health record access to all parties.

Table 11.4 EHR and PHR Comparison

	EHR	PHR
Purpose	Maintain up-to-date health information	Maintain up-to-date health information
Ownership	Healthcare provider facility	Individual
Updates	Healthcare provider or facility	Individual
Legal	Legal documents created and maintained based on federal and state laws	Not a legal document
Access	Controlled by healthcare provider or facility, requires patient authorization	Controlled by patient
Information	Health information by single provider or facility	Health information from multiple providers or facilities
Use	Healthcare provider or facility	Individual

A Networked PHR and HL7

A networked PHR is the only type of PHR that has the ability to exchange information between the PHR and an EHR system. To that end, Health Level Seven International (HL7) began to address the standard for the EHR in 2007 by developing a model known as PHR-System Functional Model (PHR-S). PHR-S identifies the features and functions of a networked PHR. These features and functions are also linked to the functions in an EHR, creating a pathway for providers, facilities, and patients to exchange information (see Figure 11.6).

Figure 11.6 Personal Health Record System

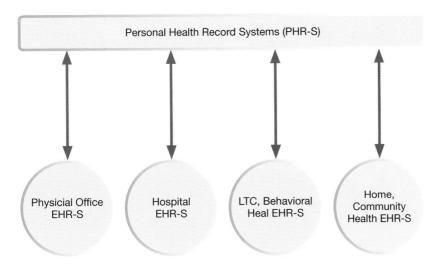

Features of a PHR-S

There are three sections of features and functions in a PHR-S: Personal Health, Supportive, and Information Infrastructure. The Personal Health section focuses on patient demographic data, clinical wellness, management of care, decision support, and management of encounters with providers. The Supportive section provides administrative and financial information related to patient medical care, including information necessary for processing claims, sharing of information for research, and quality improvement. The last section, Information Infrastructure, allows the PHR to efficiently and effectively exchange information with the EHR. Table 11.5 describes the three sections of the PHR system functions in more detail.

Table 11.5 HL7 Personal Health Record System Functional Model

Personal Health	PH.1 Account Holder Profile
	PH.2 Manage Historical Clinical Data and Current State Data
	PH.3 Wellness, Preventive Medicine, and Self Care
	PH.4 Manage Health Education
	PH.5 Account Holder Decision Support
	PH.6 Manage Encounters with Providers
Supportive	S.1 Provider Management
	S.2 Financial Management
	S.3 Administrative Management
	S.4 Other Resource Management
Information Infrastructure	IN.1 Health Record Information Management
	IN.2 Standards Based Interoperability
	IN.3 Security
	IN.4 Auditable Records

Steps in Creating a PHR

There are several steps an individual must consider before creating a PHR. First, a consumer should request a copy of his or her health records. Requesting health records entails completing a HIPAA-compliant form for a release of records from healthcare providers and facilities. Each provider may require a fee for processing the copies of the records.

While waiting for the health information, consumers should review the various types of PHRs and select the one that meets their needs. They should then organize their health information in folders or a binder until all the information has been acquired so that the transfer of information from paper to electronic will be easier. The information received in an electronic format may be copied or transferred into the PHR.

Storage

There are several ways to store health information for a PHR, such as on a flash drive, CD, secure digital card, portable hard drive, online cloud storage, computer hard drive, or even a three-ring binder. The selection of a storage device depends on the needs of the owner of the PHR. Several factors to consider include issues of portability, security, maintenance, and accessibility.

Other considerations include whether the owner of the PHR wants to:

- physically transfer data or use a web-based PHR

- store information online or use a physical storage device

- export the health data in a portable document format (PDF) that would be readable in many different programs

See Figure 11.7 for possible export formats of health information within some of these programs.

Figure 11.7 Export Formats

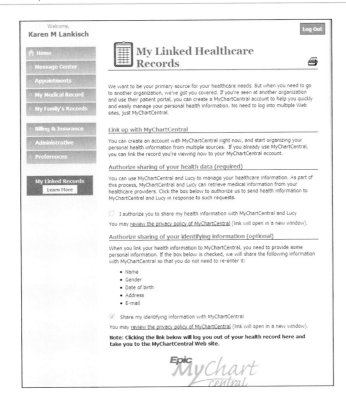

CHECKPOINT 11.2

1. List two organizations that advocate for the use of PHRs.

   a. _____

   b. _____

2. List three steps in creating a PHR.

   a. _____

   b. _____

   c. _____

Patient Portal

The concept of patient portals was created out of the growing popularity of PHRs as well as the adoption of EHR technology because it interfaces with the healthcare facility's EHR system. A patient portal provides patient access to his or her medical records, appointments, messages, billing, connection to family records, and administrative information.

During a patient visit, healthcare providers offering patient portal access will invite patients to register for access, ultimately providing them usernames and access codes. Patients can then create an account and gain access to the portal.

Many facilities are implementing patient portals to help them achieve the Stage 2 meaningful use patient engagement requirement.

Menu of a Typical Patient Portal

Many patient portal systems have similar characteristics. The menu of a typical portal includes options for messages, appointments, medical record, family record, billing and insurance, administration, and preferences. There is also an option to link records from multiple healthcare providers. The EHR Navigator has a patient portal integrated with its system, the Northstar Patient Portal. Figure 11.8 illustrates the Northstar Patient Portal menu.

Figure 11.8 Northstar Patient Portal Menu Screen

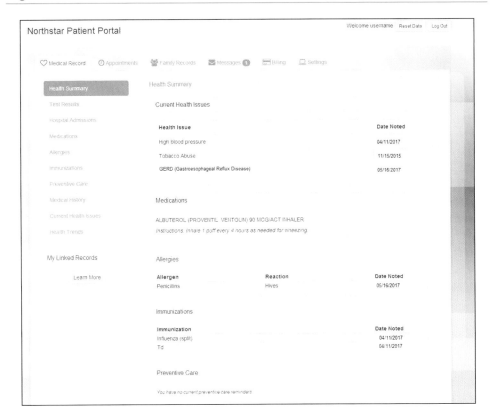

Home

The Home menu of the patient portal provides quick access to *Medical Record*, *Appointments*, *Family Records*, *Messages*, *Billing*, *Settings*, and *Link Medical Records*. The Northstar Patient Portal Home screen is shown in Figure 11.9.

Figure 11.9 Northstar Patient Portal Menu Options

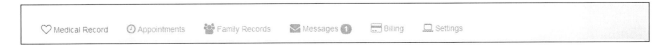

Medical Record

Medical Record allows patients to track their health information, which may include test results, current health issues, medications, allergies, immunizations, preventive care, health summary, medical history, and hospital admissions. As a user of the Northstar Patient Portal, the patient can download a summary of their health information that can be shared with someone or simply be available when traveling abroad.

Health Summary

The *Health Summary* feature of the Northstar Patient Portal provides links to current health information, medication, allergies, immunizations, and preventive care information. The *Health Summary* screen is shown in Figure 11.10.

Figure 11.10   Northstar Patient Portal Health Summary

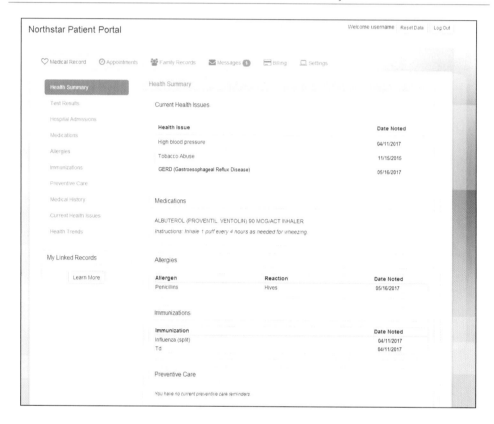

Test Results

The patient can view a list of tests and results. The healthcare provider can contact the patient if there are any issues with the test results. The *Test Results* screen is shown in Figure 11.11.

Figure 11.11   Northstar Patient Portal Test Results

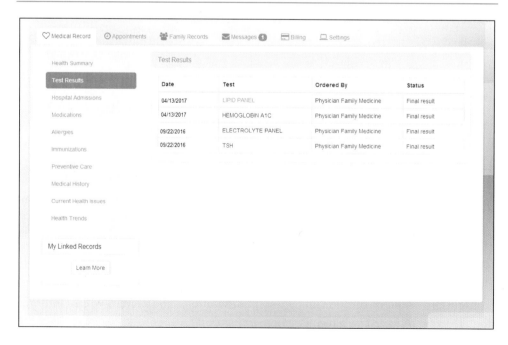

Chapter 11 The Personal Health Record and the Patient Portal

Hospital Admission

The *Hospital Admission* feature in the Northstar Patient Portal provides detailed information about hospital admissions and procedures. This screen is illustrated in Figure 11.12.

Figure 11.12   Northstar Patient Portal Hospital Admission

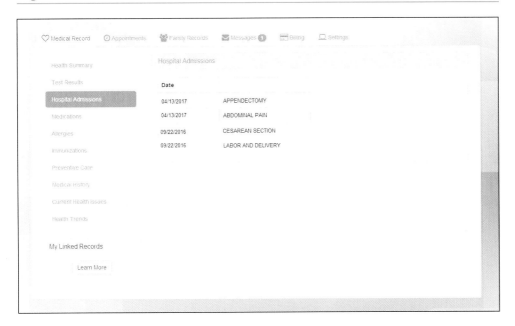

Medications

The Northstar Patient Portal includes a list of the patient's current medications and information regarding the medications, as illustrated in Figure 11.13.

Figure 11.13   Northstar Patient Portal Medications

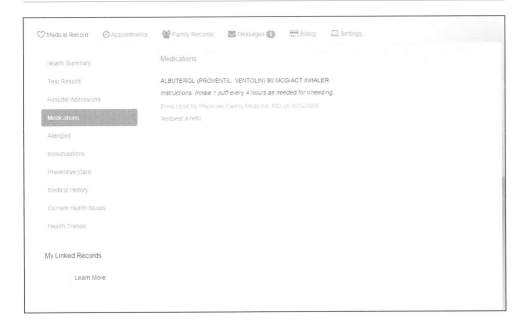

Allergies

Any allergies that impact a patient will be listed in the Northstar Patient Portal. A patient may remove or add allergies in the portal. Figure 11.14 shows the *Allergies* screen.

Figure 11.14   Northstar Patient Portal Allergies

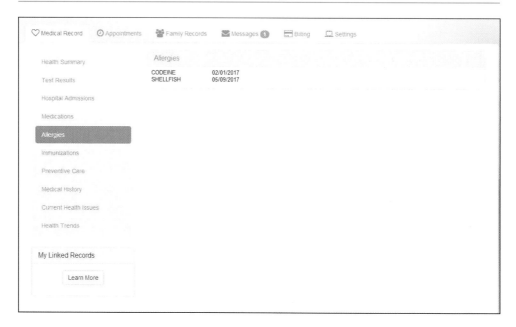

Immunizations

The portal can also track immunization information. Any additional immunizations may be entered by a provider to update the patient's immunization record. Figure 11.15 shows the *Immunizations* screen.

Figure 11.15   Northstar Patient Portal Immunizations

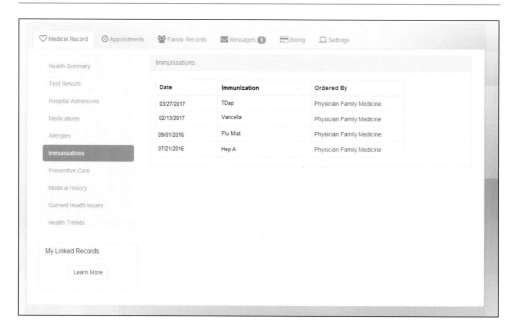

Preventive Care

A patient may view suggestions for preventive care based on age, sex, and medical history. This screen is illustrated in Figure 11.16.

Figure 11.16 Northstar Patient Portal Preventive Care

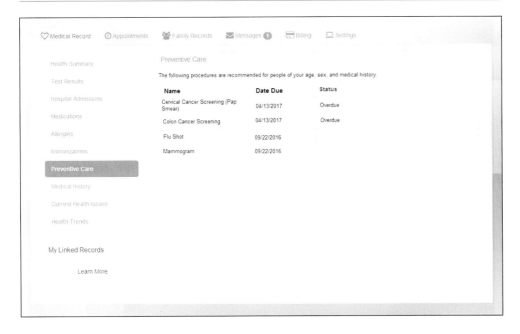

Medical History

A provider may update a patient's medical history, which can include personal notes; procedures; family, medical, and social histories; and family status. Figure 11.17 illustrates the *Medical History* screen.

Figure 11.17 Northstar Patient Portal Medical History

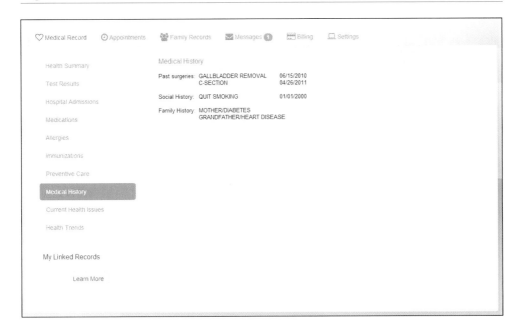

Current Health Issues

A patient's current health issues will be listed in the patient portal. Patients may monitor their health issues here. This screen is shown in Figure 11.18.

Figure 11.18 Northstar Patient Portal Current Health Issues

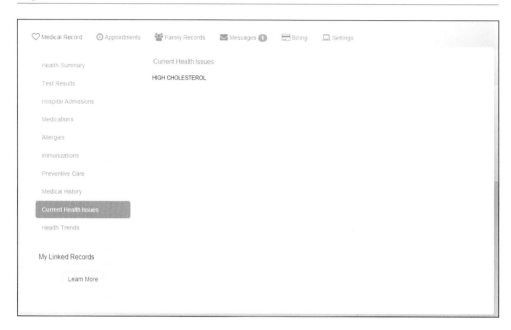

Health Trends

Patients may access their health reports through the *Health Trends* feature of the patient portal, as illustrated in Figure 11.19. Patients may access their health reports, such as a table that details a patient's blood pressure, pulse respirations, height, weight, and body mass index based on visits to the physician.

Figure 11.19 Northstar Patient Portal Health Trends

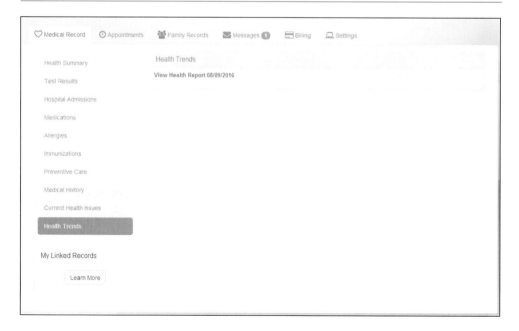

Appointments

The PHR allows a patient to view upcoming appointments, cancel appointments, or request an appointment.

View My Appointments

The *View My Appointments* feature in the Northstar Patient Portal provides a list of all the patient's appointments, detailing the day, time, healthcare provider, and location. See Figure 11.20.

Figure 11.20   Northstar Patient Portal View My Appointments

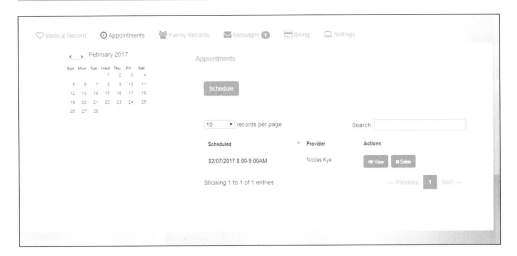

Cancel My Appointments

The portal provides a convenient way for a patient to cancel an appointment. Rather than placing a telephone call, the patient may log in to the patient portal and select the appointment he or she would like to cancel. Figure 11.21 illustrates the cancel appointment feature.

Figure 11.21   Northstar Patient Portal Cancel My Appointments

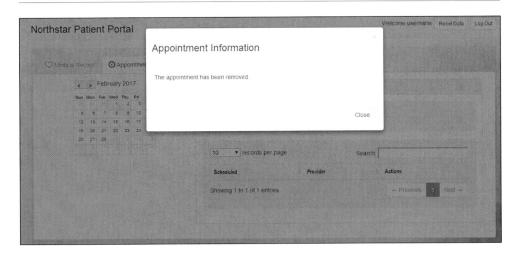

Request My Appointment

The *Request My Appointment* feature permits a patient to request an appointment. The patient may select the healthcare provider he or she would like to see or another provider he or she would be willing to see. In addition, the patient can select the reason and preferred date or days and times. In the *Notes* field, the patient can communicate any specific information necessary for the healthcare provider or facility about the requested appointment. Figure 11.22 shows the *Request My Appointment* dialog box.

Figure 11.22   Northstar Patient Portal Request My Appointment

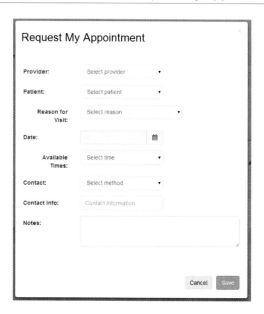

Family Records

There are times when patients may want someone in their family to have access to their health information. The *Family Records* feature allows patients to change the settings in the portal to allow family members access to all or some of their health information. The *Family Records* screen is illustrated in Figure 11.23.

Figure 11.23   Northstar Patient Portal My Family Records

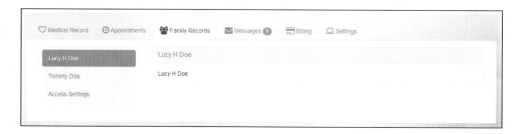

Messages

The *Messages* feature is a communication area that allows the patient and healthcare provider to communicate. Most patient portals have an *Inbox, Sent Message, Get Medical Advice, Request an Rx Refill*, and *Request a Referral*.

Get Medical Advice

There are times when a patient has a medical question and would like to ask it of his or her healthcare provider. The *Get Medical Advice* option in a patient portal provides the patient with the ability to do so. The patient may direct a question to a specific provider, or he or she can select a subject line from a drop-down list such as *Non-Urgent Medical Question*, *Prescription Question*, *Test Result Question*, or *Visit Follow-Up Question*. The *Get Medical Advice* feature is shown in Figure 11.24.

Figure 11.24 Northstar Patient Portal Get Medical Advice

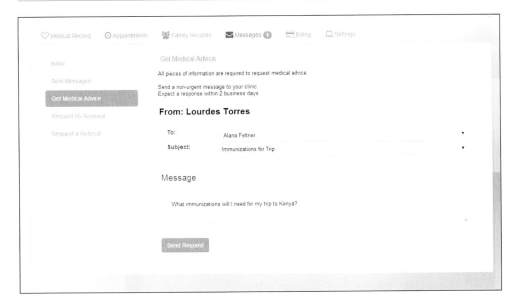

Request Rx Refill

Medications are an important part of an individual's healthcare. Depending on a prescription, healthcare providers may alter medical treatment. The Northstar Patient Portal provides information on refills, and refill history. Patients may also request refills through the patient portal. The *Request Rx Refill* feature is illustrated in Figure 11.25.

Figure 11.25 Northstar Patient Portal Request Rx Refill

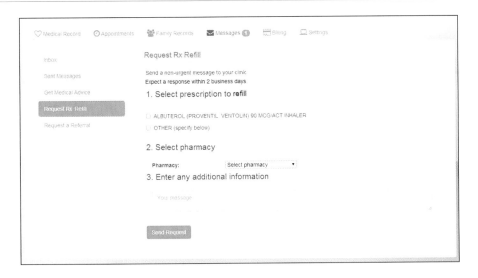

Request a Referral

Sometimes a patient may wish to request a referral to see a specialist or other physician. The Northstar Patient Portal provides an option to request a referral to another physician by filling out a form. The computer program informs the patient that up to 2 days may be required for a response. Figure 11.26 illustrates the *Request a Referral* feature.

Figure 11.26   Northstar Patient Portal Request a Referral

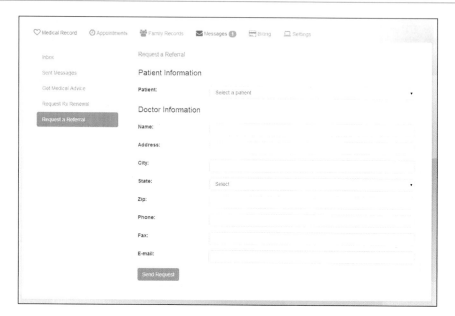

Billing and Insurance

Patients may view their billing and insurance information in the Northstar Patient Portal. The patient may track their payments, insurance payments, and outstanding balances.

Billing Account Summary

The *Billing Account Summary* feature provides a list of visits and payments and is illustrated in Figure 11.27.

Figure 11.27   Northstar Patient Portal Billing Account Summary

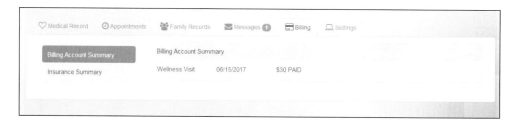

Insurance Summary

A summary of the patient's insurance coverage is listed here in the patient portal, as shown in Figure 11.28.

Figure 11.28 Northstar Patient Portal Insurance Summary

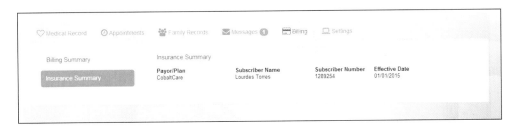

Settings

The *Settings* section of the Northstar Patient Portal includes the patient's *Profile* and *Portable PHR*.

Profile

The *Profile* section includes the patient's address, telephone, and email address as well as primary care provider and provider location. The patient may find his or her PHR identification, medical record number, or account number for billing purposes in the administrative information. The *Profile* also allows a patient to edit his or her demographic information or change his or her password. Figure 11.29 illustrates the *Profile* section.

Figure 11.29 Northstar Patient Portal Profile

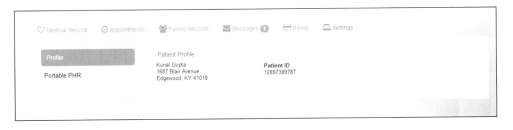

Portable PHR

A patient may print, download, or link his or her health information such as allergies, medications, current health issues, procedures, and test results to share with others. The *Portable PHR* print feature provides a printable summary of a patient's information, medical information, contacts, and insurance information. The *Portable PHR* download option allows a patient to download his or her health information to a flash drive to share with others. The downloaded information may be password-protected.

Link Medical Records

The Northstar Patient Portal provides an option to link a patient's health information, which is a useful tool if a patient is seen by another healthcare facility or provider, as the health information may be quickly and easily shared. This allows the patient to manage his or her personal health information from multiple sources. The patient also may authorize a healthcare provider or facility to send health information to other providers and facilities. Linking medical records is important because other providers and facilities may need access to health information such as medications, previous test results, previous procedures, hospital admissions, and any complications experienced. When a healthcare provider has access to this information, thus better knowing a patient's health history, the delivery and quality of care improves.

Activity 11.1   EHRNAVIGATOR

Enrolling a Patient and Exploring the Patient Portal

Go to the Course Navigator to launch Activity 11.1. As a physician, practice enrolling a patient in the Northstar Patient Portal using the EHR Navigator. Then, explore the Northstar Patient Portal as the patient.

Activity 11.2   EHRNAVIGATOR

Requesting a Refill and an Appointment in the Patient Portal

Go to the Course Navigator to launch Activity 11.2. As a patient, practice reviewing a record, requesting a prescription refill, and scheduling an appointment in the Northstar Patient Portal.

Activity 11.3   EHRNAVIGATOR

Requesting Medical Advice in the Patient Portal

Go to the Course Navigator to launch Activity 11.3. As a patient, practice requesting medical advice in the Northstar Patient Portal.

Activity 11.4   EHRNAVIGATOR

Reviewing Test Results and Adding Family History to the Patient Portal

Go to the Course Navigator to launch Activity 11.4. As a patient, practice viewing test results and adding family history to the Northstar Patient Portal.

CHECKPOINT 11.3

1. Name four features in a patient portal that you would use to improve monitoring your own healthcare.

   a. _____

   b. _____

   c. _____

   d. _____

2. Why is it important to link medical records together in a patient portal?

   _____

   _____

Chapter Summary

Individuals have started to assemble and maintain their own health information so that they have a complete picture of their health history and current health status. One way patients can accomplish this task is by creating a personal health record (PHR). A PHR allows patients to gather, track, update, and share health information. While the definition of a PHR varies somewhat among healthcare organizations, these organizations do agree that a PHR should be a collection of an individual's health information, electronically and securely accessed by an individual patient. To that end, in 2002, the Markle Foundation created a working group to develop best practices for patients and healthcare providers using PHRs.

PHRs may be one of three types: paper, computer-based, or web-based. In addition to the format of the PHR, PHRs can be classified as tethered and untethered. Tethered PHRs are linked to a healthcare provider, facility, or third-party payer. Untethered PHRs are those in which the creator of the PHR enters the health information and the record is not associated with a healthcare provider, facility, or third-party payer. Many different parties play an important role in keeping the PHR up-to-date, and patients and providers use PHRs to help them make better medical decisions, avoid duplicate tests, reduce adverse drug interactions, and support wellness and preventive care.

Aside from maintaining a complete health history of a patient, a PHR also provides additional benefits to patients and healthcare providers such as improved communication between the patient and his or her caregivers, increased patient safety, and significant cost savings for patients and providers. These benefits have not been overlooked by several healthcare organizations who endorse the use of PHRs, including the Centers for Medicare & Medicaid, the Veterans Administration, and the Office of the National Coordinator for Health Information Technology. The latter organization has determined that PHRs are key components of the electronic health record (EHR).

As PHRs have grown in popularity, many healthcare providers have created their own patient portals as part of the EHR technology. A typical patient portal includes messaging, scheduling, medical history, billing and insurance, and administrative features. The patient portal, along with the PHR, improves the delivery and quality of healthcare.

EHR Review

Check Your Understanding

To check your understanding of this chapter's key concepts, read the following true/false and multiple-choice questions and then record your answers on a separate sheet of paper. Write your answers as modeled in these examples: 1a; 2b; 6T; 7F; etc.

1. The acronym PHR stands for

   a. protected health record.

   b. personal health report.

   c. personal health record.

   d. protected health report.

2. The primary goal of the PHR is to

   a. act as a substitute for the legal medical record

   b. develop a common data set

   c. have health information available at the point of care

   d. foster communication between providers and healthcare facilities

3. Which organization defined a PHR as "an electronic universally available lifelong resource of health information needed by individuals to make health decisions. Individuals own and manage the information in the PHR, which comes from the healthcare providers and the individual. The PHR is maintained in a secure and private environment, with the individual determining rights of access."

   a. U.S. Department of Health and Human Services

   b. Healthcare Information and Management Systems Society

   c. National Committee on Vital and Health Statistics

   d. American Health Information Management Association

4. A tethered PHR is

   a. personal health information attached to a specific organization's health information system

   b. personal health information not attached to a specific organization's health information system

   c. personal health information the patient enters into the health information system

   d. protected health information not attached to a specific provider's health information system

5. Which of the following is a key benefit of the PHR for healthcare providers?

   a. An increased sense of control over health

   b. Supports understanding and appropriate use of medications

   c. Improved access to data from other providers and patients

   d. Use of aggregate data to manage employee health

6. True/False: One of several issues patients need to consider when determining the type of PHR is remote access.

7. True/False: Google Health is a PHR currently used by many patients.

8. True/False: In 2010, the Markle Foundation created Connecting for Health.

9. True/False: PHRs may be paper-, computer-, or Web-based.

10. True/False: A typical patient portal includes messaging, scheduling, billing, and record linking features.

Learn the Terms

Go to the Course Navigator to access the flashcards for Chapter 11 of *Exploring Electronic Health Records*.

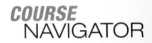

Acronyms

AHIMA: American Health Information Management Association

CMS: Centers for Medicare & Medicaid Services

HHS: Department of Health and Human Services

HIMSS: Health Information and Management Systems Society

HL7: Health Level 7 International

IOM: Institute of Medicine

NwHIN: Nationwide Health Information Network

ONC: The Office of the National Coordinator of Health Information Technology

PHR: Personal Health Record

EHR Application

Go on the Record

To build on your understanding of the topics in this chapter, complete the following short answer questions.

1. What are the benefits of having a personal health record (PHR)?

2. What are the challenges with using a PHR?

3. How do you see the future of the PHR?

4. What are the seven best practices for a PHR as described by Connecting for Health?

5. Explain the difference between a tethered and untethered PHR system.

Navigate the Field

To gain practice in handling challenging situations in the workplace, consider the following real-world scenarios and then use the guiding questions to help you formulate your responses.

1. You are a patient who wants to begin using a PHR. Using a search engine of your choice, research the various personal health records (PHRs) available from both free and subscription services. Compare and contrast the various PHRs for their features and ease of use. Select three PHRs and write a three- to four-page paper comparing the selections. After careful analysis, make a recommendation of a PHR that best fits your needs.

2. Your employer is going to begin offering a PHR. Many of your coworkers are signing up, while others have misgivings about their privacy. Would you be likely to use a PHR offered by an employer? Why or why not?

EHR Evaluation

Think Critically

Continue to think critically about challenging real-world scenarios and complete the following activities.

1. Prepare a pamphlet for patients of South Community Hospital on how to use and access the patient portal. The pamphlet should include information about the definition of a patient portal, advantages of a patient portal, features of a patient portal, and how to use and access the patient portal.

2. Investigate the patient portal system that accompanies this textbook and complete a scavenger hunt by answering questions from your instructor.

Make Your Case

Consider the following scenario and create a presentation on the following topic.

You are a member of the CobaltCare insurance company, which is promoting personal health records (PHRs) for all of its insured members. You are hosting a session on how to begin a PHR, exploring what information should be included, and how to keep the PHR current. Prepare the presentation you will share with the enrollees that attend the information session.

Explore the Technology

To expand your mastery of EHRs, explore the following online activities and complete the EHR Navigator activities.

COURSE
NAVIGATOR

Ensure you are comfortable with the functionality presented in the EHR Navigator/ Northstar Patient Portal activities, such as enrolling a patient in the patient portal, requesting a refill, requesting an appointment, requesting medical advice, reviewing test results, and adding family history. Then, complete the EHR Navigator assessments for Chapter 11 located on the Course Navigator.

Are You Ready?

Completing your training in an electronic health records (EHR) course is just one of the first steps to becoming a health information professional. However, mastering an EHR system and demonstrating knowledge of why EHRs are important will help you in any healthcare career you choose. As you continue your education and training, you may wish to refer back to this text and the tutorials in the EHR Navigator.

Beyond the Record

- The average practice takes 120 days to select its electronic health record (EHR) system.

- Approximately 40% of surveyed healthcare leaders said they are evaluating the return on investment of their EHR system.

- The northeastern United States leads the nation in facilities reaching meaningful use.

- Cerner, MEDITECH, Epic, and Allscripts were the vendors with the most meaningful use attestations in 2011.

Chart Migration Checklist

The Health Information Technology Research Center (HITRC) developed a Chart Migration and Scanning Checklist to help healthcare providers implement an EHR system. The full document is provided by the National Learning Consortium and can be found at www.healthit.gov.

Chapter 12

Implementation and Evaluation of an EHR System

To ensure it attracts creative programmers, Epic Systems, one of the largest EHR providers, has a two-story spiral slide and a statue of The Cat in the Hat in its Wisconsin office building. Workers also hold meetings in an on-site tree house.

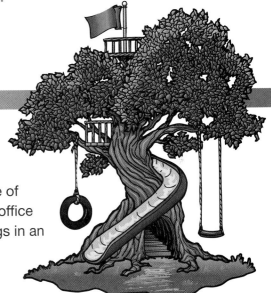

1   Scanning and Preload Checklist

To use this checklist, follow the steps below:

1. Identify who will complete the worksheet based on knowledge of chart scanning
2. Complete w
3. Review the
4. Formulate t
5. Build in che
6. Communica
7. Initiate plan

1.1   ADMINIS

1. What is you

2. Will scannin

Yes
No, if no th

3. What is the

   Scannin

   Manuall

4. How many

5. How many
   Click here t

6. How many s

7. How soon a
   in the EHR?

8. Who will be
   Click here t

9. What are the practice's goals for EHR implementation? Check all that apply to practice.

Exhibit 1 Goals

Goal	Check if 'Yes'
2.1 Become a paperless office	
2.2 Become an office with less paper	
2.3 Move paper charts off site (storage)	
2.4 Eliminate chart pulls for visits	
2.5 Eliminate chart pulls for messages	
2.6 Reduce document filing time	
2.7 Implement a document imaging management system	
2.8 Interface with lab	
2.9 Interface with hospital	
2.10 Interface with radiology	
2.11 Redesign current systems	

1.2   CHART SPECIFICS

1. Which paper charts will be scanned (Check one)?

Exhibit 2 Scanned Charts

Charts	Check if 'Yes'
All	
Patients seen in past five years	

- Define the goals of the Certification Commission for Health Information Technology.

- Explain the incentive criteria for electronic health record (EHR) systems developed by the Centers for Medicare & Medicaid Services.

- Describe how to assess a healthcare facility's readiness for the implementation of an EHR system.

- Evaluate and create a healthcare facility's goals for an EHR system.

- Examine an EHR migration plan.

- Explain the workflow analysis.

- Understand the total cost of ownership.

- Describe the evaluation process for EHR systems.

- Examine a request for proposal and an implementation plan.

- Assess stages of meaningful use.

As discussed throughout *Exploring Electronic Health Records*, the 2009 Health Information Technology for Economic and Clinical Health (HITECH) Act has accelerated the adoption of electronic health record (EHR) systems in U.S. healthcare facilities. The previous chapters discussed the advantages of EHRs, such as access to data, improved patient care, and monetary incentives for the implementation of a certified EHR system. However, system selection may be challenging because so many types of EHR systems are available. To receive a share of the $27 billion in stimulus money set aside in the HITECH Act, the EHR system must be certified by the **Office of the National Coordinator–Authorized Testing and Certification Bodies (ONC–ATCB)**, and the provider must have applied for incentive monies by 2014. The **Certification Commission for Health Information Technology (CCHIT)**, one of the ONC-ATCB certifying organizations, developed a rigorous process to examine the systems for functionality, interoperability, and security. CCHIT also provides resources to help healthcare facilities select an appropriate EHR system.

Healthcare providers interested in purchasing an EHR system must understand associated direct and indirect costs. EHR systems are complex and require careful examination, including a thorough analysis of the healthcare facility's needs and business operations. As noted earlier, an EHR is not one piece of soft-

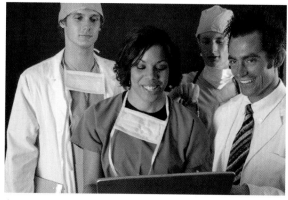

A team to analyze a facility's workflow should be made up of employees from many different departments.

ware; rather, it comprises many different applications working together to exchange and process data. EHR adoption is still in the beginning stages in most American healthcare facilities, and, although facilities typically focus the most on the dollar amount of purchasing an EHR system, this expenditure is only one part of the true cost.

Initial Steps in Implementing an EHR System

Implementing an EHR system is a time-consuming, labor-intensive project that, with proper planning, may be implemented with few disruptions. If the planning is not started long in advance of the implementation date, then the process may be challenging.

The planning stages of EHR implementation involve a series of initial steps. The first step is determining a facility's readiness to change from paper records to electronic records. Once that factor is determined, a facility needs to set goals and establish a steering committee to lay the groundwork and move the EHR planning process forward.

Assessing Readiness

Before acquiring an EHR system, it is essential to assess the readiness of the healthcare organization or facility to undergo this transition. Organizations should be advised to analyze their clinical, financial, and administrative computer applications, their technical capabilities, and their staffing resources. They should also examine their reporting needs, such as hospital utilization, gross patient revenue, and emergency visits. Several other factors, such as current technology, technical support, and facility operations must also be considered. Lastly, the organization's culture of change management and process improvement must be measured. This factor is critical to a facility's successful EHR adoption. To that end, a facility must understand the distinction between implementation and adoption. The installation of an EHR system is one thing; the willingness of staff members to embrace the technology and use its applications to the fullest extent is another thing. Consequently, adoption may take more time and effort than all of the other elements of implementation.

EXPAND YOUR LEARNING

The Agency for Healthcare Research and Quality (AHRQ) developed a free resource that helps healthcare organizations implement and evaluate an EHR system. The tool kit may be found at www.paradigmcollege.net/exploringehr/AHRQ_Toolkit.

Setting Goals

Once the readiness of a facility to implement EHR technology has been assessed, the organization must establish goals. Although these goals may differ among healthcare facilities, many organizations set goals developed from several key objectives, including:

- Improved quality of patient care
- Increased revenue
- Improved operational efficiency
- Supervised compliance
- Improved reporting

Establishing a Steering Committee

To move the EHR implementation process forward, a healthcare facility must create a cross-disciplinary steering committee whose members represent groups with a direct role or involvement in the proposed EHR system. A typical steering committee is comprised of healthcare providers, nurses, health information professionals, administrators, financial staff, and staff members of other integral departments. The committee is led by a chair or co-chairs (commonly clinicians) and is tasked with examining factors such as operational issues with the current technology infrastructure. The members then come to a consensus as to what changes need to be made to the infrastructure and draw up a plan that outlines the steps needed for successful migration to an EHR system. The committee also examines policies and procedures in support of EHR staff and resources with regard to implementation and maintenance.

The steering committee should plan to attend regularly scheduled meetings during the vendor selection process to make decisions and recommendations, as well as evaluate short- and long-term goals. During the implementation process, the committee should meet weekly to address implementation issues or challenges.

Assigning a Project Manager

It is highly recommended that, starting early in the vendor selection process, a healthcare facility hires or assigns a project manager to help implement the EHR system. The project manager may be an internal employee of the healthcare facility or an external or contracted staff person. Both types of project managers offer advantages and disadvantages.

Internal Project Manager

Hiring an internal project manager has several advantages. This individual is familiar with the culture and structure of the facility, thus allowing a better transition to an EHR system. As a permanent employee of the facility, he or she also has a vested interest in the success of the adoption process. Finally, an internal project manager is on-site and available to manage any issues that arise once implementation takes place. One disadvantage of hiring an internal person is his or her possible lack of objectivity in the decision-making processes.

External Project Manager

Hiring an external project manager also offers several advantages and disadvantages. This type of project manager or contractor is a neutral party and can, therefore, provide objectivity in implementing the migration plan. However, he or she must spend a significant portion of time learning about the organization's standards, culture, and employees—a task that certainly decelerates the EHR implementation process. In addition, an external project manager is typically hired to complete the migration process and is unavailable after that time to manage any adoption issues.

Qualities of a Project Manager

When selecting a project manager, an organization must evaluate a potential candidate for skills in communication, facilitation, negotiation, leadership delegation, and follow-up. Although he or she does not have to be a clinician, the project manager should have a good understanding of healthcare and clinical information.

Responsibilities of a Project Manager

The project manager handles all issues related to the selection and implementaiton of the EHR system. The issues may be the transition from paper to electronic records, different approaches to performing a job, or the frustration that stems from a lack of technical skills by employees or patients. The project manager should be able to visualize the end results of an organization's goals, be detailed at task monitoring, and have working knowledge of what can and cannot be accomplished. He or she will work closely with the information technology department and the vendor implementation team. Lastly, the project manager along with the vendor implementation team must identify the roles of the healthcare facility employees, create a training schedule, and monitor the training progress of the staff.

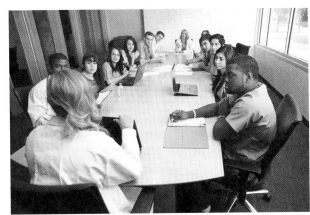

A project manager will spend time getting to know the employees and culture of an organization.

Migration Plan

In addition to the preliminary analysis, the healthcare facility should create a migration plan. A **migration plan** provides the framework to identify the basic steps that must be completed during the transition from paper health records to EHRs.

Basic Steps in a Migration Plan

A migration plan must direct a healthcare facility through these five key steps:

1. Identify requirements.

2. Create a design.

3. Analyze current systems.

4. Test the functionality.

5. Create a time line for implementation.

The first step, identifying **requirements**, asks a facility to identify the scope of the project and user needs. Creating a **design**, which is the second step, provides a blueprint that illustrates the transition process from paper health records to the new EHR system. The third step is to analyze the current systems and processes in place. This **analysis** step will examine how the healthcare facility currently uses its healthcare records and performs tasks. A workflow analysis (described in a later section) will be useful during this step. An **environmental analysis** is the process of evaluating the people and process of workflow in a healthcare organization, and is part of the analysis step. The fourth step is to **test** the functionality of the new EHR system. Finally, the last step of a migration plan is to create a timeline for **implementation**. The timeline, which is often created to look like a **Gantt chart** (a graphic representation of a project schedule), may include **schedules**, **resources**, and **dependencies**. Project managers schedule tasks for implementation, allocate resources (such as equipment and staff), and create dependencies (tasks that must occur before the next tasks can take place). Project managers often use programs like Microsoft Project to create a time line (see Figure 12.1).

Figure 12.1 Sample Time Line

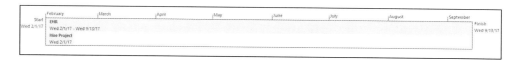

Key Considerations of a Migration Plan

Organizations that invest the appropriate amount of time and effort into a viable and sustainable migration plan will reap the rewards of successful EHR implementation. A facility's migration plan must also be fluid. There may be additional specialty software applications, such as those used by pharmacy, rehabilitation, or occupational departments that require integration into the EHR system. Healthcare staff must assess and add these applications to the implementation plan as needed.

CHECKPOINT 12.1

1. Describe the purpose of the Certification Commission for Health Information Technology.

   _____

   _____

   _____

2. Name the five key steps to electronic health record migration.

   a. _____

   b. _____

   c. _____

   d. _____

   e. _____

When preparing to evaluate and implement an electronic health record (EHR) system, one aspect of the migration plan is an environmental analysis. A key part of the environmental analysis is identifying barriers to the EHR implementation. One barrier may be the employees of the healthcare facility. For example, at Jackson Family Practice, many of the office and medical staff members are not technically savvy. Although the staff members are skilled with working with patients, some are not fond of change and are accustomed to certain processes that have historically been in place. Some were resistant to a previous migration from paper calendars to electronic scheduling. The staff eventually learned the new system, but it was a difficult process. Now that the practice is considering moving from paper health records to EHRs, staff members are concerned that learning a new technology will take time away from their patients. These are common barriers healthcare facilities face. Employees may not be confident in their technology skills, be resistant to change, or be concerned about increased time to complete tasks. If you were serving on the team assigned to complete the environmental analysis of Jackson Family Practice, how would you suggest the healthcare organization address these barriers?

Analyzing Workflow

A **workflow analysis** is an important assessment to conduct when selecting an EHR system. A workflow analysis reviews how the organization currently functions and how the paper records are used to care for patients. Workflow analysis should be considered for all back office, front office, health information management, and provider processes. Multiple stakeholders will be engaged in this process, and key internal stakeholders that comprehensively understand the flow

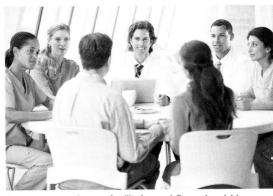

A team to analyze a facility's workflow should be made up of employees from many different departments.

of information in the facility are essential to an accurate analysis. Stakeholders may vary by facility but generally include health information managers, physicians, nurses, IT, and other department managers.

Use of a Flowchart

A **flowchart** showing all of the necessary steps in a particular procedure is an effective tool for understanding workflow analysis. The chart helps identify locations of breakdowns, insufficiencies, or bottlenecks. Armed with the knowledge that a flowchart provides, an organization or facility may be able to isolate the challenges to the flow of patient information and find a vendor that can address these workflow problems before final implementation of the EHR system.

Collection of Information

Before a facility can begin the task of gathering data for a workflow analysis, it must determine its approach. The organization may implement one of the following directives:

1. Put together a team from different departments

2. Assign staff members to perform their job requirements and analyze how work is completed

3. Conduct an internal analysis rather than working through a vendor

4. Assign overall responsibility to a project manager or internal staff person

Another approach that some facilities use to collect data is to ask departments or staff members to review how a patient is treated by "stepping into the patient's shoes." This role reversal helps them analyze the interaction between the patient and healthcare facility from the moment he or she checks in to the moment he or she leaves the facility.

Still another technique for collecting information for a workflow analysis is to ask staff members to write detailed descriptions of their tasks, actions, and sequences. Some questions may be:

1. What are the tasks or steps involved in the process?

2. Are there variations to these processes?

3. Are there acceptable reasons for process variations by your department?

4. Who completes the process?

5. How long does the process take?

6. Where are the bottlenecks where the process gets interrupted or slows down?

7. Do some tasks need to be completed more than once in a given process?

Collection of Forms

During the workflow analysis process, it is also vital to gather all the paper forms used by healthcare facility employees because these forms will now be entered electronically in an EHR system. Understanding where and how the forms are used, as well as what information is collected and communicated, is an integral part of the EHR workflow analysis.

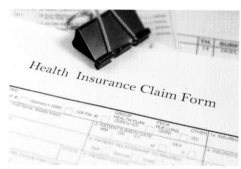

Healthcare facilities will need to gather all of the paper forms they use to perform workflow analysis.

Desired Outcome of Workflow Analysis

A workflow analysis provides an integrated framework that coordinates the processes of several departments in a healthcare facility. This workflow sequence serves:

- the facility by setting realistic expectations for the software functions
- the staff by streamlining processes and improving communication
- the patient by coordinating treatment and improving the overall quality of administered healthcare.

The workflow analysis should also reflect a sequence that aligns with the organization's goals regarding the EHR. Figures 12.2 and 12.3 show a workflow process for a medication refill—both before and after EHR system implementation.

Figure 12.2   Medication Refill Workflow Process Before EHR Implementation

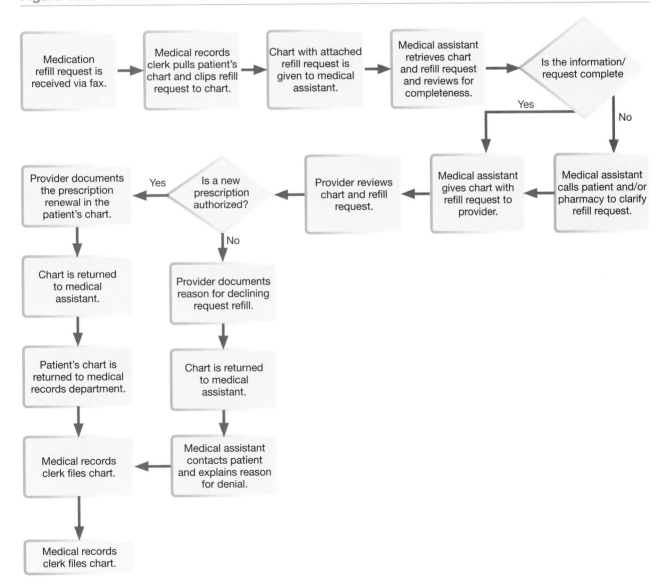

Figure 12.3 Medication Refill Workflow Process After EHR Implementation

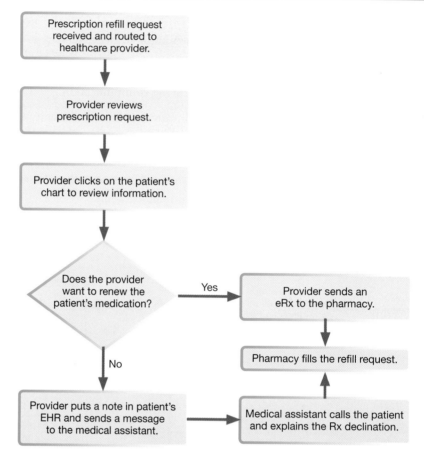

Vendor Selection

Once a facility decides to purchase an EHR system, the organization's steering committee begins the vendor selection process. This process can be a challenging and requires the input of employee representatives from several key departments of the healthcare facility. These department representatives may include management, health information staff, administrative staff, clinical staff, healthcare providers, and information technology staff. Making such an important decision regarding the EHR system should involve representatives from the entire organization. Depending on size, some facilities may choose to hire consultants to assist with the vendor selection process.

One helpful suggestion is to think of working with an EHR system vendor as a long-term relationship. The healthcare facility must be certain that it can work effectively with the selected vendor because both parties will be entering a closely collaborative relationship. To determine if an EHR vendor fits the needs of a facility, the steering committee should consider the following questions:

- Does the vendor have the support staff, financial resources, and capabilities to meet the needs of the organization?

- Does the vendor have the management expertise to ensure the completion of all tasks related to EHR implementation?

- Is continued research and development in technology and health information a priority for the vendor?

- Is the vendor knowledge-able of the requirements for government certification and regulations of EHR systems?

- Does the vendor have a functional product with the ability to adapt to changes required by the healthcare industry?

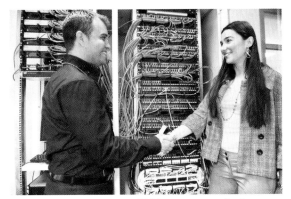

Positive support from an EHR system vendor is an important part of a collaborative relationship.

- Does the vendor offer technical and training support for healthcare personnel?

- Has the vendor received positive reviews by other healthcare organizations?

Healthcare facilities have many choices when selecting an EHR system. They may choose to build their own, use several applications from a variety of vendors, or choose an **integrated system**. No matter which option a facility pursues, the organization must select a certified EHR system to receive federal incentives. A **best-of-breed** EHR system is when the healthcare organization goes to market to find a vendor or vendors to supply the clinical applications needed. The healthcare facility then chooses various vendors evaluated to be the best in the particular area of healthcare and integrates them into an entire EHR system.

CCHIT Certification

In 2006, CCHIT started certifying EHR systems. The organization began by providing a comprehensive, practical definition of an EHR system's required capabilities, which was established by a voluntary, consensus-based process that included a diverse group of stakeholders. As a result, the U.S. federal government recognizes CCHIT as a certifying organization of EHR systems. Some certified EHR inpatient systems include NextGen Ambulatory EHR, GE Healthcare, EpicCare Inpatient and EpicCare Ambulatory, and Allscripts.

CCHIT certification is based on more than 400 criteria encompassing functionality, interoperability, and security. Table 12.1 gives an overview of the CCHIT certification criteria categories. The kind of certification awarded to a facility depends on the type of facility: ambulatory, inpatient, emergency department, or behavioral health (see Table 12.2). CCHIT also offers certifications for long-term, post-acute care centers, and electronic prescribing (e-prescribing) EHR systems.

Each healthcare facility will determine the criteria important for their facility. CCHIT awards different types of certifications based on the type of facility. The certifications are illustrated in Table 12.2.

In addition, CCHIT offers certifications for long-term, post-acute care centers, and electronic prescribing EHR systems.

EXPAND YOUR LEARNING

You may find a full list of certified products on CCHIT's website at www.paradigmcollege.net/exploringehr/cchit.

Table 12.1 CCHIT Certification Criteria

Criterion	Description
Patient Record	Creates unique records with unique identifiers, demographic information, and provider information, and ensures compatibility with records of other systems
Diagnosis Data	Accurately and discretely captures, manages, and accesses patient compliance information
Medications	Accurately and discretely tracks medication usage and history and suggests, prescribes, and administers medications, taking into account patient complaints, allergies, and drug interactions for potential adverse reactions
Document Management	Makes and modifies notes, captures vital signs, manages authorizations and advance directives, and integrates images and documents from external sources as necessary
Patient Education	Generates and records patient instructions based on condition, severity, and/or patient history, and modifies that information or customizes it to the patient
Testing	Integrates with diagnostic tests and laboratory results, including ordering, receiving, tracking, graphic ability, and compatibility with external sources
Disease Management	Tracks the patient condition for preventive care, providing automatic alerts based on standard and customizable warning criteria
Administration	Includes clinical task assignment, interprovider communication scheduling, and report generation
Concurrent Use	Allows multiple providers to simultaneously use the same or different settings
Security	Provides HIPAA compliance, including authentication and selective access control with the office environment

Table 12.2 CCHIT Certifications

Certification	Description
Ambulatory	Meets all the criteria for outpatient facilities. In addition to the standard certification, ambulatory certification may have add-on certification for the following specialties: behavioral, cardiovascular, pediatric, dermatology, clinical research, oncology, and obstetrics
Inpatient	Focuses heavily on medication orders and orders sets (standardized list of orders for a specific diagnosis), including the ability to administer medications safely and effectively. CCHIT encourages inpatient systems to test against all Office of the National Coordinator–Authorized Testing and Certification (ONC-ATC) Body criteria for eligible hospitals at no additional charge
Emergency Department	Focuses on laboratory messaging; must to meet criteria for bed management, discharge instructions, and transfers to other departments
Behavioral Health	Manages clinical documents, notes, assessments, and treatment plans that change over time; may have qualified under an ambulatory EHR with a behavioral add-on or as a stand-alone behavioral health certification.

Features of an Effective EHR System

Selecting an EHR system is a difficult task, with significant pressure on the steering committee to select a system that demonstrates profitability and improved clinical quality. Essential essential features of an effective EHR system include:

- CCHIT certification
- Operating system
- Web-based or on-site server
- Backup, downtime, and disaster recovery
- Data management and reporting systems

- Functionality
- Security
- Interoperability
- Payer interface
- License agreement
- Maintenance and support

As part of the vendor evaluation process, the steering committee should request an on-site or online demonstration. After the demonstration, the committee should evaluate the EHR system based on a previously developed assessment tool. See Figure 12.4 for a sample demonstration request and evaluation tool. The evaluation tool should include the essential features similar to the list provided in Figure 12.5.

Once the steering committee narrows down the short list of potential EHR systems, the committee should request a quote from the vendor. This quote is often referred to as a **request for proposal (RFP)**, which is typically executed near the end of the vendor selection process. The RFP includes requirements, services, vendor information, and a bid or quote for the EHR system. For example, after the committee recommends the top three EHR systems, an RFP will be sent to each of those vendors. The facility and its committee will receive system requirements and services along with bids or quotes from the vendors and will compare each of them. After the committee selects the EHR system, the healthcare facility will enter an agreement with the chosen vendor.

Consider This

You are a member of the steering committee at Cincinnati Grace Physicians. Your commitee has developed an electronic health records (EHR) checklist and has requested demonstrations from four different EHR vendors. However, one of the committee members has a relative that works for one of the proposed vendors. Several members of the committee are concerned that the member will try to persuade the rest of the committee to select the vendor where the relative is employed. What measures should the committee implement to ensure an objective evaluation of all four EHR vendors?

VENDOR RATING TOOL

For each EHR product you are considering, assign a ranking from 1 to 5 (with 5 being best) for each of the criteria listed in the functionality and vendor characteristics categories below. Total the rankings for each vendor to determine a combined score for each category, then assign an overall ranking. For the cost section, supply a dollar amount for each criteria listed and then rank each vendor based on your assessment of its total initial and total annual costs. Next, consider the relative importance of the three categories and assign a percentage to each (e.g., functionality = 40 percent, cost = 20 percent and vendor characteristics = 40 percent). Finally, use these percentages to calculate the weighted scores for each vendor.

FUNCTIONALITY	VENDOR 1	VENDOR 2	VENDOR 3	VENDOR 4	VENDOR 5
Quality/presence of features we prioritized (see demo rating summaries)					
Ease of use (e.g., minimizes typing, is intuitive, simple layout)					
Speed (network/hardware configuration, minimizes keystrokes)					
Individual user flexibility • Multiple note creation options (transcribe, voice, template) • Provider can modify/create own templates • Provider can create own macros					
Preloaded templates and patient education					
Combined functionality score (total the rankings for each vendor)					
A Overall functionality ranking					

COST	VENDOR 1	VENDOR 2	VENDOR 3	VENDOR 4	VENDOR 5
Initial hardware and network upgrades					
Initial interfaces					
Initial software					
Total initial cost					
Annual software maintenance (includes upgrades and support)					
Annual interface upgrades					
Total annual cost (excludes initial costs)					
B Overall cost ranking					

VENDOR CHARACTERISTICS	VENDOR 1	VENDOR 2	VENDOR 3	VENDOR 4	VENDOR 5
Training					
Support					
Implementation					
Software upgrades					
Company stability					
Combined vendor characteristics score (total the rankings for each vendor)					
C Overall vendor characteristics ranking					

D Functionality		%
E Cost		%
F Vendor characteristics		%
		should total 100%

OVERALL RANKING	VENDOR 1	VENDOR 2	VENDOR 3	VENDOR 4	VENDOR 5
G Weighted functionality score ($(A \times D) \div 100$)					
H Weighted cost score ($(B \times E) \div 100$)					
I Weighted vendor characteristics score ($(C \times F) \div 100$)					
Weighted overall score ($G + H + I$)					
Final Ranking					

Source: American Academy of Family Physicians. Used with Permission.

EHR DEMONSTRATION RATING FORM

Each person who observes vendor demonstrations should complete a form like the one below. The form you use should list the functionality that your selection group decided was most important to your practice. To analyze the results, assign 1 point to strongly disagree, 2 to disagree, 3 to unsure, 4 to agree, and 5 to strongly agree. Calculate average scores for each function and print a summary score sheet for each vendor.

PRODUCT: _____

DATE: _____

EVALUATOR: _____

Please evaluate the product based on all the information you have available at this time. If you need more information, please note that in your comments.

I. FUNCTIONALITY: This product performs the following functions with little user effort:

	Strongly disagree	Disagree	Unsure	Agree	Strongly agree
Results reporting (lab/X-ray)					
Progress/consult notes					
E/M coding					
Telephone message documentation and tasking					
Chart documentation (problem list, medication list, allergies, vital signs, health maintenance, trending lab values, etc.)					
Order entry (lab/X-ray)					
Prescription writer					
Formularies					
E-fax to outside physicians					
Remote access (e.g., to off-site transcription or physician's home)					
Referral management					
Charge capture without manual entry					
E-mail (encrypted)					
Health maintenance alerts					
Medical decision support tools					
Patient education materials					
Security (passwords, audit trails)					

Comments: _____

_____

_____

II. OVERALL EASE OF USE AND FLEXIBILITY

	Strongly disagree	Disagree	Unsure	Agree	Strongly agree
This product allows individual user-specific customization					
This product minimizes user data input					
This product offers multiple note creation options					

Comments: _____

_____

_____

Source: American Academy of Family Physicians. Used with Permission.

Total Cost of Ownership

Total cost of ownership is more than just the price of purchasing an EHR system. A healthcare organization must examine all relevant costs to make an informed decision, including accounting, opportunity, and economic costs. A facility will also incur many additional expenditures associated with EHR implementation.

Accounting Costs

An **accounting cost** is the total amount of money paid out for products, goods, or services. The accounting costs of an EHR system include the hardware, software, productivity loss, implementation, vendor or technical support, and software licenses. Hence, the accounting cost is the direct cost of the EHR system.

Opportunity Costs

An **opportunity cost** is the value of a decision. Something must be given up for the benefit of something else. For instance, an opportunity cost could include the consequence of not implementing an EHR system and losing patients to healthcare facilities that have one. Accounting worksheets do not show opportunity costs.

Economic Costs

An **economic cost** is the combination of accounting and opportunity costs. It includes the cash outlays related to the implementation of the EHR and is what is given up following the EHR implementation decision.

Additional Financial Considerations

Healthcare providers interested in purchasing an EHR system must understand that, in addition to accounting and opportunity costs, there are additional financial expenditures that must be considered:

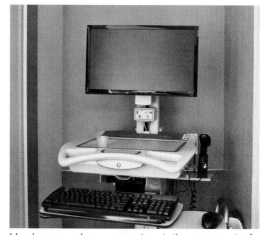

Hardware such as computer stations are part of the cost of implementing an EHR.

- The healthcare facility may have to hire additional staff trained in health informatics.

- The technical support staff may need to hire additional employees or outsource the job functions.

- The healthcare facility must conduct and assess workflow analysis.

- The healthcare facility must provide training for all healthcare employees.

- Data dictionaries and templates must be created, developed, and reviewed.

Other factors that must be considered are as follows:

- Hardware—initial cost, maintenance, and other ongoing expenses

- Software—license fees, electronic claims and remittance, electronic prescribing costs

- Implementation and training—cost of installing, building, testing, and training

- Maintenance—annual fees for upgrades, support, training, and customization

- Downtime and recovery—depending on the type of EHR system (web-based or on-site server), the vendor should communicate its plans for downtime and data backup and storage (such as cloud, online, disk, or tape)

Once an EHR system has been purchased, installed, and implemented, the healthcare facility continue to perform regular maintenance on the system. For example, the software must be updated with information on the latest evidence-based medicine, new and recalled drugs, new disease terminology, and new processes and workflows of external factors such as reimbursement or patient needs.

CHECKPOINT 12.2

1. Name four financial considerations when purchasing an electronic health records (EHR) system.

   a. _____

   b. _____

   c. _____

   d. _____

2. Name the three costs included in the total cost of EHR ownership.

   a. _____

   b. _____

   c. _____

Return on Investment

When preparing to make a decision about implementing an EHR system, a healthcare facility may perform a **cost–benefit analysis** to determine the return on investment. **Return on investment (ROI)** is a performance measurement that calculates the benefit or gain of an investment. The healthcare facility will need to pinpoint the payback period by comparing the cash flow (cash inflow minus cash outflow) with the cost of the investment to determine how long it takes to achieve a positive difference. If the payback period is longer than five years, the investment may not be worth it. Therefore, the healthcare organization may look at a less expensive EHR system to achieve a payback period of two to five years.

Internal rate of return (IRR) and net present value (NPV) should also be calculated. The **internal rate of return (IRR)** is a calculation used to measure the profitability

EXPAND
YOUR LEARNING
The American Society of Health Informatics Managers provides a free, downloadable return on investment (ROI) calculator. The calculator, found at www.paradigmcollege .net/exploringehr/ ROI_calculator, provides the necessary framework for assessing the ROI of an EHR system.

of an investment—in this case, the EHR system. The **net present value (NPV)** is the present value of future cash flows minus the purchase price of goods or services. The NPV measures the excess or shortfall of cash flows once the financial obligations are met. If the IRR or NPV for an EHR system is greater than the IRR or NPV of other EHR systems considered, then the EHR system is considered a good investment. Many healthcare organizations are recognizing that an EHR system must not be considered as a cost of doing business, but rather as a necessary component of healthcare delivery.

Most vendors provide an ROI analysis; however, this analysis requires a careful interpretation of the results. Typically, a vendor assigns a monetary value to every benefit, whether or not actual savings will result, so it is important for the steering commitee of the facility to scrutinize these numbers.

Consider This

Many times, healthcare organizations state that the implementation of an EHR system had a significant return on investment (ROI). To view one perspective on this issue, go to www.paradigmcollege.net/exploringehr/ ROI. Read the following case about Coastal Medical, the 2012 Ambulatory HIMSS Davies Award of Excellence, and their view of ROI and EHR implementation. What did the article say were the three key areas that benefited from implementing an EHR system?

Costs vs. Benefits of EHR Implementation

The costs and benefits associated with EHR implementation depend on a number of factors. To meet the meaningful use provision of EHRs required by the U.S. Department of Health & Human Services (HHS), a healthcare facility must make such an investment, and, depending on the type of healthcare facility, the total cost will vary. For example, a small community hospital working with a single vendor may spend $3 million; a medium-sized hospital that selects a "best-of-breed" system may spend $10 million to $15 million; and a large hospital may spend up to $100 million.

The size of the facility, complexity of the practice, implementation strategy, and types of services offered or performed factor in to the total cost of EHR implementation.

The benefits of EHR use depend on a variety of factors in the areas of efficiency, finance, quality, and compliance. The benefits in these areas are listed below:

- Efficiency
  - Reduces duplication of tests
  - Increases accuracy in patient information
  - Allows healthcare providers and services to view automated transfers

- Financial
  - Offers internal and external savings
  - Decreases malpractice insurance costs
- Quality
  - Provides reminders about preventive care
  - Eliminates illegible medication prescriptions
  - Standardizes data and quality of patient care
- Compliance
  - Creates reports
  - Complies with requirements from The Joint Commission and the Centers for Medicare & Medicaid Services (CMS)
  - Determines eligibility for Medicaid and Medicare programs

A healthcare facility must determine the overall costs and benefits in order to justify the investment. The real key, after all the numbers have been crunched, is the level of acceptance from a facility's staff. If its employees do not embrace the EHR system, then the facility will find its path to implementation difficult.

EHR Implementation

Implementation is as important as the selection of the EHR system. One of the factors that often contributes to implementation failure is fear and a lack of support from management; therefore, leadership is an essential aspect of implementation. The steering committee of the facility must identify leaders in each department who will champion the EHR system. These leaders should encourage adaptability and flexibility in their discussions with co-workers and act as a link between the departments and steering committee to provide staff feedback and suggestions for implementation.

The steering committee must devise a plan to train and manage the healthcare facility staff and to create security levels for staff members. The plan should contain the time line of when to begin training, how the training will take place, and how quickly the healthcare facility will be ready to switch over to the EHR system. As previously discussed in Chapter 3, the security level assigned to each healthcare facility staff member is based on the job requirements. Employees of the healthcare facility can only access portions of the EHR system directly related to their positions.

Roll Out Process

With the EHR system selected, the project manager in place, and the implementation plan created, the **rollout** process can begin. The rollout process occurs in three phases: organizational, training, and operational.

Organizational Phase

The first phase is organizational, which entails the plan for installation of the EHR system. This phase is usually complete once the rollout begins. As part of this phase, the healthcare staff converts all paper records to electronic records. As healthcare delivery systems begin the conversion process, there may be portions of patient records on paper and other portions stored electronically. As you learned in Chapter 2, this type of record is known as a hybrid health record. Healthcare providers with a small patient population may convert to an EHR system in a shorter time frame. However, a provider with a larger patient population, such as a major hospital, may take longer to fully convert to an EHR system; therefore, larger organizations may use a hybrid health record for a considerably longer period than their smaller counterparts.

Training Phase

The second phase is training and heavily emphasizes learning, fine tuning, customizing, and testing of the EHR system.

Operational Phase

The rollout process ends with the operational phase, which includes the launch of the EHR system and continual training while maintenance begins. A successful EHR launch depends on the efforts put into the other phases. Prior to the "go live" date, the EHR system must be tested many times, including its hardware, software, backup, networking, connectivity, and recovery components. Most healthcare organizations choose to complete pilots prior to going live. A **pilot** is a test run of the EHR system. In addition, during the pilot, users can identify issues or problems that they encounter.

Preparation Phase

A few weeks prior to the "go live" date, all staff members should be trained for the required functionalities and assessed for mastery. **Functionality testing** often requires a facility to use a test environment before implementing the EHR system facilitywide. Key users, who are selected because of their expertise and knowledge, run the system to ensure it works as described and meets the needs of the facility. Lastly, the healthcare facility should notify its patients that its facility is implementing an EHR system and inform them of the "go live" date. This notification prepares patients for upcoming changes, including any potential delays in scheduling, billing, or wait times.

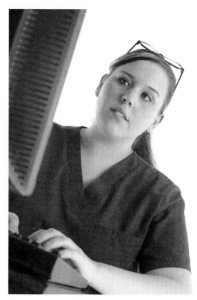

Staff members will be trained on the system prior to the "go live" date.

"Go Live" Date

Healthcare organizations have different approaches to going live. Some facilities choose a phased implementation in which one function of the EHR system is made available at a time. This staggered approach allows for the organization to resolve issues and receive feedback on individual features or applications. Alternatively, an organization can choose a "big bang" approach, making all EHR functions immediately available to all users. This approach speeds up implementation but runs the risk of creating multiple problems or delays.

It is important that every member of the organization be prepared for the "go live" date of the EHR system. If a healthcare facility is using a commercial product, then the vendor will usually provide a customized checklist. The checklist may include determining healthcare provider schedules, planning downtime to catch up, informing users where they can go to receive help, informing third parties in case there is a delay or need to provide additional support to the healthcare facility, and planning for end-of-day debriefing.

Consider This

One aspect of electronic health record (EHR) implementation is to plan for an information technology (IT) outage. Boulder Community Hospital in Boulder, CO, learned this lesson when it experienced a computer system outage, leaving patients frustrated. To learn more about this incident and the measures taken to rectify the situation, go to www.paradigmcollege.net/exploringehr/outage

How would you handle an IT outage that meant the EHR system would be unavailable?

Meaningful Use

As you learned in Chapter 1, the adoption of EHR systems is based on the idea of meaningful use, which connects all parts of the EHR into a system that can effectively communicate and deliver electronic healthcare services. To qualify a system as succeeding in this standard, a practitioner must demonstrate that the EHR system is used in a significant and measurable manner.

Stages of Meaningful Use

As you remember from Chapter 1, the HITECH Act, funded by the American Recovery and Reinvestment Act of 2009 [ARRA], outlined three main components of Stage 1 meaningful use:

- Use of a certified EHR in a meaningful manner (such as e-prescribing)
- Use of a certified EHR for electronic exchange of health information to improve quality of care
- Use of certified EHR system to submit clinical quality measure (CQM) and other measures

The criteria for meaningful is divided into three stages and spans four years, 2011–2015. Stage 1 (2011–2012) sets the baseline for electronic data capture and information sharing. Stage 2 (established in October 2012) and Stage 3 (expected to be implemented in 2015) will continue to expand on this baseline.

EHR Incentive Payments

There are several ways for a healthcare facility to qualify for ARRA-funded EHR incentive payments and meet meaningful use requirements, including the following:

- Meet the guidelines of Medicaid EHR Incentive Program

  - Eligible professionals, eligible hospitals, and critical access hospitals may qualify for incentive payments if they demonstrate meaningful use of certified EHR technology and in the first year of participation and every year thereafter.

- Meet the guidelines of Medicare EHR Incentive Program

  - Eligible professionals and eligible hospitals may qualify for incentive payments if they adopt, implement, upgrade, or demonstrate meaningful use in their first year of participation. They must successfully demonstrate meaningful use for subsequent participation years.

- Adopt an EHR system

  - Acquire and install certified EHR technology

- Implement an EHR system

  - Begin using certified EHR technology

- Upgrade an EHR system

  - Expand existing technology to meet certification requirements

Activity 12.1	EHRNAVIGATOR

Generating an Attestation Report

Go to the Course Navigator to launch Activity 12.1. As an IT manager, practice generating an attestation report.

Chapter Summary

The transition from paper health records to electronic health records (EHRs) can be a challenge. Each organization must be thoughtful as it determines how to initiate this process.

A healthcare organization must first assess its readiness to adopt an EHR system before it selects a system to meet its needs. The organization should form a steering committee, set goals, and create a migration plan. A migration plan should identify the EHR requirements, create a design, analyze current systems, test the new system, and set an implementation date for the EHR system. The committee should also conduct a workflow analysis for each area of the organization and prepare a cost–benefit analysis to present to the administration.

Once these initial steps have been taken, the steering committee should then review potential vendors based on the organization's criteria. These vendors should be selected by reviewing a list of EHR systems that have been certified for functionality, interoperability, and security by the Certification Commission for Health Information Technology. They may use vendor demonstrations and issue proposal requests to help them determine EHR system selection.

Upon system selection, it is necessary to establish a rollout process and a "go live" date. Internal leaders from all areas of the organization are necessary to champion the newly selected system and enhance buy-in. A healthcare organization that follows this process enhances the probability of successful EHR implementation.

EHR Review

Check Your Understanding

To check your understanding of this chapter's key concepts, read the following multiple-choice and true/false questions and then record your answers on a separate sheet of paper. Write your answers as modeled in these examples: 1a; 2b; 6T; 7F; etc.

1. For a healthcare organization to receive stimulus funds, the electronic health record (EHR) system must be certified by the:

   a. Office of the National Coordinator-Authorized Testing and Certification Bodies

   b. American Health Information Management Association

   c. American Medical Association

   d. Centers for Medicare & Medicaid Services

2. The first step in selecting an EHR system is to:

    a. establish goals.

    b. assess readiness.

    c. form a steering committee.

    d. create a budget.

3. The accounting costs of an EHR system may include any of the following *except*:

    a. Hardware, software, vendor support, software licenses

    b. Software, productivity loss, implementation, vendor support

    c. Hardware, software, technical support, project management

    d. Productivity loss, implementation, technical support, software license

4. Return on investment is a/an:

    a. formula that calculates the cost of the EHR system.

    b. analysis of the cost benefit of an EHR system.

    c. performance measurement that calculates the expense of an investment.

    d. performance measurement that calculates the benefit of an investment.

5. Benefits of adopting an EHR system include all of the following *except*:

    a. Financial

    b. Analysis

    c. Quality

    d. Compliance

6. True/False: The five key steps of a migration plan are identify the requirements, create a design, analyze current systems, test functionality, and create a time line for implementation.

7. True/False: A workflow analysis reviews how an organization will function in the future and how EHRs are used.

8. True/False: A facility that selects an EHR vendor or vendors from the market to meet its need is adopting a "best-of-breed" system.

9. True/False: A request for proposal (RFP) is a request for demonstration by an EHR vendor.

10. True/False: The rollout process is the planning phase of the EHR system selection.

Learn the Terms

Go to www.paradigmcollege.net/exploringehr/Chapter12_Flash_Cards to access flash-cards for Chapter 12 of *Exploring Electronic Health Records*. Use the password paradigm to access the flashcards.

COURSE
NAVIGATOR

Acronyms

AHRQ: Agency for Healthcare Research and Quality

ARRA: American Recovery and Reinvestment Act of 2009

ASHIM: American Society of Health Informatics Managers

CCHIT: Certification Commission for Health Information Technology

CMS: Centers for Medicare & Medicaid Services

HHS: U.S. Department of Health & Human Services

HITECH Act: Health Information Technology for Economic and Clinical Health Act

HITRC: Health Information Technology Research Center

IRR: internal rate of return

IT: information technology

NPV: net present value

ONC-ATCB: Office of the National Coordinator-Authorized Testing and Certification Bodies

RFP: request for proposal

ROI: return on investment

EHR Application

Go on the Record

To build on your understanding of the topics in this chapter, complete the following short answer questions.

1. Describe the importance of selecting an EHR system certified by the Certification Commission for Health Information Technology (CCHIT).

2. Explain how an organization may assess its readiness to move to an EHR system.

3. Describe the key areas of a workflow analysis.

4. Discuss the key players on an EHR selection committee and how their roles affect EHR selection.

5. Compare three areas (accounting, opportunity, and economic costs) of the total cost of ownership and how those areas may affect EHR selection.

Navigate the Field

To gain practice in handling challenging situations in the workplace, consider the following real-world scenarios and then use the guiding questions to help you formulate your responses.

1. You are testing HealthWest Physician Practice's EHR system. Suddenly, the computer screen goes blank. You now realize you should have had an EHR system downtime plan to continue so the practice may keep operating. Go to www.paradigmcollege.net/exploringehr/downtime_plan and review the article. Then prepare a plan for HealthWest Physician Practice. After reviewing the article, prepare the appropriate guidelines for your healthcare facility to implement during this EHR system downtime.

2. You work for St. Stephen's Hospital and are leading the EHR steering committee. The committee has met and is in the RFP preparation phase. Your task is to write the introduction of the RFP. Be sure to include an overview of the healthcare organization, the opportunity, and the facility's goals in this introduction.

EHR Evaluation

Think Critically

Continue to think critically about challenging real-world scenarios and complete the following activities.

1. You are the EHR Implementation Specialist at Northstar Physicians. You are assigned the task of migrating the paper records to the EHR Navigator. Research migration plans for converting paper records to electronic records. Create a checklist that identifies which documents and information will need to be migrated to EHR Navigator.

2. As part of the EHR selection team, you have been given the task to research three certified complete Inpatient EHR Systems. You may use www.paradigmcollege.net/exploringehr/cchit as one source to locate complete Inpatient EHR Systems. You are to prepare a report comparing and contrasting the three systems. Write a two- to three-page report that would be submitted to the EHR selection committee making a recommendation based on your analysis of the three products.

Make Your Case

Consider the following scenario and create a presentation on the following topic.

You are the chair of the EHR system steering committee. Your team has met and reviewed the entire vendor selection process. Now you must present your findings and a recommendation to the administrators of your healthcare facility. Include the team's process in contacting vendors and examining the EHR systems, its recommendation, and the time line for implementation.

Explore the Technology

To expand your mastery of EHRs, explore the following online activities and complete the EHR Navigator assessments.

COURSE
NAVIGATOR

Ensure you are comfortable with the functionality presented in the EHR Navigator activities, such as running a meaningful use report. Then, complete the EHR Navigator assessment for Chapter 12 located on the Course Navigator.

1. Visit www.paradigmcollege.net/exploringehr/ehr_guidelines and then prepare a presentation on the recommended EHR guidelines.

2. Create a chart that analyzes the patient registration workflow.

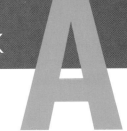

Checkpoint Answer Key

Checkpoint 1.1

1. An electronic version of patient files within a single organization that allows healthcare providers to place orders, document results, and store patient information for one facility.

2. The patient health information gathered from the EMRs of multiple healthcare delivery organizations that is electronically stored and accessed.

3. a. EMR belongs to a single healthcare provider or organization whereas EHR integrates EMRs from multiple providers.

   b. EHRs contain subsets of patient information from each visit that a patient has experienced.

   c. EHRs are interactive and can share information among multiple healthcare providers.

Checkpoint 1.2

1. The ability of one computer system to communicate with another computer system.

2. Level 3: Semantic interoperability level.

3. Health Level 7 (HL7).

Checkpoint 1.3

1. a. Improved documentation.

   b. Streamlined and rapid communication.

   c. Immediate and improved access to patient information

2. a. High cost.

   b. Privacy and security.

   c. Inexperience in implementation and training.

   d. Significant daily process changes.

Checkpoint 2.1

1. Data includes the descriptive or numeric attributes of one or more variables. Data collected and analyzed becomes information. A record is a collection, usually in writing of an account or an occurrence.

2. Administrative data includes demographic information; clinical data is information such as admission dates, office visits, laboratory test results, evaluations, or emergency visits; legal data is composed of consents for treatments and authorizations for the release of information; financial data includes the patient's insurance and payment information.

Checkpoint 2.2

1. The source-oriented record is the most common used by healthcare facilities. It organizes the health documents into sections that contain information from a specified department or type of service.

2. S(subjective) O (objective) A (assessment) P (plan).

Checkpoint 2.3

1. Answers may vary, and could include five of the following: admission record, history and physical, progress notes, laboratory tests, diagnostic tests, operative notes, pathology reports, physician orders, consents, consultations, emergency department encounters, and discharge summary.

2. Answers may vary, and could include five of the following: demographic information, contact information, history and physical, immunization records, problem lists, allergy lists, prescription lists, progress notes, assessment, consultations, referrals, treatment plans, patient instructions, laboratory tests and results, consents, communication, external correspondence, and financial information.

Checkpoint 3.1

1. a. input
   b. processing
   c. output
   d. storage
2. A LAN is a group of computers connected through a network confined to a single area or small geographic area. The network is secure and reliable. The networked computer system allows computer workstations to work and communicate together.

Checkpoint 3.2

1. a. Monthly calendar
   b. Weekly calendar
   c. Daily calendar

2. The messages feature allows you to communicate with other system users in your organizations using a HIPAA-compliant feature. It improves the collaboration and continuity of patient care.

Checkpoint 3.3

1. Answers may vary, and could include four of the following: medical diagnoses, treatments, procedures, allergies, medical history, medications, test results, and reports.

2. An integrated laboratory feature enables healthcare facilities and providers to connect with national and regional laboratories or to maintain an existing laboratory partner. Integrating laboratories into an EHR system gives you the ability to create laboratory orders and view results from any computer at any time, with abnormal results flagged and organized for easy review.

Checkpoint 4.1

1. Answers may vary, and could include four of the following: acute care setting such as a hospital; ambulatory care settings such as surgery centers, physician offices, clinics, group practices, emergency departments, therapeutic services, dialysis clinics, birthing centers, cancer treatment centers, home care, correctional facilities, and dentist offices; other healthcare settings, such as long-term care facilities, behavioral health settings, rehabilitation facilities, and hospice care.

2. If a patient goes to an ambulatory care facility for a procedure and complications occur, requiring the patient to be admitted to an acute care facility.

Checkpoint 4.2

1. a. Personal/Family
   b. Workers' Compensation
   c. Third-Party Liability
   d. Corporate
   e. Research

2. If two insurance plans cover a child, then the birthday rule is applied. The birthday rule specifies that the insurance of the parent whose birthday falls first in a calendar year will be the primary insurance. It helps to determine which insurance should be used as the primary insurance.

Checkpoint 5.1

1. a. Open Hours

    b. Time Specified

    c. Wave

    d. Modified Wave

    e. Cluster

2. Meetings, holidays, lunch hours, surgical schedules, physician rounds, or emergencies.

Checkpoint 5.2

1. Patient portals are available 24-hours a day and allow the patient to view a provider's calendar. The portal allows patients to enter demographic, insurance, medical history, and current health information prior to the first appointment, reducing the resources necessary from the healthcare facility.

2. a. Select the patient

    b. Select Add Appointment

    c. Select Calendar

Checkpoint 5.3

1. a. Change in patient condition

    b. Change in isolation status

    c. Patient preference

2. The patient tracker offers a real-time, at-a-glance view of a patient's current status and location. It improves the healthcare facility's work flow and increases patient satisfaction.

Checkpoint 6.1

1. True

2. False

3. Covered entities

Checkpoint 6.2

1. Answers may vary, and could include three of the following: impermissible uses and disclosures of PHI, lack of safeguards of PHI, lack of patient access to his or her PHI, uses or disclosures of more than the minimum necessary PHI, lack of administrative safeguards of electronic PHI.

2. A civil violation is when a person mistakenly obtains or discloses individually identifiable health information in violation of HIPAA. A criminal violation is when a person knowingly obtains or discloses individually identifiable health information in violation of HIPAA.

Checkpoint 6.3

1. a. General Rules

    b. Administrative Safeguards

    c. Physical Safeguards

    d. Technical Safeguards

    e. Organization Requirements

    f. Policies and Procedures and Documentation Requirements

2. Technical Safeguards

3. Administrative Safeguards

Checkpoint 7.1

1. Answers may vary, and could include three of the following: EHR documentation is more legible than handwritten paper records, documentation may be more timely, diagnostic reports automatically interface to the EHR, electronic physician queries are potentially answered in a timelier manner, EHRs that use templates may contain more complete information if completion of all data items in the templates is required, physicians may be more likely to document more information in an EHR, coders can access a record at any time, records can be accessed by more than one individual at a time, coders do not have to wait for a discharged chart to be physically collected from the nurses station,

and coders do not have to wait for the HIM staff to assemble and analyze the discharged chart before having access for coding.

2. a. Cloned notes

   b. Automatic population of "normal"

Checkpoint 7.2

1. True

2. Medical transcription service organizations

3. Accurate, complete, and reliable clinical documentation in an EHR.

Checkpoint 8.1

1. Because it requires less personnel time, avoids repetitive request of information from patients, and may allow for more consistent data entry.

2. The history is the subjective element and has the following components: history of present illness, past medical history, allergies, medications currently prescribed, family and social histories. The physical examination is the objective element of the H&P, and consists of a physical examination of body systems, an assessment of the patient and his or her condition, and a treatment plan.

Checkpoint 8.2

1. Answers may vary, but could include three of the following: improved prescribing accuracy and efficiency; a decreased potential for medication errors and prescription forgeries; improved billing; less risk for potential medication errors due to a healthcare provider's handwriting, illegible faxes, or misinterpretation of prescription abbreviations.

2. a. Laws governing the dispensing of controlled substances

   b. Lack of interoperability between healthcare facility software and pharmacy software

Checkpoint 9.1

1. Answers may vary, and could include three of the following: reimbursement, research, decision making, public health, quality improvement, resource utilization, and healthcare policy and payment.

2. October 1, 2014

3. 2020

Checkpoint 9.2

1. a. Efficient concurrent and final coding

   b. Accuracy in code assignments

   c. Improved access to health records

2. False. Upcoding is illegal. Unintentional upcoding is considered abuse, and intentional upcoding is considered fraud.

Checkpoint 10.1

1. Health information technology that integrates with the EHR and assists healthcare providers with decision-making tasks such as determining diagnoses, choosing the best medications for the patient, and selecting proper diagnostic tests.

2. a. Knowledge-based

   b. Non-knowledge-based

3. Answers may vary and may include three of the following advantages: reduced risk of medication errors; reduced risk of misdiagnosis, increased direct patient care time for healthcare providers; access to state-of-the-art data, research, clinical pathways, and guidelines; reduction of unnecessary diagnostic tests; faster diagnoses, resulting in faster treatments; and prescriptions for lower cost medications. The potential disadvantages may include three of the following: costs of maintaining the CDSS with up-to-date medical research, clinical pathways, guidelines, and medication costs; potential over-reliance on computer technology; perception by healthcare providers as a threat to clinical knowledge and skills; and harmful outcomes if software is not thoroughly and continuously updated.

Checkpoint 10.2

1. EHRs play a major role in quality improvement activities. Reporting capabilities in EHR systems provide healthcare organizations with important statistics and can identify opportunities to improve patient care.

2. Answers may vary, but could include three of the following for inpatient facilities: infection rates; ventilation wean success rates; lengths of stay; fall rates; morbidity and mortality rates; types and frequency of diagnostic tests per diagnosis-related group; and medication errors. The examples for outpatient facilities may include three of the following: mammography, diabetes, and colorectal screenings; and routine physical examinations.

Checkpoint 11.1

1. Answers may vary, but could include low cost, private, secure, and safe at home rather than in cyberspace.

2. Answers may vary, but could include difficulty in assembling, organizing, and updating. There is no established format, and a paper PHR may lack the necessary details to provide a complete picture of a patient's health status. Security may also be an issue. Finally, in an emergency, a paper record may be unavailable or difficult to decipher.

Checkpoint 11.2

1. a. The Veterans Administration

   b. The Centers for Medicare & Medicaid Services (CMS)

2. a. Request a copy of your health records.

   b. Review the various types of PHRs and select one that meets your needs.

   c. Organize your health information.

Checkpoint 11.3

1. Answers may vary, but could include four of the following: Medical Record, Health Summary, Test Results, Hospital Admission, Medications, Allergies, Immunizations, Preventive Care, Medical History, Current Health Issues, Health Trends, View My Appointments, Cancel My Appointments, Request My Appointment, My Family Records, Message Center, Get Medical Advice, Request Rx Refill, Request a Referral, Billing and Insurance, Billing Account Summary, Insurance Summary, Settings, or Portable PHR.

2. Linking medical records is important because other providers and facilities may need access to health information such as medications, previous test results, previous procedures, hospital admissions, and any complications experienced. When a healthcare provider has access to this information, thus better knowing a patient's health history, the delivery and quality of care may improve.

Chapter 12.1

1. CCHIT developed a rigorous process to examine EHR systems for functionality, interoperability, and security. CCHIT also provides resources to help healthcare facilities select an appropriate EHR system.

2. a. Identify requirements

   b. Create design

   c. Analyze current systems

   d. Create a timeline for implementation

Checkpoint 12.2

1. Answers may vary, but could include four of the following: the healthcare facility may have to hire additional staff trained in health informatics; the technical support staff may need to hire additional employees or outsource the job functions; the healthcare facility must conduct and assess workflow analysis; the healthcare facility must provide training for all healthcare employees; data dictionaries and templates must be created, developed, and reviewed.

2. a. Accounting costs

   b. Opportunity costs

   c. Economic costs

Sample Paper Medical Record

A medical record, in any form, is the legal record of the care and treatment provided to a patient. In this textbook, *Exploring Electronic Health Records*, you have read about and have experienced hands-on activities using the EHR. In these hands-on activities you accessed the EHR Navigator as many different healthcare professionals including a physician, nurse, IT administrator, admissions clerk, front desk clerk, health information management professional, etc.

Now that you have experienced an EHR, perhaps you would benefit from a review of a sample paper medical record. The average medical record is generally more than 200 pages long. The sample paper medical record included in this appendix is significantly smaller and is meant to provide you with exposure to a paper medical record.

The paper medical record in this appendix includes:

- Facesheet
- Consent to Treat
- Informed Consent for Invasive, Diagnostic, Medical & Surgical Procedures
- Notice of Acknowledgment of Advance Directive
- Discharge Summary
- Consultation Report
- History and Physical
- Operative Report
- Physician's Orders
- Progress Notes
- Lab Results
- Radiology Report
- Nurse's Notes
- Physical Therapy Evaluation
- Speech Evaluation
- Patient Continuum of Care Transfer Form
- Medication Administration Record

The health care providers involved in the completion of this paper medical record include:

- Admission Clerk
- Attending Physician
- Consulting Physician
- Surgeon
- Laboratory Technician
- Radiologist
- Nurses
- Physical Therapist
- Speech Therapist

NORTHSTAR MEDICAL CENTER

NORTHSTAR
Medical Center

Facesheet

PATIENT INFORMATION

Patient's Last Name	First	Middle Initial	Type of Care:	☒In Patient ☐ Same Day Surgery
Walker	Marjorie	R	☐ Maternity ☐ Surgery ☐ Outpatient	

Race	Marital Status	Religion	Primary Language	Date of Birth (mm/dd/yyyy)	Date of Scheduled Visit
Caucasian	M	Mormon	English	06/03/1956	

Physician's Last Name	First Name	☒Female	Social Security No.
Chaplin	Patrick	☐ Male	000-00-0000

Patient's Street Address	Apt. No.	City	State	Zip
3370 Oakwood Ave		Cincinnati	OH	45203

Home Phone	Work Phone	Cell Phone	Visit Reason or Diagnosis	Admission Date
(513) 555-1632	(513) 555-1818	(513) 555-0823	Left Leg Wound	03/18/2012

Temporary Address	Apt. No.	City	State	Zip

Patient's Current Employer Name	Employer Address	City	State	Zip
Rapid Printing	6240 Parkland Drive	Cincinnati	OH	45201

Employer Phone	Patient's Occupation	Employment Status: ☐ Not Employed ☒Full Time
(513) 555-1818	Pre-Press Operator	☐ Part Time ☐ Student ☐ Retired and Date:

Full Name of Emergency Contact	Relationship	Home Phone	Work Phone
Fulton Walker	Husband	(513) 555-1632	(513) 555-1471

Have you ever been a patient at Northstar Medical Center? ☒Yes ☐ No	If yes, when was your last visit? 02/06/1980	Under what name? Buehler

Guarantor

Last Name	First	Middle Initial	Relationship	Date of Birth (mm/dd/yyyy)
Walker	Marjorie	R	Self	06/03/1956

Street Address	Apt. No.	☐ Female	Marital Status	Social Security No.
3370 Oakwood Ave		☐ Male	M	000-00-0000

City	State	Zip	Home Phone	Work Phone	Cell Phone
Cincinnati	OH	45203	(513) 555-1632	(513) 555-1818	(513) 555-0823

Employer Name	Employer Address	City	State	Zip
Rapid Printing	6240 Parkland Drive	Cincinnati	OH	45201

Employer Phone	Occupation	Employment Status: ☐ Not Employed ☒Full Time
(513) 555-1818	Pre-Press Operator	☐ Part Time ☐ Student ☐ Retired and Date:

Insurance Information

Primary Insurance Name	Name of Insured exactly as appears on card
Cobalt Blue	Marjorie Ruth Walker

Insurance Billing Address	City	State	Zip	Phone No.
PO Box 690	Seattle	WA	98119	(800) 475-755X

Policy No.	Group No.	Plan Code	State	Effective Date	Expiration Date
189624733	9985	3	OH	01/01/2012	12/31/2012

Subscriber's Full Name	Subscriber's Soc. Sec. No.	Subscriber's Date of Birth	☒Female
Marjorie Ruth Walker	000-00-0000	06/03/1956	☐ Male

Subscriber's Employer name (if self-employed, company name)	Relation to Insured	Subscriber's Employment Status: ☐ Not Employed
Rapid Printing	Self	☒Full Time ☐ Part Time ☐ Student ☐ Retired and Date:

Subscriber's Employer Address	City	State	Zip	Phone No.
6240 Parkland Drive	Cincinnati	OH	45201	(513) 555-1818

<table>
<tr><td rowspan="8">Insurance Information</td><td colspan="2">Medicare Number</td><td colspan="2">Patient's name as appears on card</td><td colspan="2">Effective Date (mm/dd/yyyy)
_____

_____</td><td>☐ Part A (Hospital Benefit)

☐ Part B (Medical Benefit)</td></tr>
<tr><td colspan="2">Medicaid Number</td><td colspan="2">Patient's name as appears on card</td><td colspan="2">Effective Date</td><td>State</td></tr>
<tr><td colspan="4">Secondary Insurance Name
NA</td><td colspan="3">Name of Insured exactly as appears on card</td></tr>
<tr><td colspan="3">Insurance Billing Address</td><td>City</td><td>State</td><td>Zip</td><td>Phone No.
(   )</td></tr>
<tr><td colspan="2">Policy No. (for BCBS, include 3 letter prefix)</td><td>Group No.</td><td>Plan Code</td><td>State</td><td>Effective Date</td><td>Expiration Date</td></tr>
<tr><td colspan="2">Subscriber's Full Name</td><td colspan="2">Subscriber's Soc. Sec. No.</td><td colspan="3">Subscriber's Date of Birth (mm/dd/yyyy)   ☐ Female   ☐ Male</td></tr>
<tr><td colspan="2">Subscriber's Employer name (if self-employed, company name)</td><td colspan="2">Relation to Insured</td><td colspan="3">Subscriber's Employment Status: ☐ Not Employed
☐ Full Time ☐ Part Time ☐ Student ☐ Retired and Date:</td></tr>
<tr><td colspan="2">Subscriber's Employer Address</td><td>City</td><td>State</td><td>Zip</td><td colspan="2">Phone No.
(   )</td></tr>
<tr><td rowspan="3">Worker's Compensation</td><td colspan="2">Is this visit the result of an accident?

☐ Yes   ☐ No</td><td colspan="2">☐ Employment
☐ Automobile
☐ Other</td><td colspan="2">Date of Accident:
(mm/dd/yyyy)</td><td>Claim No.</td></tr>
<tr><td colspan="2">Letter of Authorization

☐ Yes   ☐ No</td><td colspan="2">Claim Adjuster / Contact Name</td><td colspan="2">Phone No.
(   )</td><td>Insurance Name</td></tr>
<tr><td colspan="2">Insurance Address</td><td colspan="2">City</td><td>State</td><td>Zip</td><td>Phone No.
(   )</td></tr>
</table>

Advance Directive

Do you have an Advance Directive, such as a Living Will or Durable Power of Attorney for Health Care?   ☒ Yes   ☐ No
Please specify the type: <u>Living Will</u>
*** *If yes, please bring a copy at the time of your admission****

Self-Pay

* If insured but your procedure is not covered or verified by your plan, a deposit is required at the time of admission.

* If you do not have insurance, please call our *Northstar Financial Services at 513-555-122X* before your scheduled arrival date to discuss financial arrangements.

Additional Information

Do you need special accommodations, such as Translation, Visual Aid, etc.?   ☐ Yes   ☐ No

*** If yes, please specify so that prior arrangements can be made for the day of your visit. ***

☐ Language Interpreter _____   ☐ Sign Language Interpreter   ☐ Visual aid   ☐ Other: _____

NORTHSTAR MEDICAL CENTER

NORTHSTAR
Medical Center

Walker, Marjorie
PT#1772571 MRN#585120
DOB: 06/03/1956 Age: 56   Sex: F
Physician: Chaplin, Patrick
Admit: 03/18/2012

CONSENT TO TREAT

Thank you for selecting Northstar Medical Center to provide for your healthcare needs. We are committed o providing exceptional healthcare. The first step pin this process is to provide information regarding patient rights, risks and responsibilities. The second step is to obtain your consent to treat the patient. The admitting staff can answer any questions you may have in regards to the following agreement.

I agree to the following

1. **Consent to Treat**: I consent to the treatment or admission of ____3/18/12____ at Northstar Medical Center for services or supplies that have been or may be ordered by a licensed professional healthcare provider. I understand that treatment may include but is not limited to: radiological examinations, laboratory procedures, physical therapy, anesthesia, nursing care or medical and surgical treatment. Your case may be attended by vendors and clinical students. I understand that all licensed professional healthcare providers that render service to the patient are responsible and liable for their own acts, orders and omissions. I acknowledge that the hospital has not made nor can it make a guarantee of the outcome of treatment.

2. **Financial Agreement**: I agree to pay for all services and supplies rendered to the patient in accordance with the rates and financial policies in effect at the time of service. I agree to pay interest fees on any unpaid balance after 30 days of discharge or date of service.

3. **Assignment of Insurance Benefits**: I assign and authorize payment directly to Northstar Medical Center of any healthcare benefits that the patient is entitled to receive. This assignment will not be withdrawn or voided at any time unless I pay the account in full. I understand that I am responsible for any and all charges not covered by my insurance policy(s).

4. **Assignment of Physician Benefits**: I am aware that physician services by Radiologist, Pathologist, Anesthesiologist, as well as medical, surgical and emergency care are not billed by the hospital but are billed separately. I understand that I am under the same obligation to those providers as stated in this agreement unless otherwise agreed to in writing with those providers. I authorize payment of any medical benefits for such claims to the appropriate provider.

5. **Release of Medical Information**: I authorize the hospital or any professional healthcare provider who rendered services to the patient to release any medical or other information necessary to process claims.
   - ☑ I acknowledge that I have received a copy of the Privacy Notice
   - ☐ I decline to accept a copy of the Privacy Notice

6. **Personal Valuables and Belongings**: I understand that the hospital maintains a safe for the protection of valuables. I agree that the hospital is not responsible for the loss or damage of any article or personal property unless they are deposited in the safe.

7. **Advance Directive/Living Will**: Northstar Medical Center honors the patient's right to formulate, review or revise their Advance Directives or Living Will and can refer you to resources for assistance if necessary
   - ☑ I have provided a copy of my Advance Directive or Living Will and request that it be put in my chart as part of my Medical Record
   - ☐ I have received information with regard to my right to make Advance Healthcare Directives
   - ☐ My Advance Directive or Living Will is suspended for this elective procedure
   - ☐ I have not provided nor do I have an Advance directive or Living Will and I decline information on Advance Directives
   - ☐ I understand if my Advance Directive or Living is not present in my medical record its directives will not be followed.

   Action taken by registrar _____

8. **Right to Donate Organs**: The patient understand that they have a right to donate organs and they have discussed their decision with their family. Should circumstances arise please do the following:
   - ☐ Speak with the family regarding the matter
   - ☐ The patient does NOT wish to donate. Please DO NOT speak to the family in regards to the matter.
   - ☑ I wish to donate my organs.

I understand and accept the terms of this agreement and certify that I am duly authorized by the patient or by law to execute the above agreement in their behalf

Patient _Marjorie Walker_ Date _3/18/12_ Time _6:32_

_____   _____   _____
Patient's Guardian or Representative   Relationship   Witness

Northstar Medical Center
Informed Consent for Invasive, Diagnostic, Medical & Surgical Procedures

Patient Name __Walker, Marjorie__

Date of Birth __6/3/56__

Medical Record # __585120__

I hereby authorize __Dr. Stillwater__ and/or ____—____ and/or such assistants and associates as may be selected by him/her/they to perform the following procedure(s)/treatment(s) upon myself/the patient

Procedure(s)/Treatment(s) __Excisional debridement, Lft Leg__

The procedure has been explained to me and I have been told the reasons why I need the procedure. The risks of the procedure have also been explained to me. In addition, I have been told that the procedure may not have the result that I expect. I have also been told about other possible treatments for my condition and what might happen if no treatment is received.

I understand that in addition to the risks describe to me and about this procedure there are risks that may occur with any surgical or medical procedure. I am aware that the practice of medicine and surgery is not an exact science, and that I have not been given any guarantees about the results of this procedure.

I have had enough time to discuss my condition and treatment with my health care providers and all of my questions have been answered to my satisfaction. I believe I have enough information to make an informed decision and I agree to have the procedure. If something unexpected happens and I need additional or different treatment(s) from the treatment I expect, I agree to accept any treatment which is necessary.

I agree to have transfusion of blood and other blood products that may be necessary along with the procedure I am having. The risks, benefits and alternatives have been explained to me and all of my questions have been answered to my satisfaction. If I refuse to have transfusions I will cross out and initial this section and sign a Refusal of Treatment form.

I agree to allow this facility to keep, use or properly dispose of, tissue, and parts of organs that are removed during this procedure.

___Marjorie Walker___   ___3/18/12___

Signature of Patient or Parent/Legal Guardian of Minor Patient   Date

---

If the patient cannot consent for him/herself, the signature of either the health care agent or legal guardian who is acting on behalf of the patient, or the patient's next of kin who is asserting to the treatment for the patient, must be obtained.

_____   _____

Signature of Patient or Parent/Legal Guardian of Minor Patient   Date

_____   _____

Signature and Relationship of Next of Kin   Date

Witness:

I, _____, am a facility employee who is not the patient's physician or authorized health care provider named above and I have witnessed the patient or other appropriate person voluntarily sign this form

_____

Signature and Title of Witness

NORTHSTAR MEDICAL CENTER

NORTHSTAR
Medical Center

Walker, Marjorie
PT#1772571   MRN#585120
DOB: 06/03/1956   Age: 56   Sex: F
Physician: Chaplin, Patrick
Admit: 03/18/2012

NOTICE OF ACKNOWLEDGEMENT ADVANCE DIRECTIVE

PATIENT NAME: _Walker, marjorie_ DOB: _6/3/56_

An Advance Directive is a legal document allowing a person to give directions about future medical care or to designate another person(s) to make medical decisions if he or she should lose decision making capacity. Advance Directives are the following written instruments: The Living Will and The Durable Power of Attorney for Heath Care. The instrument may be revoked and a notation of the date and time must be made to the patient's medical record.

Do you have an Advance Directive?

A. Directive to Physicians (Living Will)   Yes ___✓___ No _____

B. Durable Power of Attorney for Health Care   Yes ___✓___ No _____

Is it up to Date?   Yes ___✓___   No _____

Where is a copy located?   _With me_

Principal Agent: _Fulton Walker_

Address: _3370 Oakwood_

Phone #:   _513-555-1632_

Alternate Agent: _Anne Walker_

Address: _1530 Eastland_

Phone #:   _513-555-4445_

Marjorie Walker   _3/18/12_
Signature of Patient or Representative   Date

NORTHSTAR MEDICAL CENTER

NORTHSTAR

Medical Center

Walker, Marjorie
PT#1772571   MRN#585120
DOB: 06/03/1956   Age: 56   Sex: F
Physician: Chaplin, Patrick
Admit: 03/18/2012

Discharge Summary

Date of Discharge: 3/27/2012

Discharge Diagnosis:

1. Left leg wound, S/P MVA, left shin degloving injury
2. Anxiety
3. Hematoma, right thigh
4. Paroxysmal atrial fibrillation

History of Present Illness: This is a 56-year-old white female who on 2/23/12 was involved in a motor vehicle accident when she was driving from Florida to Cincinnati. She was admitted to a Chattanooga, Tennessee hospital and she had suffered multiple rib fractures and also suffered a left nondisplaced fibular fracture and an avulsion and degloving injury on the left shin. She also had possible suprapubic ramus fracture and a fracture of the sternum and a slight laceration of the liver and spleen and she was transfused 19 units of packed red blood cells for acute blood loss anemia. The patient was on Coumadin at the time for atrial fibrillation and she had to be reversed. She also went into a-fib with rapid rate needing Cardizem to reverse it.

She was then transferred to Northstar Medical Center and was pretty stable at the time. She had a lot of pain and then she was seen by Orthopedics for that left tib fib fracture and they said she was okay for weight-bearing and she was see by wound care, physical therapy and occupational therapy. The patient stayed in sinus rhythm throughout. She was maintained on Coumadin and her hemoglobin stayed in the 9 and 10 range and she had later complained of a lot of pain in the right leg and a Doppler had shown some small hematomas, however, the pain and hematomas resolved on their own.

The large wound on her left shin was treated by Dr. Stillwater, Plastic Surgeon. She underwent several debridements of this area and will later likely undergo a skin graft after the wound has healed more.

On the day of discharge, 31 minutes was spent on discharge planning and all medications were discussed with her in detail. Patient is discharged to home with home health care.

Dictated by: Patrick Chaplin, MD

NG
D: 3/27/12 1535
T: 03/28/2012 1124

NORTHSTAR MEDICAL CENTER

NORTHSTAR

Medical Center

Walker, Marjorie
PT#1772571   MRN#585120
DOB: 06/03/1956 Age: 56   Sex: F
Physician: Chaplin, Patrick
Admit: 03/18/2012

CONSULTATION REPORT
PLASTICS AND RECONSTRUCTIVE SURGERY

CHIEF COMPLAINT: Left leg wound

HISTORY OF PRESENT ILLNESS: This is a 56-year-old white female who on 2/23/12 was involved in a motor vehicle accident when she was driving from Florida to Cincinnati. She was admitted to a Chattanooga, Tennessee hospital and she had suffered multiple rib fractures and also suffered a left nondisplaced fibular fracture and an avulsion and degloving injury on the left shin. She also had possible suprapubic ramus fracture and a fracture of the sternum and a slight laceration of the liver and spleen and she was transfused 19 units of packed red blood cells for acute blood loss anemia. The patient was on Coumadin at the time for atrial fibrillation and she had to be reversed. She also went into a-fib with rapid rate needing Cardizem to reverse it.

PAST MEDICAL/SURGICAL HISTORY:
Significant for:
1. Hypertension
2. Rheumatoid arthritis
3. Depression
4. Osteopenia
5. Hyperlipidemia
6. History of perforated diverticulum, for which she required surgery and had a colostomy, and it was reversed.
7. History of hysterectomy
8. Hypothyroidism
9. Bilateral knee replacements
10. The patient does not report that she has congestive heart failure.
11. She does report that she had an angiogram for evaluation of atrial fibrillation, and she does not have any coronary artery disease.

ALLERGIES:
None

MEDICATIONS:

Prior to this accident included:

1. Methotrexate.
2. Misoprostol
3. Remicade
4. Methimazole

CURRENT MEDICATIONS:

That she was on when transferred from a Chattanooga, Tennessee hospital are as follows:

1. Keflex 500 mg every 8 hours for 5 days
2. Ipratropium as needed
3. Coumadin per pharmacy protocol
4. Lovenox 110 mg subcutaneously every twelve hours, to discontinue when INR is more than 2
5. Atenolol 50 mg every 12 hours
6. Vicodin 5/325 mg every four hours as needed for pain.
7. Paxil 20 mg daily

FAMILY HISTORY:

Positive for father dying of leukocytosis at age of 54. Mother had myocardial infarction at the age of 67. Sister has Parkinson disease and another sister died of colon cancer.

PHYSICAL EXAMINATION:

GENERAL:

She is awake, alert and oriented, in no acute distress.

VITAL SIGNS:

Stable. Her blood pressure this morning is 126/64, temperature 98.6, pulse 72.

HEAD, EYES, EARS, NOSE AND THROAT:

Shows pupils equal, round, and reactive to light and accommodation. Mucous membranes are moist.

NECK:

Shows no thyromegaly.

LUNGS:

Clear to auscultation.

HEART:

Regular rate and rhythm, a few missed beats.

ABDOMEN:

Shows no organomegaly.

EXTREMITIES:

Dorsalis pedis pulses bilaterally are 2+. There is a vacuum-assisted closure on the left upper skin extending to the knee. Large left lower leg wound with fairly well vascularized red granulation tissue in the bulk of the wound. There is a deep cavity on the medial aspect in the area of the recently evacuated hematoma. There are sutures in place which the patient was unaware and fibrin covering necrotic tissue on the lateral aspect of the wound space. There is no purulent discharge or evidence of infection. Remainder of the left lower extremity shows no other clinically significant lesions.

LABORATORY DATA:

From 3/17/12, her albumin was 2.4, total protein was 5.2. Her CBC from 3/16/12 shows a white cell count of 9.6, hemoglogin 9.7, platelets 252,000. INR was 1.4.

ASSESSMENT AND PLAN:

The patient needs protein repletion. She will ultimately need the sutures removed and the fibrinous exudate debrided from the lateral aspect of the wound. Would recommend resuming negative pressure wound therapy including packing, black GranuFoam dressing into the current hematoma cavity. The patient will ultimately require skin graft reconstruction.

It is always a pleasure seeing and treating your patients. We look forward to seeing and treating other patients in the future.

Dictated by Frank Stillwater, MD

KR
D: 03/20/12 1904
T: 03/20/12 23:50

NORTHSTAR MEDICAL CENTER

NORTHSTAR

Medical Center

Walker, Marjorie	
PT#1772571	MRN#585120
DOB: 06/03/1956 Age: 56	Sex: F
Physician: Chaplin, Patrick	
Admit: 03/18/2012	

HISTORY AND PHYSICAL

HISTORY OF PRESENT ILLNESS:
History of Present Illness: This is a 56-year-old white female who on 2/23/12 was involved in a motor vehicle accident when she was driving from Florida to Cincinnati. She was admitted to a Chattanooga, Tennessee hospital and she had suffered multiple rib fractures and also suffered a left nondisplaced fibular fracture and an avulsion and degloving injury on the left shin. She also had possible suprapubic ramus fracture and a fracture of the sternum and a slight laceration of the liver and spleen and she was transfused 19 units of packed red blood cells for acute blood loss anemia. The patient was on Coumadin at the time for atrial fibrillation and she had to be reversed. She also went into a-fib with rapid rate needing Cardizem to reverse it.

She has been transferred to Northstar Medical Center and is stable at this time. Dr. Stillwater from Plastics will be consulted to address her wound on her left shin. PT, OT and Wound Care will be ordered. We will monitor her atrial fibrillation and labs for anemia.

PAST MEDICAL/SURGICAL HISTORY:

Significant for:

1. Hypertension
2. Rheumatoid arthritis
3. Depression
4. Osteopenia
5. Hyperlipidemia
6. History of perforated diverticulum, for which she required surgery and had a colostomy, and it was reversed.
7. History of hysterectomy
8. Hypothyroidism
9. Bilateral knee replacements
10. The patient does not report that she has congestive heart failure.
11. She does report that she had an angiogram for evaluation of atrial fibrillation, and she does not have any coronary artery disease.

ALLERGIES:

None

MEDICATIONS:

Prior to this accident included:

1. Methotrexate.
2. Misoprostol
3. Remicade
4. Methimazole

CURRENT MEDICATIONS:

That she was on when transferred from a Chattanooga, Tennessee hospital are as follows:

1. Keflex 500 mg every 8 hours for 5 days
2. Ipratropium as needed
3. Coumadin per pharmacy protocol
4. Lovenox 110 mg subcutaneously every twelve hours, to discontinue when INR is more than 2
5. Atenolol 50 mg every 12 hours
6. Vicodin 5/325 mg every four hours as needed for pain.
7. Paxil 20 mg daily

FAMILY HISTORY:

Positive for father dying of leukocytosis at age of 54. Mother had myocardial infarction at the age of 67. Sister has Parkinson disease and another sister died of colon cancer.

PHYSICAL EXAMINATION:

GENERAL:
She is awake, alert and oriented, in no acute distress.

VITAL SIGNS:
Stable. Her blood pressure this morning is 126/64, temperature 98.6, pulse 72.

HEAD, EYES, EARS, NOSE AND THROAT:
Sclerae are anicteric. Mucous membranes are moist.

NECK:
There is no carotid bruit.

LUNGS:
Clear to auscultation.

HEART:
Regular rate and rhythm, a few missed beats.

ABDOMEN:
Soft, nontender.

EXTREMITIES:
Dorsalis pedis pulses bilaterally are 2+. There is a vacuum-assisted closure on the left upper skin extending to the knee.

LABORATORY DATA:
From 3/17/12, her albumin was 2.4, total protein was 5.2. Her CBC from 3/16/12 shows a white cell count of 9.6, hemoglogin 9.7, platelets 252,000. INR was 1.4.

ASSESSMENT AND PLAN:
1. Status post MVA with multiple injuries. Pain control is an issue. Patient will be scheduled for PT and OT Therapy
2. Avulsion/degloving injury of the left shin with large wound. Plastic surgery will be consulted.
3. History of paroxysmal atrial fibrillation. Will follow and monitor.

_____
Patrick Chaplin, MD

KK
Dictated: 3/18/12 14:45
Trans: 3/18/12 18:30

NORTHSTAR MEDICAL CENTER

NORTHSTAR

Medical Center

Walker, Marjorie
PT#1772571   MRN#585120
DOB: 06/03/1956   Age: 56   Sex: F
Physician: Chaplin, Patrick
Admit: 03/18/2012

OPERATIVE REPORT

DATE OF OPERATION: 03/23/12

PREOPERATIVE DIAGNOSIS: Left leg wound

POSTOPERATIVE DIAGNOSIS: Left leg wound

PROCEDURE PERFORMED: Excision, necrotic tissue, left leg wound, 3.0 cm in length. Application of a Kerlix stack and less than 50 sq. cm negative pressure wound therapy dressing.

SURGEON: Frank Stillwater, MD

ASSISTANT: Karen Tweedle, MD

OPERATIVE PROCEDURE: The patient was properly prepped and draped under local sedation. A 0.25% Marcaine was injected circumferentially around the necrotic wound. A wide excision and debridement of the necrotic tissue taken down to the presacral fascia and all necrotic tissue was electrocauterized and removed. All bleeding was cauterized with electrocautery and then a Kerlix stack was then placed and a pressure dressing applied. The patient was sent to recovery in satisfactory condition.

Dictated by Frank Stillwater, MD

GR
D: 3/23/12 11:14
T: 3/23/12 15:10

NORTHSTAR MEDICAL CENTER

Walker, Marjorie
PT#1772571   MRN#585120
DOB: 06/03/1956   Age: 56   Sex: F
Physician: Chaplin, Patrick
Admit: 03/18/2012

Date/Time	PHYSICIAN"S ORDERS	Nurse's Initials
3/10/12 930AM	CBC, BMP in am PT/INR c a.m. labs *Patrick Chaplin MD*	
3/19/12 8AM	U/A, c+s today *Patrick Chaplin MD*	
3/19/12 9AM	D/c oxycontin Vicodin 5/500mg i po q 4-6° prn pain. *Patrick Chaplin MD*	

NORTHSTAR MEDICAL CENTER

NORTHSTAR
Medical Center

Walker, Marjorie
PT#1772571   MRN#585120
DOB: 06/03/1956   Age: 56 Sex: F
Physician: Chaplin, Patrick
Admit: 03/18/2012

Date/Time	Progress Notes
3/18/12 9 15 AM	FP Feels better today less N/V. Appetite better. Up to hallway c̄ assistance. Vss AF Lys - CTAB heart - reg rate no mur Abd - soft NT NABS Ext - ∅ c<c wound vac in place ① leg labs pending A/P - ① wound left leg consult surgery ② PAF coumadin / PT protocol ③ High protein diet Ann Turell M

NORTHSTAR MEDICAL CENTER

NORTHSTAR

Medical Center

Walker, Marjorie
PT#1772571　　　　MRN#585120
DOB: 06/03/1956　Age: 56　　　　Sex: F
Physician: Chaplin, Patrick
Admit: 03/18/2012

*****************************COMPLETE BLOOD COUNT*****************************

TEST:	WBC	WBC	HGB	HBG	HCT	HCT	PLATELET	PLT	RBC
UNITS:	THOU/mcL	THOU/mcL	g/dl	g/dl	%	%	THOU/mcL	THOU/mcL	THOU/mcL
REF RANGE:	3.9-10.5	3.6-10.5	12.0-15.5	12.0-15.2	36-47	36-46	140-375	140-375	3.80-5.20

03/25/2012

	0530		6.0 CBCR [NS]		9.7L [NS]	29L [NS]		302 [NS]	

03/24/2012

	1115		7.4 CBCR [NS]		9.9L [NS]	30L [NS]		323 [NS}	

03/23/2012			7.8 CBCR [NS}		10.1L [NS]	30L [NS]		311 [NS]	

03/22/2012			7.1 [NS]		8.4L [NS]	27L [NS]		331 [NS]	

03/21/2012	9.4 [NS]		9.8L [NS]		31L [NS]		370 [NS]		3.32L [NS]

03/20/2012	7.9 [NS]		10.0L [NS]		32L [NS]		397H [NS]		3.32L [NS]

---FOOTNOTES---

[NS]　Tested at Northstar Medical Center

End of Report

NORTHSTAR MEDICAL CENTER

NORTHSTAR

Medical Center

Walker, Marjorie
PT#1772571   MRN#585120
DOB: 06/03/1956   Age: 56   Sex: F
Physician: Chaplin, Patrick
Admit: 03/18/2012

*****************************COAGULATION***********************************

TEST: PROTIME   INR

UNITS: Seconds

REF RANGE: 9.0-11.4   0.8-1.2

_____

03/18/2012

+ 0615   16.9 H 1.6   H
                 [NS]   (a)
                         (b)
                         (c)
                         [NS]

---FOOTNOTES---
(a)   INR Therapeutic Ranges:
(b)   Routine Anticoagulation: 2.0 to 3.0
(c)   Aggressive Anticoagulation: 2.5 to 3.5
[NS]   Tested at Northstar Medical Center

_____

End of Report

NORTHSTAR MEDICAL CENTER

NORTHSTAR

Medical Center

Walker, Marjorie
PT#1772571   MRN#585120
DOB: 06/03/1956   Age: 56   Sex: F
Physician: Chaplin, Patrick
Admit: 03/18/2012

Ordered by: Patrick Chaplin, MD
*All clinical times shown on this page are in
Knee 2 Views – Right 32017251
Site: Northstar Medical Center Radiology
Rad# X081134773
Unit# M000048880
Location: NSMC14CD
Account#: V1030767632B
Req#11-4104931
Order# RAD20120318-0349
Primary Insurance:
Procedure: Knee 2 views – Right 32017251
Admitting Diagnosis: Left Lower Extremity Wound
Reason for exam: Change in Status
Impression
Impression/Conclusion below

Report
Two Views Right Knee 3/20/12

Indication: Motor Vehicle Accident

Comparison: None

Findings: Right total knee arthroplasty is in place. The lateral view was somewhat oblique. No large joint
effusion or fracture. There is mild soft tissue swelling

Impression:

No evidence of fracture or gross complication with right total knee arthroplasty in place

Dictated by: Michael Zuckerman MD
Signed by: Michael Zuckerman MD 3/21/2012

End of Report

NORTHSTAR MEDICAL CENTER

Walker, Marjorie
PT#1772571   MRN#585120
DOB: 06/03/1956   Age: 56 Sex: F
Physician: Chaplin, Patrick
Admit: 03/18/2012

Nurse's Notes (Include observations, medications, and treatment when indicated.)

Date/Time	
3/19/12 0816	Assessment complete as noted, sitting up in bed, IVPB infusing s̄ difficulty, dsg dry and intact, foley draining clear yellow urine, denies pain or SOB @ this time will continue to monitor wound care — B. Cullars, RN
3/19/12 1930	pt resting in bed. A+O x3 VSS LSCTA per nurse assess. foley draining clear yellow urine. Denies any further issues @ this time. SOB noted previously currently subsided. will cont to monitor. Call light in reach — J. Hurley, RN
3/20/12 0730	VSS. Denies any pain or discomfort at this time. Assessment completed per flow sheet - no changes noted from previous shift. Able to make needs known. Call light is in reach. Will monitor — J. Smith, RN

Appendix B Sample Paper Medical Record

NORTHSTAR MEDICAL CENTER

NORTHSTAR
Medical Center

Walker, Marjorie
PT#1772571   MRN#585120
DOB: 06/03/1956   Age: 56 Sex: F
Physician: Chaplin, Patrick
Admit: 03/18/2012

Nurse's Notes (Include observations, medications, and treatment when indicated.)

Date/Time	
3/18/2012 @ 1300	Received pt via ACLS transport. Pt transferred from stretcher to bed. Pt did not bring any personal belongings. Admission assessment completed. VSS & WNL. Dr. Chaplin notified of pt's arrival - orders received. Pt informed of POC & instructed on safety to include use of call light & bed side controls. Will continue to monitor. S. Schmidt RN.
3/18/2012 2015	Assessment complete + charted. Pt is A+O x4, lungs CTA, +BS x4, no noted edema, heart sounds regular in rhythm. Pt has #20 @ FA dated 3/17 c̄ a dsg that is CD+I. VSS + hardly unchanged from admit. Pt has no needs or questions at this time & denies any pain. Call light left within reach, will continue to monitor. ─────── S Salath RN

NORTHSTAR MEDICAL CENTER

NORTHSTAR
Medical Center

```
Walker, Marjorie
PT#1772571  MRN#585120
DOB: 06/03/1956 Age: 56    Sex: F
Physician: Chaplin, Patrick
Admit: 03/18/2012
```

Physical Therapy Ankle Evaluation

DX (L) leg wound, s/p mva. wound care ___ Date 3/19/12

PMH Rib fx, fibular fx, degloving injury (L) shin, sternum fx, anemia, anxiety, paroxysmal A Fib,

Physician Patrick Chaplin ___ Onset 2/23/12 ___

Initial Evaluation X ___ Re-Evaluation___ Pain Rating___ Funct. Rating___ Involved: R L

SUBJECTIVE: Pain with X squatting X walking ___ sitting NA running NA stairs

Pt reports 5/10 (L) leg pain. Pt reports ↑ pain 7/10 ē amb ē RW ē squatting. Pt states she lives ē husband & receives his help to get in & out of care. Currently able to live on 1st floor. Reports she is unable to climb 10 steps ē IHR upstairs to her bedroom. Currently has transport w/c, RW, cane (SPC)

Occupation/Social Hx: Pt is a 3rd grade math teacher

Work Duties: standing, walking, bending, squatting, sitting on floor,

Pt. Goals: Pt reports she would like to amb ↑↓ 10 steps IHR to bedroom, & be able to squat down to floor for return to work

OBJECTIVE:

Gait: ___antalgic Trendelenburg R L ___Crutches X Walker___Cane___No AD ☐
___FWB___PWB___TTWB___NWB X WBAT

Other___

Observation: (In Standing) (WNL) R L

Knee: ___

Effusion: **R** none ☒ min ☐ mod ☐ severe ☐   **L** none ☒ min ☐ mod ☐ severe ☐

Foot: Pes Cavus R L   Pes Planus (R)(L)   Hallux Valgus R L

Other___

ROM/ Strength:

	Active R		Active L		Passive R		Passive L		Strength R		Strength L	
DF.	4/5	P	3+/5	P	WFL	P	WFL	P		P		P
PF	4/5	P	4/5	P		P		P		P		P
INV	NT	P	NT	P		P		P		P		P
EV		P		P		P		P		P		P
1st MTP Ext		P		P		P		P		P		P
						P		P				

Girth Measurements: (From mid-patella)   WNL   Bruising   Temp. (WNL) Warm

	R	L
Around Malleoli	NT	NT
Figure 8		

(L) leg
(L) thigh

1

Palpation: ® thigh tenderness anterior ⓛ anterior shin tenderness _____

Resting BP: 124 / 76   Resting HR: 71

Name: Marjorie, Walker _____   DOB: 6/3/56

Flexibility: (NT= normal, T= tight, VT= very tight): very tight BLE hamstring _____

Special Tests: (+ or —)

	R	L		R	L
Anterior Drawer	NT	NT	Eversion Stress Test	NT	NT
Spring Test	+	+	Inversion Stress Test	+	+

Unilateral Stance Time: R _3_ Sec. L _0_ Sec.

Unilat. Heel
Raise X 5:   R WNL ☐   painful ☐   weakness/↓ control ☒   Unable to perform ☐
                  L WNL ☐   painful ☒   weakness/↓ control ☐   Unable to perform ☒
6" step test: R WNL ☐   painful ☐   weakness/↓ control ☐   Unable to perform ☒
                  L WNL ☐   painful ☐   weakness/↓ control ☐   Unable to perform ☒
Single leg squat: R WNL ☐   painful ☐   weakness/↓ control ☐   Unable to perform ☒
                  L WNL ☐   painful ☐   weakness/↓ control ☐   Unable to perform ☒

Treatment: Pt perf BLE therex SLR, ABD/ADD, heel slide 2 x 15. amb 100' x 2 c̄ RW
↓ stance time LLE. Pt amb ↑↓ 1 6" step BHR BLE lead c̄ minA.

ASSESSMENT: _____ See Initial Eval Summary/ Plan of Care
Pt demo ↓ BLE strength, ↓ balance ↓ safety awareness Pt demo ↓ Ⓘ c̄ amb
↓ step length RLE, ↓ stance time LLE, forward head & shoulders Pt reports ↑ pain c̄
squatting & walking Pt will benefit from skilled PT to ↓ pain ↑ ability to
squat to floor Ⓘ ↑ amb ↑↓ 10 steps IHR to bedroom.

Rehabilitation Potential: (Excellent) Good   Fair   Poor

STG/LTG: X   See Initial Eval Summary/ Plan of Care

PLAN: (Circle) # Rx/ wk _____ ~ # wks _____

☒ Strengthening   ☒ Stretching   ☐ Joint Mobs   ☒ Moist Heat/ Cold Pack
☐ Bracing/ Taping ☐ Ultrasound   ☐ EStim   ☒ Gait Training
☒ Other: _neuro re-ed_

Avg. Pain Rating 6/10   Self Reported Functional Rating _____   Foot Function Index: _____

Therapist Signature: _Josilea Thomas PT_   Date: 3/19/12 Time: 4:05pm
                     Allim Bummingry PT

2

NORTHSTAR MEDICAL CENTER

NORTHSTAR
Medical Center

Walker, Marjorie
PT#1772571   MRN#585120
DOB: 06/03/1956   Age: 56   Sex: F
Physician: Chaplin, Patrick
Admit: 03/18/2012

SPEECH EVALUATION FORM

Nature of the communication problem: Speech consulted 2° "slurred speech"
per RN report

Speech/language therapy in the past?   YES___   NO ✓

Where? N/A _____   For what reason? N/A

Brief description of problem:
Pt initially admitted to OSH 3-9-12 following MVA, transferred to Northstar
Medical Center for continued wound care, nutritional support and therapy

Any pain associated with this problem? YES___ NO ✓
Description:
Pt denies pain.

Was this onset gradual or sudden? Describe:
Sudden, following brain trauma sustained in MVA

Mental Status (check all that apply):
        ✓   alert
        ✓   responsive
        ✓   cooperative
        ✓   confused
        ____ lethargic
        ✓   impulsive
        ____ uncooperative
        ____ combative
        ____ unresponsive

Oral Motor, Respiration, and Phonation
Lips
        WNL, mild, mode severe impairment
        Observation at rest (WNL, Edema, Erythema, Lesion): Ⓡ - droop, drooling
        Symmetry, range, speed, strength, tone:
                Pucker   reduced
                Retraction   reduced
                Alternating pucker/retraction   reduced speed/coordination

Involuntary movement (e.g., chorea, dystonia, fasciculation, myoclonus, spasms, tremor):

not observed

Tongue
    WNL, mild, (mode) severe impairment
    Observation at rest (WNL, Edema, Erythema, Lesion): lingual fasciculations
    Symmetry, range, speed, strength, tone:
        Protrusion   reduced range + strength
        Retraction   reduced strength
        Lateralization   reduced range + speed
    Involuntary movement   as noted above

Jaw
    WNL, (mild), mode severe impairment
    Observation at rest: rests in slightly open position
        Symmetry, range, speed, strength, tone:
        Opening   reduced oral aperture
        Closing   reduced strength
        Lateralization   reduced ROM
        Protrusion   NT
        Retraction   NT
    Involuntary movement   not observed

Soft Palate
    WNL, mild, (mode) severe impairment
    Observation at rest (WNL, Edema, Erythema, Lesion): WNL
    Symmetry, range, speed, strength, tone: ↓ speed, Ø asymmetry
    Elevation   reduced upon phonation
    Sustained elevation   reduced upon phonation
    Alternating elevation/relaxation   reduced range + speed
    Involuntary movement   not present

Respiration/Phonation
Observations/formal measures administered: _____

Activity	Stimulus	Quality	Duration	Loudness	Steadiness
Phonation		WNL Breathy (circled) Hoarse Harsh Strained- Strangled	2 secs WNL Mildly impaired Moderately impaired Severely impaired (circled)	WNL Monoloudness (circled) Excessive loudness Variable loudness	
Oral reading		WNL Breathy (circled) Hoarse Harsh Strained- Strangled	WNL Mildly impaired Moderately impaired Severely impaired (circled)	WNL Monoloudness (circled) Excessive loudness Variable loudness	
Conversation		WNL Breathy (circled) Hoarse Harsh Strained- Strangled	WNL Mildly impaired Moderately impaired Severely impaired (circled)	WNL Monoloudness (circled) Excessive loudness Variable loudness	

Findings

_____Motor speech within normal limits

_____(Mild, mild-moderate, moderate, moderate-severe, severe)apraxia characterized by:

_____

___✓___(Mild, mild-moderate, moderate (circled), moderate-severe, severe) dysarthria characterized by:
_____moderate dysarthria 2° breathy vocal quality (suspect vocal cord involvement), reduced strength + range of motion for oral
Recommendations: (check all that apply) structures, and hypernasality during all speech tasks.

_____✓___ Speech-language pathology treatment
           Frequency: 3-5 x/week Duration: 4 weeks
_____Augmentative-Alternative Communication or Speech Generating Device evaluation
_____Other suggested referrals:
_____Neurology
___✓__Otolaryngology
_____Pulmonology
_____Other

X Allison Binny MA CCC-SLP

NORTHSTAR MEDICAL CENTER

Patient Continuum of Care Transfer Form

Walker, Marjorie
PT#1772571   MRN#585120
DOB: 06/03/1956   Age: 56   Sex: F
Physician: Chaplin, Patrick
Admit: 03/18/2012

Patient Last Name: Walker | Patient First Name: Marjorie

Transfer to: Spring Care | Attending Physician: Chaplin

Reason for Transfer: Wound Care | DATE/TIME: 3/18/12 650

❑ Attempted Treatment in SNF unsuccessful?

☒ Please list ALLERGIES (meds, dyes, food): Latex, Demerol

❑ NKA

Relative / Guardian Notified: Yes ☒ No ❑ Phone Number:

Name of Relative Notified: Jennifer DeCapua

Transfer Ambulance: Life Care

VITAL SIGNS TAKEN   Yes ☒ No ❑   Time Taken: 1230 AM ❑ PM ☒

Respirations: 24	Blood glucose: 118 Time: 1210
O2 Sat: 96%	VRE: Yes ❑ No ☒ Hx of ❑
Pulse: 84	MRSA: Yes ❑ No ☒ Hx of ❑
BP: 118/82	C. Diff: Yes ❑ No ☒ Hx of ❑
Temp: 99.2 (A)	ANY pending cultures? Yes ❑ No ☒
Height: 5'10"	If Yes, what?
Weight: 163 Lbs ☒ Kg ❑	MDRO?

ATTACHMENTS (Please check)

☒ Face Sheet
☒ History & Physical
❑ Discharge Summary
☒ MAR
❑ Wound Assessment & Tx Sheet
☒ Labs
❑ Code Status
❑ MD Orders
☒ X-rays
❑ MD Progress Notes
❑ Nurse's Notes (last 5 days)
❑ Other:
❑ Other:

ISOLATION PRECAUTIONS? Yes ❑ No ☒ | **TYPE:** Contact ❑   Droplet ❑   Airborne ❑   Other: ❑

VACCINATION HISTORY	SKIN OR PRESSURE ULCER CONCERNS
Pneumococcal Vaccine: Yes ☒ DATE: 3-16-12 Refused ❑	**HIGH risk for skin breakdown**PLEASE TURN** Yes ❑ No ❑
Flu Vaccine: Yes ☒ DATE: 11-7-10 Refused ❑	Current Skin Breakdown: Yes ❑ No ❑
Tetanus: Yes ❑ DATE: Refused ❑	Most Recent Treatment Time: AM ❑ PM ❑
TB Skin Test: Negative ❑ Positive ❑ DATE:	Please Treat at (time): AM ❑ PM ❑
OR Chest X-ray ☒ Result Date: 1	Treat with (product name): Dakins Solution virig BIL
Comments:	To (what area): (B) LE

MEDICATION INFORMATION	SAFETY CONCERNS		
See Attached Medication Reconciliation	History of Falls Yes ❑ No ☒	Risk for Falls Yes ❑ No ☒
Prefers meds with: applesauce	Behavior Issues Yes ❑ No ☒	Explain:
Pain Meds in past 24 hours Yes ☒ No ❑	RESTRAINT Use: Yes ❑ No ☒	
Level on **Pain Scale** at time of transfer :	Type of Restraint Used:	
(Please circle level) 1 2 3 (4) 5 6 7 8 9 10	When Used:	

DIET & FEEDING	ELIMINATION	
Current Diet: Diabetic 2000 kcal ADA	Bladder Incontinence ❑	DATE of UTI (within 14 days):
Needs Assistance ❑	Feeds Self ❑	Feeding Tube ❑	Catheter: Yes ❑ No ❑	Date Inserted or Last Changed:
Thickened Liquid ❑ Consistency?	Bowel Incontinence: Yes ❑ No ❑	Colostomy: Yes ❑ No ❑
Supplement ❑ If so, name:	Date of Last BM:	

IMPAIRMENTS/DISABILITIES: (Please check all that apply)	PATIENT EQUIPMENT/BELONGINGS: (Check all sent with resident)
Speech ❑ Contractures ❑ Mental Confusion ❑ Vision ☒	None ❑ Right Hearing Aid ❑ Left Hearing Aid ❑
Hearing ❑ Amputation ❑ Paralysis ❑ Language Barrier ❑	Glasses ❑ Upper Denture ❑ Lower Denture ❑
COMMENTS: wears glasses	Jewelry ❑ Please list:
Report Called to: Jane Elson RN	Other (i.e., prosthesis):

| Nurse Name (Print): Karen Scheitlin RN | Nurse Signature: Karen Scheitlin RN | Phone #: 862-4444 | Date/Time: 3/18/12 7:00 |

NORTHSTAR MEDICAL CENTER

NORTHSTAR
Medical Center

Walker, Marjorie
PT#1772571   MRN#585120
DOB: 06/03/1956   Age: 56   Sex: F
Physician: Chaplin, Patrick
Admit: 03/18/2012
Allergies: No Know Drug Allergy

Medication Administration Record

No:	Medication	Start/Stop	Adm	07:00 to 18:59	19:00 to 6:69	00:00 to 00:00
0286618	ATENOLOL 50 MILLIGRAM PO EVERY 12 HOURS ONE DOSE= 50 MILLIGRAM = 1 TABLETS TENORMIN (Atenolol Tab 50 MG) ****FLOOR STOCK****	03/18/2012 at 2200 03/27/2012 at 1000		1000	2200	
0286621	COZAAR 50 MILLIGRAM PO ONCE DAILY ONE DOSE= 50 MILLIGRAM = 1 TABLETS LOSARTAN (COZAAR) (Losartan Potassium Tab 50 MG) ****FLOOR STOCK****	03/18/2012 at 2200 03/27/2012 at 1000		1000		
0286631	DOCUSATE SODIUM 100 MILLIGRAM PO TWICE DAILY ONE DOSE= 100 MILLIGRAM = 1 CAPSULE USED FOR COLACE (Docusate Sodium Cap 100 MG) ****FLOOR STOCK****	03/18/2012 at 2200 03/27/2012 at 1000		1000	2200	
0286619	FLECAINIDE ACETATE 100 MILLIGRAM PO EVERY 12 HOURS ONE DOSE= 100 MILLIGRAM = 1 TABLETS USED FOR TAMBOCOR (Flecainide Acetate Tab 100 MG)	03/18/2012 at 2200 03/27/2012 at 1000		1000	2200	
0286630	LORazepam 0.5 MILLIGRAM PO TWICE DAILY ONE DOSE= 0.5 MILLIGRAM = 1 TABLETS ATIVAN (Lorazepam Tab 0.5 MG) ****FLOOR STOCK****	03/18/2012 at 2200 03/27/2012 at 1000		1000		
0286629	KLOR-CON M10 10 MILLIEQUIV PO ONCE DAILY ONE DOSE= 10 MILLIEQUIV = 1 TABLETS (Potassium Chloride Microencapsulated Crys CR Tab 10 mEq) ****FLOOR STOCK****	03/18/2012 at 2200 03/27/2012 at 1000		1000	2200	
0286628	FUROSEMIDE 40 MILLIGRAM PO ONCE DAILY ONE DOSE= 40 MILLIGRAM = 1 TABLETS LASIX 40MG TAB (Furosemide Tab 40 MG) ****FLOOR STOCK****	03/18/2012 at 2200 03/27/2012 at 1000		1000		
0286970	OXYCONTIN 10 MILLIGRAM PO EVERY EVENING ONE DOSE= 10 MILLIGRAM = 1 TABLETS (Oxycodone HCl Tab SR 12HR 10 MG) ****FLOOR STOCK****	03/18/2012 at 2200 03/27/2012 at 2200			2200	
0286627	PARoxetine HCL 20 MILLIGRAM PO ONCE DAILY ONE DOSE= 20 MILLIGRAM = 1 TABLETS PAXIL 20 MG TAB (Paroxetine HCl Tab 20 MG) ****FLOOR STOCK****	03/18/2012 at 2200 03/27/2012 at 1000		1000		

Signatures	Init	Shift	Signatures	Init	Shift
			Ryan Goldman RN		
			Sylvia Yang RN		

abuse unintentional upcoding

accounting cost the total amount of money paid out for products, goods, or services

Accreditation Association for Ambulatory Health Care (AAAHC) a specialty accrediting organization

addressable the portions of the privacy and security standards that the covered entities must address to determine if it is a reasonable and appropriate safeguard in the entity's environment

administrative data includes demographic information about the patient such as the patient's name, address, date of birth, race, primary language, religion, and marital status

Administrative Safeguards a section of the Security Rule that includes the assignment or delegation of security responsibility to an individual and the need for security training for employees and users

admission date the day and time the patient is admitted to the acute care facility

admission/registration clerks a staff member generally responsible for entering insurance information into the EHR system at the time the patient is admitted to an inpatient hospital or scheduled for treatment at an outpatient facility or physician's office; also known as *patient access specialists*

advance directive a document that provides information about how the patient would like to be treated if he or she is no longer able to make his or her own medical decisions

alert fatigue a condition that arises when too many alerts cause physicians to disregard them

American College of Surgeons (ACS) an organization that developed a hospital standardization program establishing the minimum standards for reporting care and treatment

American Health Information Management Association (AHIMA) a professional organization that provides resources, education, and networking with other professionals, focusing on the quality of health information used in the delivery of healthcare

American Recovery and Reinvestment Act of 2009 (ARRA) an economic stimulus package signed into law by President Barack Obama

analysis the third step in the migration plan; this step examines how the healthcare facility currently uses its healthcare records and performs tasks

assignment of benefits a patient authorization form that allows his or her health insurance or third-party provider to reimburse the healthcare provider or facility directly

Association for Healthcare Documentation Integrity (AHDI) a professional organization that sets and upholds standards for education and practice in the field of clinical documentation that ensure the highest level of accuracy, privacy, and security for the U.S. healthcare systems to protect public health, increase patient safety, and improve quality of care for healthcare consumers

attestation report a listing of meaningful use criteria demonstrating the results of the percentage of compliance of each measure

automated data collection when the data from the initial patient encounter is automatically copied over to each new patient encounter

automatic method the entry of results that allows those results to be immediately available

back-end speech recognition the most common type of speech recognition used in healthcare; requires the healthcare provider to use a digital dictation system that sends the dictation through a speech recognition machine and into a draft document, which is then routed along with the original voice recording to an editor, who edits it and saves it to the EHR; also known as *deferred speech recognition*

bar coding technology a process that allows the user to quickly scan charts as they move from location to location

behavioral health setting a facility that provides care to patients with psychiatric diagnoses

best-of-breed an EHR system provided by a vendor or vendors that supplies the clinical applications needed

birthday rule a rule which specifies that the insurance of the parent whose birthday falls first in a calendar year will be the primary insurance for a child

breach an impermissible use or disclosure under the Privacy Rule that compromises the security or privacy of PHI such that the use or disclosure poses a significant risk of financial, reputational, or other harm to the affected individual

Centers for Medicare & Medicaid Services (CMS) a federal agency that oversees federal healthcare programs, including Medicare Conditions of Participation (CoPs)

Certification Commission for Health Information Technology (CCHIT) one of the ONC-ATCB certifying organizations; developed a rigorous process to examine the systems for functionality, interoperability, and security; CCHIT also provides resources to help healthcare facilities select an appropriate EHR system

Certified Professional in Healthcare Information & Management Systems (CPHIMS) a certification offered by HIMSS; eligibility requires a bachelor's degree and five years of associated information and management systems' experience, three years of which must be in healthcare

Chart tracking software software that is part of, or integrated into, the EHR system and can help track and locate paper health records

checking out the procedure for a patient leaving an outpatient facility

chief complaint a narrative articulated by the patient as his or her reason for seeking health services

claim scrubber a software program that checks bills for thousands of edits and billing rules before the bills are sent to insurance companies

classification system a standardized coding method that organizes diagnoses and procedures into related groups to facilitate reimbursement, reporting, and clinical research

clinical coders people who assign or validate diagnostic and procedural codes to represent the patient's diseases or conditions and the treatment rendered

clinical data information such as admission dates, office visits, laboratory test results, evaluations, or emergency visits

clinical decision support system (CDSS) a computer system, usually integrated with the EHR system, that assists healthcare providers with decision-making tasks such as determining diagnoses, choosing the best medications to order for a patient, and selecting proper diagnostic tests

clinical encoder a software program that helps coding professionals navigate coding pathways with the end result of assigning codes and diagnostic-related groups (DRGs)

clinical inputs the data entered into the patient record related to the patient's clinical status, whether they are in an EHR or a paper record

clinical outputs clinical data that can be extracted from a patient record and compiled in a meaningful way

clinical results reporting an EHR function that allows healthcare providers to view laboratory and diagnostic test results immediately, as long as there is an interface between the clinical results system and the EHR

cloned notes identical notes resulting from copying and pasting from one encounter or visit to another; also known as *cloned progress notes* or *copycat charting*

cloud storage data stored on virtual servers

cluster type of schedule in which similar appointments are scheduled together at specific times of the day

co-payment the amount that an insured individual must pay for healthcare services received, typically office visits, urgent care visits, or emergency department encounters

Community Health Accreditation Program (CHAP) a specialty accrediting organization

computer protocol a standardized method of communicating or transmitting data between two computer systems

computer-assisted coding (CAC) programs that automatically assign diagnosis and procedure codes based on electronic documentation, which can increase the productivity of a coder by up to 20%

concurrent coding the process of coding while a patient is still receiving treatment in a hospital

Consolidated Health Informatics (CHI) an initiative that created standards adopted by federal agencies and healthcare vendors doing business with the U.S. federal government to ensure efficient communication among agencies and EHR systems

controlled substance a drug declared by U.S. federal or state law to be illegal for sale or use but may be dispensed under a healthcare provider's prescription

Controlled Substances Act of 1970 legislation that placed tight controls on the pharmaceutical and healthcare industries and outlined the five schedules of controlled substances based on potential for harm

core data elements the data elements that are necessary for the master patient index and include patient identification number, patient name, date of birth, Social Security number, address, etc.

cost–benefit analysis a process of looking at the costs and benefits and determining the return on investment of implementing an EHR system

covered dependent a person who is covered by the guarantor or subscriber's health insurance

covered entities entities that have to comply with HIPAA Privacy and Security Rules; include healthcare providers, health plans, and healthcare clearinghouses transmitting health information in an electronic format

Current Dental Terminology (CDT) a classification system used to code dental procedures

Current Procedural Terminology (CPT) one of the most widely used classification systems in the United States used to code outpatient procedures for facility coding, as well as all physician services rendered

data collection the process of gathering information through a combination of manual and automated collection methods within an EHR

data integrity the accuracy, completeness, and reliability of clinical documentation in the EHR

data mining the process of searching and examining data to organize and reorganize it into useful information, patterns, and trends

data stewardship the authority and responsibility associated with collecting, using, and disclosing health information in its identifiable and aggregate forms

data the descriptive or numeric attributes of one or more variables

de-identified health information health information that neither identifies an individual nor provides a reasonable basis to identify an individual

deductible the amount an insured individual must pay out of pocket before the insurance will pay

deferred speech recognition the most common type of speech recognition used in healthcare; requires the healthcare provider to use a digital dictation system that sends the dictation through a speech recognition machine and into a draft document, which is then routed along with the original voice recording to an editor, who edits it and saves it to the EHR; also known as *back-end speech recognition*

demographic information information provided by the patient that includes name, date of birth, address, phone number, email address, etc.

design the second step in the migration plan; this step creates a blueprint for how the healthcare facility will transition from paper-based records to the new EHR system

Diagnostic and Statistical Manual of Mental Disorders, Fifth Edition (DSM-5) a classification system used to classify psychiatric disorders

diagnostic-related groups (DRGs) a patient classification system that groups hospital patients of similar age, sex, diagnoses, and treatments

Digital Imaging and Communications in Medicine (DICOM) a standard that allows images and associated information to be accessed and transferred from manufacturers' devices and medical staff workstations

discharge the procedure for a patient leaving an inpatient facility

discharge date the day and time the patient leaves the facility

discharge disposition the patient's destination following a stay in the hospital

Discharged Not Final Billed (DNFB) patient accounts that are not able to be final billed to the insurance company or responsible party due to a lack of final coding, insurance verification, or other data errors

e-prescribing a process that allows a physician, nurse practitioner, or physician assistant to electronically transmit a new prescription or renewal authorization to a pharmacy; also known as *electronic prescribing*

economic cost the combination of accounting and opportunity costs

electronic health records (EHRs) a computer system used to improve healthcare delivery; EHRs replace traditional paper medical records and make health information accessible to healthcare providers across the world with only a few keystrokes

electronic medical record (EMR) an electronic version of patient files within a single organization

electronic protected health information (ePHI) protected health information in electronic format

enterprise identification number (EIN) an identifier used by an organization to identify a patient across various healthcare settings

enterprise master patient index (EMPI) a systemwide database that maintains patient identifier information across an EHR system for all healthcare settings, allowing a healthcare organization to compile the patient's information into one index using registration, scheduling, financial, and clinical information

enterprise storage a centralized system (online or offline) that businesses use for managing and protecting data

established patient a patient who has received professional services from a healthcare provider or a provider in the same group and/or specialty within the past three years

facility identifier an identifier that indicates the healthcare setting where the patient is seeking care

File Import an interface that sends documents to the facility's network and an EHR program imports the reports into the EHR system; also known as *File Monitor Utility*

financial data information that includes the patient's insurance and payment information for healthcare services

flow chart a document that demonstrates a workflow process

fraud intentional upcoding

front-end speech recognition a technology that allows the dictator to dictate, edit, and sign the report in the same process because the transcribed words appear directly on the screen as the healthcare provider is dictating

functionality testing a process that requires a facility to use a test environment before implementing the EHR system facilitywide

functionality the ability to create and manage EHRs for all patients in a healthcare facility

Gantt chart a graphic representation of a project schedule

general consent a form used in acute care facilities that gives the healthcare provider the right to treat a patient

General Rules a section of the Security Rule that includes general requirements that all covered entities must meet; establishes the flexibility of approach that covered entities have when implementing the standards and identifying the standards required and the standards addressable

guarantor the person or financial entity that guarantees payment on any unpaid balances on the account

guarantor account a record that saves the information about the guarantor, including the guarantor's name and address

health information management (HIM) professionals that plan information systems, develop health policy, identify current and future information needs, and practice the maintenance and care of health records

Health Information Technology for Economic and Clinical Health (HITECH) Act an act enacted in February 2009 as part of the ARRA that promoted the nationwide implementation of EHR technology

Health Insurance Portability and Accountability Act of 1996 (HIPAA) a comprehensive federal law passed in 1996 to protect all patient-identifiable medical information

Health Level Seven International (HL7) the most common communication protocol that focuses on the exchange of clinical and administrative data; also an international group of collaborating healthcare subject-matter experts and information scientists

health record an accumulation of information about a patient's past and present health

Healthcare Common Procedure Coding System (HCPCS) a classification system used to code ancillary services and procedures

healthcare delivery (HCD) system a healthcare facility

healthcare facility an organization, such as a hospital, clinic, dental office, outpatient surgery center, birthing center, or nursing home, that performs healthcare services

Healthcare Information and Management Systems Society (HIMSS) an organization that focuses on using information technology and management systems to improve the quality and delivery of healthcare

healthcare operations activities including quality assessment and improvement, competency assurance activities, conducting or arranging for medical reviews, audits, or legal services, specified insurance functions, business planning, development, management, and administration and business management and general administrative activities

hibernation mode a privacy feature in an EHR system that prevents disclosure of PHI

Hippocrates considered one of the most important figures in medical history; he was among the first to describe and document many diseases and medical conditions

History and Physical Examination (H&P) a report that helps identify and treat patient diagnoses; consists of two main elements: a subjective element and an objective element

history the subjective element of an H&P that includes history of present illness, past medical history, allergies, medications currently prescribed to the patient, and family and social histories

hospice care palliative, or short-term, care provided to terminal patients within acute care or home care settings

hospital acquired diagnoses and conditions that developed when the patient was an inpatient in the hospital

hybrid health record a patient record that is stored on paper and electronically

ICD-9-CM/PCS and **ICD-10-CM/PCS** used in the United States to code diagnoses and procedures for inpatients and diagnoses for all healthcare providers, including hospital outpatients, physician offices, dental offices, skilled nursing facilities, and outpatient centers, among others

implementation the fifth step in the migration plan; this step creates a timeline for the implementation, and is often created to look like a Gantt chart

indemnity plan a type of insurance plan in which insured patients have the freedom to obtain healthcare from the providers of their choice in exchange for higher premiums, deductibles, and out-of-pocket expenses

indexing the process of assigning a code to each type of document that is part of the paper medical record and associating the code with the location in the EHR where the document should digitally reside

individually identifiable health information information including demographic data that identifies an individual

information data collected and analyzed

information processing cycle the sequence of events that includes four components: input, processing, output, and storage

Inpatient Prospective Payment System (IPPS) the first diagnostic-related group (DRG) system that was implemented in 1983 to reimburse acute care hospitals for the treatment of Medicare patients

inpatients patients who occupy a hospital bed for at least one night in the course of treatment, examination, or observation

input device a device used to enter data into an EHR system; includes keyboard, mouse, scanner, microphone, camera, stylus, and touchscreen

input the first component of the information processing cycle; data entered by the user of an EHR system (e.g., the patient's first name, last name, identification number)

Institute of Electrical and Electronics Engineers 1073 (IEEE 1073) a professional organization that addresses the interoperability of medical devices

Institute of Medicine of the National Academies (IOM) a nonprofit organization that developed a committee to explore EHRs

insurance verifier the person who confirms the patient's insurance coverage with the insurance company

insured patients patients who participate in some type of healthcare insurance plan

integrated health record a health record format that is organized either in chronologic or reverse chronologic order

integrated system the combination of systems an organization already uses and the new EHR system

interface a device or program that provides communication flow between two or more computer systems

internal rate of return (IRR) a calculation used to measure the profitability of an investment

International Classification of Diseases (ICD) one of the most widely used classification systems used to code diagnoses and procedures for inpatients and diagnoses for all healthcare providers

interoperability the ability of an EHR system to exchange data with other sources of health information, including pharmacies, laboratories, and other healthcare providers

interoperability the ability of one computer system to communicate with another computer system

isolation status the precautions that must be taken by healthcare staff and visitors to avoid the spread of bacterial or viral infections

Joint Commission an independent, not-for-profit organization that accredits and certifies a variety of healthcare organizations; formerly known as the Joint Commission on Accreditation of Healthcare Organizations (JCAHO)

legal data information composed of consents for treatment and authorizations for the release of information

levels of conceptual interoperability model (LCIM) a model that defines the hierarchy of interoperability

limited data set protected health information from which certain specified direct identifiers of individuals and their relatives, household members, and employers have been removed

local area network (LAN) a group of computers connected through a network confined to a single area or small geographic area such as a building or hospital campus

Logical Observation Identifiers Names and Codes (LOINC) a database and universal standard for the electronic transfer of clinical laboratory results

long-term care facility a facility in which patients typically reside more than 30 days

longitudinal a patient's record that will continue to develop over the course of care

managed care plan a type of insurance plan offered by a carrier who has negotiated and contracted with healthcare providers to provide healthcare services for their subscribers

manual data collection a process initiated by a staff member upon initial patient contact with a healthcare facility done without the aid of an automatic system

manual method the entry of results that needs to be manually scanned into the EHR for access

master patient index (MPI) a database created by a healthcare organization to assign a unique medical record number to each patient served, thus allowing easy retrieval and maintenance of patient information; also known as a *patient list*

meaningful use the set of standards that governs the use of EHRs and allows eligible providers and hospitals to earn incentive payments by meeting specific criteria

MEDCIN a naming system primarily used in physicians' offices

medical transcription service organizations (MTSOs) companies that contract their medical transcription services

medical transcription the process of typing medical reports from voice-recorded formats, dictated by physicians and other healthcare providers

migration plan a plan that provides the framework to identify the basic steps of how the healthcare facility will move from a paper-based record system to an EHR system

minimum necessary a concept required by the Privacy Rule that states that covered entities must make reasonable efforts to limit the use, disclosure of, and requests for the minimum amount of protected health information necessary to accomplish the intended purpose

minimum standards a set of requirements for reporting care and treatment

modified wave type of schedule in which patients arrive at planned intervals in the first half hour; then, in the second half hour, the healthcare provider catches up

National Committee for Quality Assurance (NCQA) an independent, nonprofit organization that focuses on healthcare quality

National Committee on Vital and Health Statistics (NCVHS) an advisory body to the U.S. Department of Health and Human Services; the NCVHS completed a review of core health data elements and developed a list and definitions of the 42 core elements that can be used in a variety of healthcare settings

Nationwide Health Information Network (NwHIN) a set of standards that enable the secure exchange of health information over the Internet

net present value (NPV) the present value of future cash flows minus the purchase price of goods or services

new patient a patient who has not received any services from a healthcare provider or a provider in the group in the same specialty within the past three years

no-shows patients who do not show for their scheduled appointments

nomenclature a common system of naming things

noncovered entities entities that do not have to comply with HIPAA Privacy and Security Rules; these include workers' compensation carriers, employers, marketing firms, life insurance companies, pharmaceutical manufacturers, casualty insurance carriers, pharmacy benefit management companies, and crime victim compensation programs

objective element the portion of the history and physical report that includes the physical examination

Office for Civil Rights (OCR) the agency responsible for enforcing the HIPAA Privacy and Security Rules

Office of the National Coordinator for Health Information Technology (ONC) the U.S. federal body that recommends policies, procedures, protocols, and standards for interoperability

Office of the National Coordinator-Authorized Testing and Certification Body (ONC-ATCB) a body that certifies EHR systems

open hours type of schedule typically used in an urgent care setting in which patients are seen throughout certain time frames or on a first-come, first-served basis

opportunity cost the value of a decision

optional data elements the data elements that are optional for the master patient index, and include marital status, telephone number, mother's maiden name, place of birth, advance directive decision-making, organ donor status, emergency contact, allergies, and problem list

Organizational Requirements a section of the Security Rule that includes standards for business associate contracts and other arrangements and the requirements for group health plans

outpatients patients who do not spend more than 24 hours in a healthcare facility

output device a device that displays the results from EHRs; includes computer monitor, digital device screen, and printer

output the third component of the information processing cycle; data produced that provides meaningful information for the user

patient portal a web-based site that gives patients access to their health records

payment the activities of a health plan to obtain premiums, to determine or fulfill responsibilities for coverage and provision of benefits, and to furnish or obtain reimbursement for healthcare delivered to an individual

personal health record (PHR) an emerging health information technology initiative that gives patients a tool to improve the quality of their healthcare; these records are updated and maintained by the patient

physical examination the objective element of the H&P; this procedure is conducted by the nursing or medical staff and consists of a physical examination of body systems, an assessment of the patient and his or her condition, and a treatment plan

Physical Safeguards a section of the Security Rule that includes mechanisms necessary to protect electronic systems and the data they store from threats, environmental hazards, and unauthorized intrusion

physician query a request, typically from a coder or a case manager, to add documentation to the health record that clarifies a diagnosis or procedure performed

Policies and Procedures and Documentation Requirements a section of the Security Rule that addresses the implementation of reasonable and appropriate policies and procedures to comply with the Security Rule standards

present on admission (POA) diagnoses and conditions that the patient already had when they were admitted to the healthcare organization

Problem-Oriented Medical Record (POMR) a medical record format that takes a systematic approach to documentation

problem-oriented record (POR) a health record format that focuses on assessment of the clinical documentation by healthcare providers and the creation of a plan that addresses the patient's health concerns

processing the second component of the information processing cycle; takes data and makes the information usable within the system

progress notes the portion of the health record in which healthcare providers of all disciplines document the patient's progress or lack thereof in relation to the established goals of the care plan

PROMIS (Problem-Oriented Medical Information System) a software program developed at the University of Vermont under a federal grant in the 1970s

protected health information (PHI) all individually identifiable health information held or transmitted by a covered entity or its business associate, in any form or media, whether electronic, paper, or oral

record a collection, usually in writing, of an account or an occurrence

registrar the healthcare personnel at the admission or registration desk that is the initial contact for a patient

rehabilitation facility a facility that offers acute care and ambulatory care, typically serving patients recovering from accidents, injuries, or surgeries

Remittance Advice (RA) a document that lists the patient's information and amount paid by Medicare or other payer to the physician practice

remote coders coders who work from home

request for proposal (RFP) a document that includes requirements, services, vendor information, and a bid or quote for the EHR system

required standards the portions of the standards with which each covered entity must comply

requirements the first step in the migration plan; this step asks a facility to identify the scope of the project and user needs

Resolution Agreement a contract signed by the federal government and a covered entity in which the covered entity agrees to perform certain obligations (e.g., staff training regarding privacy and confidentiality, audits of all releases of health information to ensure compliance) and to send reports to the federal government for a certain time period (typically three years)

return on investment (ROI) a performance measurement that calculates the benefit or gain of an investment

revenue cycle management all administrative and clinical functions that contribute to the capture, management, and collection of patient service revenue

review of systems (ROS) an examination of each body system that includes physical assessment of general appearance; vital signs; head, ears, eyes, nose, and throat (HEENT); respiratory; cardiovascular; abdominal; gastrointestinal; genitourinary; musculoskeletal; and neurologic

Security Rule the standards developed to address the security provisions of HIPAA; also known as *Security Standards for the Protection of Electronic Protected Health Information*

Security Standards for the Protection of Electronic Protected Health Information the standards developed to address the security provisions of HIPAA; also known as *Security Rule*

security the standard that prevents data loss and ensures that patient health information is private

self-pay patients patients who do not have any type of insurance coverage and must pay for healthcare services themselves

semantic interoperability level the level that allows the meaning of data to be shared and information interpreted

SNOMED-CT a standardized vocabulary of clinical terminology used by healthcare providers for clinical documentation and reporting; considered the most comprehensive healthcare terminology in the world

sole practitioner a single, independent healthcare practice

source-oriented record (SOR) the health record format used most by healthcare facilities; organizes health documents into sections that contain information collected from a specific department or type of service

speech recognition a technology widely used in many industries that translates spoken word into text

storage device a place where data for the EHR may be stored, such as on a dedicated server at the healthcare facility or on a server provided by a vendor; if an EHR system is networked, then the storage may exist on the healthcare system's server

storage the fourth component of the information processing cycle; patient information is stored so that it can be retrieved, added to, or modified for later use

structured data a format in which data is stored in a database rather than in an unstructured or free-form format; examples include date of birth, sex, and race

subjective element the portion of the history and physical report that relies on patient narrative

subscriber the person whose insurance coverage is used for acute or ambulatory care

superbill a document that records the diagnosis and treatment for each patient at each visit; also known as an *encounter form*

syndromic a group of symptoms that, when grouped together, are characteristic of a specific disorder or disease

syntactic interoperability level the level that introduces a common data format for information exchange, but the meaning of the data cannot be interpreted

Technical Safeguards a section of the Security Rule that covers the automated processes used to protect data and control access to data

template a preformatted file that provides prompts to obtain specific, consistent information

test the fourth step in the migration plan; this step tests the functionality of the new EHR system

tethered PHR a PHR system where the health information is attached to a specific organization's health information system

time specified type of schedule used in an acute care setting in which patients are given a specific date and time to arrive at a facility

total cost of ownership a financial estimate that helps determine the direct and indirect costs of the EHR system

treatment plan a plan a healthcare practitioner decides on to treat a patient's diagnoses

treatment the provision, coordination, or management of healthcare and related services for an individual by one or more healthcare providers, including consultation among providers regarding a patient, and referral of a patient by one provider to another

U.S. Department of Health & Human Services (HHS) a federal United States federal agency that protects the health of Americans; it has undertaken efforts to create and adopt health informatics standards

UHDDS core data elements the data elements that include patient identifier; date of birth; sex; ethnicity; address; healthcare setting identification; admission date; type of admission; discharge date; attending physician identification; surgeon identification; principal diagnosis; other diagnoses; qualifier for other diagnoses; external cause of injury code; birth weight of neonate; significant procedures and dates; disposition of patient; expected source of payment; total charges

Uniform Ambulatory Care Data Set (UACDS) the data set that ensures that all healthcare settings and providers are gathering identical types of information on each patient

Uniform Hospital Discharge Data Set (UHDDS) a set of items used for reporting inpatient data in acute care hospitals

unstructured data a format in which data is stored in a free-form format rather than in a database; examples include progress notes, test interpretations, and operative reports

upcoding an illegal maneuver that encourages physicians to document simply for the purpose of claiming a higher paying diagnostic-related group (DRG) and, therefore, increased reimbursement

uploading the process of transmitting a file from one computer to another or to a portal

vendors a company that provides an EHR system to a healthcare organization

Veterans Administration the federal department that provides a government-run military benefit system

wave type of schedule in which patients are scheduled to arrive at the beginning of the hour, and the number of appointments is determined by dividing the hour by the length of an average visit or procedure

wide area network (WAN) a network that covers a broader area than a LAN, spanning regions, countries, or the world

workflow analysis a process that reviews how an organization currently functions and how paper records are used to care for patients

workplan an annual report created by the OIG that establishes areas of healthcare documentation and billing practices to be addressed and audited during the year

workstation a computer paired with input and output devices

Archived Messages, 75, 76f
Ask Customer Service, 286, 286f
Assignment of Benefits form, 112, 112f
Association for Healthcare Documentation Integrity (AHDI), 181
    overview of, 43
automated data collection, 197
automatic method of clinical results reporting, 207
automatic population of Normal, 180

B

back-end speech recognition, 182
backup system, requirements for, 88
bar coding technology, 175–176
behavioral health setting, 99
Bertillon, Jacques, 216, 220
Bertillon Classification of Causes of Death, 216, 220
best-of-breed EHR system, 312
Billing Account Summary feature, 286, 286f
billing and reimbursement
    Billing Account Summary feature, 286, 286f
    claim scrubber, 234
    cloned progress notes and issues of reimbursement, 202
    co-payment, 230–231
    deductible, 231
    Explanation of Benefits (EOB), 231, 231f
    improved accuracy and efficiency with EHR system, 232–233
    insurance plans and, 230
    Insurance Summary feature, 287, 287f
    insurance verifier, 230
    posting payments, insurance appeals, and collections, 231–232
    process overview, 230–232
    Remittance Advice (RA), 234
    revenue cycle management, 229–230, 229f
    superbill, 233–234, 233f
Billing feature, 80, 80f
birthday rule, 108
blocking off time EHR schedule, 126, 126f
breach, 156
    Privacy Rule notification requirements, 156–157

C

Calendar
    Daily Calendar, 79, 79f
    Hours feature, 76, 77f
    overview, 76, 77f
    Weekly Calendar, 77, 78f
canceling appointments, 133
Cancel My Appointments feature, 283, 283f
CCHIT. *See* Certification Commission for Health Information Technology (CCHIT)

Centers for Disease Control and Prevention, reportable laboratory results, 209
Centers for Medicare & Medicaid Services (CMS), 10
    advocate of personal health record, 272
    definition of clinical decision support, 243
    MEDCIN and, 219
    overview of, 44
    Security Standards Matrix, 160–162, 161f
Certification Commission for Health Information Technology (CCHIT), 296
    criteria, 306t
    kinds of certifications, 306t
    overview of, 305
    scheduling standards, 124
Certified Healthcare Technology Specialist (CHTS), 16
Certified Professional in Healthcare Information & Management Systems (CPHIMS), 16
Charts feature
    Add Chart Note, 83, 84f
    administrative feature of, 80, 81f
    clinical features of, 83, 84f
    Patient Chart, 80, 81f
    Patient History, 83, 84f
    patient list, 80, 81f
chart tracking, 175–176
chart tracking software, 175
checkout procedure, 135
chief complaint, 199
Chunyu Yi, 24
Cignet Health, 154
claim scrubber, 234
classification systems, 219–224
    CDT coding, 223
    CPT coding, 222–223
    defined, 219
    DSM-5 coding, 223
    ICD coding, 220–222
    overview of, 219–220
    purposes of, 220
clinical coders, 218
clinical data
    characteristics of, 29f
    defined, 26
    example of, 29f
clinical decision support system (CDSS), 242–248
    accurate data and, 250
    alert fatigue, 246
    alerts, 245–246, 245t
    benefits and disadvantages of, 244
    common uses of, 245, 245t
    cost reduction, 245t, 248
    defined, 242, 243
    diagnosis, 245t, 247
    knowledge-based, 243–244, 243f
    meaningful use requirement, 248–249

non-knowledge-based, 243
    preventive care, 245t, 247–248
    provider efficiency, 245t, 248
    quality improvement activities, 249–250
    role of EHR system, 242
    treatment options, 245t, 247
clinical encoder, 224–225
    accurate code assignment, 226–227
    physician query, 227
clinical features of EHR navigator, 83–87
    Charts feature, 83, 84f
    Diagnostic Test Results tab, 86, 87f
    eRx feature, 84, 85f
    Labs feature, 85, 85f
    Manage Orders feature, 86, 86f
clinical inputs, 196
clinical outputs, 197
clinical results reporting
    automatic method, 206–207
    defined, 206
    manual method of, 207
    patient safety goals and, 206
    timeframe for, 206
cloned progress notes
    coding and reimbursement issued, 202
    defined, 201
    problems with, 179, 201
cloud storage, 59
cluster scheduling method, 128
coders, 218
    remote, 228
coding
    accuracy in code assignment, 226–227
    advantages of coding from EHR, 176–177
    automatic population of Normal, 180
    CDT coding, 223
    classification systems for, 176, 219–224
    cloned notes, 179, 202
    code assignment, 224–225
    computer-assisted coding (CAC) programs, 227
    concurrent coding, 226
    CPT coding, 222–223
    data integrity and, 180
    defined, 176
    with diagnostic-related groups (DRGs), 224–225
    disadvantages of coding from EHR, 179–180
    Discharged Not Final Billed (DNFB) accounts, 226
    DSM-5 coding, 223
    EHR and, 226–228
    hospital-acquired diagnosis and conditions, 227
    ICD coding, 220–222
    from manuals, 224
    nomenclature systems, 219
    physician query, 227

Photo credits

xx *top*, © iStockphoto/UygarGeographic; *bottom* © iStockphoto/sqback; **1** *top*, © Shutterstock/ilterriorm; *bottom* © Shutterstock/Rene Jansa; **2** © iStockphoto/dra_schwartz; **4** © Shutterstock/Monkey Business Images; **6** © Wikipedia; **8** © http://www.hartsteve.com used with permission; **11** © Cartoonstock/Bacall, Aaron; **13** © iStockphoto/Pamela Moore; **14** © iStockphoto/francisblack; **22** *top* © Shutterstock/sheff; *bottom left* © Shutterstock/PENGYOU91; *bottom right* © Shutterstock/SPb photo maker; **23** *top* © Shutterstock/yanugkelid; *middle* © Shutterstock/Feng Yu; *bottom* © Shutterstock/Marc Dietrich; **24** © iStockphoto/spxChrome; **25** *top* © iStockphoto/imagestock; *bottom* © Shutterstock/Smart7; **28** © Shutterstock/alexskopje; **37** © iStockphoto/babyblueut; **38** © istock/BanksPhotos; **40** © iStockphoto/Snowleopard1; **46** *top* © iStockphoto/joeynick; *bottom* © Wikipedia; **48** © iStockphoto/alexsl; **56** *top* © Shutterstock/Andrey_Popov; *bottom* © Shutterstock/alexmillos; **57** *top* © Shutterstock/megainarmy; *bottom* Courtesy of Karen Lankisch; **59** © iStockphoto/CostinT; **60** © Shutterstock/planet5D LLC; **61** © Shutterstock/Ohmega1982; **64** © Shutterstock/PaulPaladin; **88** © Practice Fusion used with permission; **94** *top* © iStockphoto/Franck-Boston; *bottom* © iStockphoto/SocjosensPG; **95** © Shutterstock/Christine Langer-Pueschel; © Shutterstock/Anan Kaewkhammul; **96** © iStockphoto/JerryPDX; **97** © iStockphoto/uchar; **99** *top* © iStockphoto/Steve Debenport; *bottom* © Paradigm Education Solutions; **105** © Shutterstock/Tyler Olson; **109** © Shutterstock/racorn; **122** *top* © Shutterstock/wavebreakmedia; *middle* © iStockphoto/Spiderstock; *bottom* © iStockphoto/exdez; **123** Public Domain; **124** ©iStockphoto/ DenGuy; **128** © iStockphoto/Mark Bowden; **129** © Shutterstock/Monkey Business Images; **132** © iStockphoto/annedde; **135** © Paradigm Education Solutions; **136** © iStockphoto/vm; **142** *top* © Shutterstock/Piotr Marcinski; *bottom* © Shutterstock/Africa Studio; **143** *top* © iStockphoto/DNY59; *bottom* © iStockphoto/dra_schwartz; **147** © Shutterstock/zimmytws; **148** © iStockphoto/leezsnow; **152** Public Domain; **153** © cartoonstock/mban1505; **154** © Shutterstock/nyasha; **155** Public Domain; **158** © Shutterstock/Robert A. Levy Photography, LLC; **161** Public Domain; **170** *top* © Shutterstock/mast3r; *bottom* © Shutterstock/Emanuel; **171** © Shutterstock/Deyan Georgiev; **175** © iStockphoto/Vasiliki Varvaki; **176** © Shutterstock/Jim Lopes; **177** © iStockphoto/skodonnell; **178** Courtesy of Darline Foltz; **181** *top* © iStockphoto/lovleah; *bottom* © iStockphoto/diego_cervo; **182** © HIPAA Cartoons; **187** © iStockphoto/lbodvar; **194** © Shutterstock/Radu Razvan; **195** *top* © Shutterstock/Daboost; *middle* © Shutterstock/ilterriorm; *bottom* © Shutterstock/Brian A Jackson; **197** © iStockphoto/Sportstock; **198** © iStockphoto/LajosRepasi; **203** © Paradigm Education Solutions; **206** © iStockphoto/GlobalStock; **208** *top* © HIPAA Cartoons; *bottom* © iStockphoto/PhotoEuphoria; **216** *top* © HIPAA Cartoons; *bottom* © Shutterstock/PRILL; **217** *top* © Shutterstock/KITSANANAN; *middle* Courtesy of Diana Fischer; *bottom* Courtesy of Kyle Meerkins; **218** © iStockphoto/pkline; **223** © iStockphoto/bjones27; **224** © Shutterstock/Keith Bell; **228** © Shutterstock/elwynn; **232** © iStockphoto/row lbodvar; **240** Courtesy of Darline Foltz; **241** *top* © Shutterstock/Bombaert Patrick; *middle* © Shutterstock/Pete Saloutos; *bottom* © Shutterstock/Feng Yu; **242** *top* © Shutterstock/iofoto; *bottom* © iStockphoto/svetikd; **246** © iStockphoto/stevecoleimages; **247** © iStockphoto/Sproetniek; **249** © Shutterstock/StockLite; **256** *top* © iStockphoto/exdez; *middle* © iStockphoto/dra_schwartz; *bottom* © iStockphoto/Devonyu; **257** *top* © iStockphoto/hudiemm; *bottom* Courtesy of Karen Lankisch; **263** © iStockphoto/andhedesigns; **264** © iStockphoto/Christopher Futcher; **294** © Shutterstock/My Life Graphic; **295** *top* © iStockphoto/XonkArts; *bottom* Public Domain; **296** © iStockphoto/Bryngelzon; **299** © iStockphoto/Steve Debenport; **301** © Shutterstock/Monkey Business Images; **302** © Shutterstock/zimmytws; **305** © Shutterstock/dotshock; **308** © American Academy of Family Physicians used with permission; **309** © American Academy of Family Physicians used with permission; **310** © Shutterstock/Denise Lett; **314** © iStockphoto/donald_gruener